VITAMINS AND HORMONES

VOLUME 40

VITAMINS AND HORMONES

ADVANCES IN RESEARCH AND APPLICATIONS

Editor-in-Chief

G. D. AURBACH

Metabolic Diseases Branch
National Institute of Arthritis,
Diabetes, Digestive and Kidney Diseases
National Institutes of Health
Bethesda, Maryland

Editor

DONALD B. McCORMICK

Department of Biochemistry
Emory University School of Medicine
Atlanta, Georgia

Volume 40
1983

ACADEMIC PRESS A Subsidiary of Harcourt Brace Jovanovich, Publishers

New York London
Paris San Diego San Francisco São Paulo Sydney Tokyo Toronto

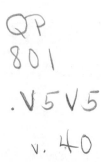

ACADEMIC PRESS, INC.
111 Fifth Avenue, New York, New York 10003

United Kingdom Edition published by
ACADEMIC·PRESS, INC. (LONDON) LTD.
24/28 Oval Road, London NW1 7DX

LIBRARY OF CONGRESS CATALOG CARD NUMBER: 43-10535

ISBN 0-12-709840-2

PRINTED IN THE UNITED STATES OF AMERICA

83 84 85 86   9 8 7 6 5 4 3 2 1

Contents

Biosynthesis of Ubiquinone

ROBERT E. OLSON AND HARRY RUDNEY

Synthesis and Analysis of the Pteroylpolyglutamates

CARLOS L. KRUMDIECK, TSUNENOBU TAMURA, AND ISAO ETO

Vitamin A and Cancer

DAVID E. ONG AND FRANK CHYTIL

Hypothalamic–Hypophysial Vasculature and Its Relationship to Secretory Cells of the Hypothalamus and Pituitary Gland

JOHN C. PORTER, JANICE F. SISSOM, JUN ARITA, AND MARIANNE J. REYMOND

Growth and Somatomedins

K. HALL AND V. R. SARA

Calciferols: Actions and Deficiencies in Action

STEPHEN J. MARX, URI A. LIBERMAN, AND CHARLES EIL

Contributors to Volume 40

Numbers in parentheses indicate the pages on which the authors' contributions begin.

JUN ARITA, *Cecil H. and Ida Green Center for Reproductive Biology Sciences, Departments of Obstetrics and Gynecology and Physiology, The University of Texas Health Science Center at Dallas, Southwestern Medical School, Dallas, Texas 75235* (145)

FRANK CHYTIL, *Department of Biochemistry, Vanderbilt University School of Medicine, Nashville, Tennessee 37232* (105)

CHARLES EIL, *Endocrinology Branch, Department of Medicine, National Naval Medical Center and Uniformed Services University of the Health Sciences, Bethesda, Maryland 20814* (235)

ISAO ETO, *Department of Nutrition Sciences, University of Alabama, Birmingham, Alabama 35294* (45)

K. HALL, *Department of Endocrinology, Karolinska Hospital, S-104 01 Stockholm, Sweden* (175)

CARLOS L. KRUMDIECK, *Department of Nutrition Sciences, University of Alabama, Birmingham, Alabama 35294* (45)

URI A. LIBERMAN, *Metabolic Diseases Branch, National Institute of Arthritis, Diabetes, and Digestive and Kidney Diseases, National Institutes of Health, Bethesda, Maryland 20205, and Beilinson Medical Center, Tel Aviv University Medical School, Tel Aviv, Israel* (235)

STEPHEN J. MARX, *Metabolic Diseases Branch, National Institute of Arthritis, Diabetes, and Digestive and Kidney Diseases, National Institutes of Health, Bethesda, Maryland 20205* (235)

ROBERT E. OLSON, *University of Pittsburgh School of Medicine, Pittsburgh, Pennsylvania 15261* (1)

DAVID E. ONG, *Department of Biochemistry, Vanderbilt University School of Medicine, Nashville, Tennessee 37232* (105)

JOHN C. PORTER, *Cecil H. and Ida Green Center for Reproductive Biology Sciences, Departments of Obstetrics and Gynecology and Physiology, The University of Texas Health Science Center at Dallas, Southwestern Medical School, Dallas, Texas 75235* (145)

MARIANNE J. REYMOND, *Cecil H. and Ida Green Center for Reproductive Biology Sciences, Departments of Obstetrics and Gynecology and Physiology, The University of Texas Health Science Center at Dallas, Southwestern Medical School, Dallas, Texas 75235* (145)

HARRY RUDNEY, *Department of Biological Chemistry, College of Medicine, University of Cincinnati Medical Center, Cincinnati, Ohio 45267* (1)

V. R. SARA, *Karolinska Institute's Department of Psychiatry, St. Göran's Hospital, S-112 81 Stockholm, Sweden* (175)

JANICE F. SISSOM, *Cecil H. and Ida Green Center for Reproductive Biology Sciences, Departments of Obstetrics and Gynecology and Physiology, The University of Texas Health Science Center at Dallas, Southwestern Medical School, Dallas, Texas 75235* (145)

TSUNENOBU TAMURA, *Department of Nutrition Sciences, University of Alabama, Birmingham, Alabama 35294* (45)

Preface

With Volume 40, the editorship of *Vitamins and Hormones* is transferred once again to the hands of successors. It is forty years, virtually to the day, since R. S. Harris and K. V. Thimann wrote the Preface to Volume 1. That first volume contained chapters authored by C. H. Best, George Wald, Roger Williams, George Minot, Thaddeus Reichstein, and Gregory Pincus. The high standards thus established were sustained by succeeding editors, and we are particularly indebted to Dr. Paul Munson, who with Egon Diczfalusy, Robert E. Olson, and John Glover performed so outstandingly in fostering the scientific and literary excellence of this serial publication. A challenging, awesome tradition has been set by the earlier editors for us to uphold! We note that to this day Dr. Thimann continues to make important suggestions for topics and authors for this serial publication.

We have modified somewhat the editorial format that has been the standard for *Vitamins and Hormones* since its inception. Instead of a group of two or more coeditors and consultant editors, we have instituted an editorial board of outstanding scientists to assist the Editors in policy and proposals for articles. But this does not portend any significant change in editorial policy or tenor of the series. We will strive to keep our readers supplied with the best reviews of current and interesting areas related to nutrition and endocrinology.

In this volume we believe this goal is achieved. D. E. Ong and F. Chytil develop a comprehensive review on the relationships between vitamin A nutritional status and the development and growth of malignant tumors, a subject of investigation that may have important practical as well as research interest. Hormonal control of cell growth is treated in the chapter by K. Hall and V. R. Sara who discuss growth and the somatomedins. They provide an excellent review of the chemistry, biology, and secretion of the insulin-like growth factors and clarify much of the confusion concerning the biological role and nomenclature of these substances. C. L. Krumdieck, T. Tamura, and I. Eto discuss the synthesis and role of side chain polyglutamate function in translocation and actions of the pteroylpolyglutamates. Regulation of side chain length may be a factor in the control of one carbon metabolism. R. E. Olson and H. Rudney provide a thorough overview of the biosynthesis of the ubiquinones and discuss enzymatic and metabolic control of this pathway.

J. C. Porter, J. F. Sissom, J. Arita, and M. J. Reymond have prepared a classic exposition on the hypothalamic–hypophysial vasculature and propose how abnormalities in vasculature could lead to abnormal physiological control of secretion of pituitary hormones. The closing chapter by S. J. Marx, U. A. Liberman, and C. Eil is a definitive review of defects in the actions of vitamin D and its metabolites. This aspect of vitamin D has not been presented in earlier volumes and includes descriptions of a fascinating series of metabolic abnormalities that lead to rickets and related disorders.

We wish to thank the staff of Academic Press for their most able services in producing this volume and, in particular, for smoothing the transition to new editors.

G. D. AURBACH
DONALD B. McCORMICK

VITAMINS AND HORMONES

VOLUME 40

Biosynthesis of Ubiquinone

ROBERT E. OLSON

University of Pittsburgh School of Medicine, Pittsburgh, Pennsylvania

HARRY RUDNEY

*Department of Biological Chemistry, College of Medicine,
University of Cincinnati Medical Center, Cincinnati, Ohio*

I. Introduction

Ubiquinone was discovered in Morton's laboratory in Liverpool in 1955 as a nonsaponifiable lipid with a striking ultraviolet absorption spectrum at 272 nm (Festenstein *et al.*, 1955). In 1957, Crane at the University of Wisconsin reported the isolation of the same compound

1

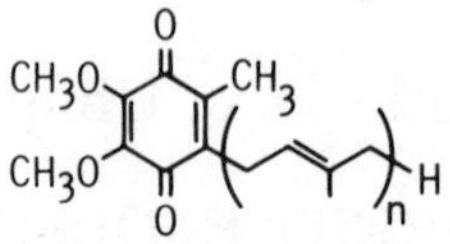

FIG. 1. The structure of ubiquinone-n, n = numbers of isoprenyl groups in side chain.

from lipid extracts of beef heart mitochondria. Because the new compound appeared to be a quinone and was catalytic in mitochondrial hydrogen transport, Crane named the compound "Q" (Crane et al., 1957). This subject was last reviewed 16 years ago in Vitamins and Hormones (Rudney and Raman, 1966; Olson, 1966).

Ubiquinone serves as a lipid-soluble electron carrier in the membrane-bound electron transport chains of both prokaryotes and eukaryotes. Eighty-five percent of cell ubiquinone is located in the mitochondria or equivalent membrane system. The structure of ubiquinone is shown in Fig. 1 and the dimensions of various ubiquinone homologs with respect to a typical membrane bilayer are shown in Fig. 2. During respiration, reducing equivalents entering the electron transport chain are transferred through a series of redox components from pyridine nucleotides and flavoproteins to ubiquinone, and thence via the cytochromes (b, c, c_1, a, and a_3) to oxygen (Green and Fleischer, 1968). Ubiquinone provides a linkage between the 2-electron transport enzymes and the 1-electron cytochrome system through semiquinone formation. Oxidation and reduction of ubiquinone in the respiration chain have been studied by Hatefi and Quiros-Perez (1959), Green and Lester (1959), and Pumphrey and Redfearn (1959). Acetone extraction of the endogenous ubiquinone disrupts electron transport. Moreover, readdition of ubiquinone-9 to ubiquinone-depleted mitochondria restores both cyanide and antimycin sensitivity to levels approaching the unextracted systems (Lester and Fleischer, 1959,1961).

The proposal by Mitchell (1961,1966), that ATP synthesis from electron transport resulted from generation of a proton gradient across the inner membrane of the mitochondria, revolutionized concepts of oxidative phosphorylation. Central to the chemiosmotic hypothesis of oxidative phosphorylation is the protonmotive ubiquinone Q cycle, which accounts for the release and uptake of protons by ubiquinone during its

---

FIG. 2. Space-filling models illustrating the dimensions of reduced ubiquinone-10 and shorter homologs compared to a phospholipid bilayer which is 60–70 Å in width. The phospholipid to the upper left is 18:0, 18:2-phosphatidylcholine, the one to the lower left is 16:0, 18:1-phosphatidylethanolamine (Trumpower, 1981).

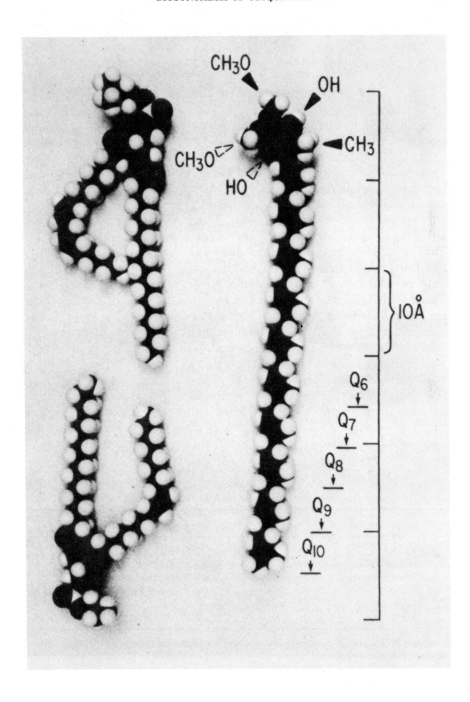

oxidation and reduction in electron transport (Mitchell, 1966, 1967; Trumpower, 1981).

II. Distribution of Ubiquinones

In the ubiquinones isolated from natural sources, the number (n) of isoprenyl units usually varies from 6 to 10. In animals the main homolog is Q-10, although some rodents and fish possess Q-9. Very small amounts of ubiquinones with less than 6 prenyl units have been detected in some microorganisms. In *Escherichia coli,* Daves *et al.* (1967) have identified all of the members from Q-1 to Q-8, in *Rhodospirillum rubrum,* all members from Q-1 to Q-10, and in yeast, all members from Q-1 to Q-6. This distribution of the major homologs is summarized in Table I, and was reviewed in detail by Crane (1965), Pennock (1966), and Collins and Jones (1981). Another ubiquinone type, so far found only in filamentous fungi (Lavate *et al.,* 1962, 1965; Gale *et al.,* 1963a,b), is Q-10(H_2) in which the isoprenoid unit farthest from the ring is reduced (Lavate *et al.,* 1965). Partially reduced ubiquinones containing fewer than 10 C_5 residues have not yet been discovered in nature. The dihydroubiquinone-9, tentatively identified in rat liver, was probably an ethoxy-Q-9 formed during saponification (Edwin *et al.,* 1960b). Several derivatives of Q-10, containing an epoxy group in the isoprenoid side chain, have been obtained from *R. rubrum* lipid extracts (Friis *et al.,* 1967a). Although these epoxides might be artifacts of isolation, this appears unlikely since oxygen atoms have also been found in the side chains of plastoquinones and menaquinones.

TABLE I
NATURALLY OCCURRING UBIQUINONES[a]

Source	Ubiquinones
Yeasts	Q-6, Q-7
Bacteria	Q-8, Q-9, Q-10
Plants	Q-9, Q-10
Fungi	Q-7, Q-8, Q-9, Q-10, Q-10(H_2)
Invertebrates	Q-9, Q-10
Vertebrates	Q-10, (Q-9)[b]

[a]The most commonly occurring ubiquinones are listed; trace amounts of other homologs are frequently present.

[b]Among vertebrates, only the tissues of the rat, mouse, and walleyed pike have been reported to contain Q-9.

III. Assembly of Ubiquinones from Precursor Molecules

A. Isoprenyl Side Chain

Studies on the biosynthesis of the ubiquinones, a homologous series now known to extend from ubiquinone-1 to -10, began in both microorganisms and mammals soon after the determination of its structure. The idea that Q was an essential nutrient was soon dispelled by finding that elimination of ubiquinone from the diet had no effect on tissue levels (Olson *et al.*, 1961; Gloor and Wiss, 1959; Dialameh and Olson, 1959). Olson and Dialameh (1960) and Olson *et al.* (1961) reported that [1-^{14}C]acetate and [2-^{14}C]mevalonate were incorporated into ubiquinone-9 in the rat. Rats and mice differ from most mammals in having ubiquinone-9 instead of ubiquinone-10 as the principal homolog in their tissues.

Nutritional considerations led Olson *et al.* (1961) to propose the hypothesis that the benzoquinone moiety of Q should be derived from the phenylamino acids and the side chain from acetate via mevalonate. These predictions were realized in studies of the incorporation of acetate, mevalonate, phenylalanine, and tyrosine into ubiquinone in rat liver slices. Subsequent degradation of the diacetyl derivative of dihydroubiquinone-9 by ozonolysis showed that acetate carbon was found exclusively in the side chain and phenylalanine carbon was found predominantly in a ring fragment (3',6'-dimethoxy-2-methylphenylacetic acid) (Bentley *et al.*, 1961; Olson *et al.*, 1965).

It seemed possible at that time that homogentisate, a metabolite of tyrosine, was an intermediate in the biosynthesis of Q with retention of the β-carbon atom as the 5-methyl group in Q. When the substrates [3-^{14}C]phenylalanine and [3-^{14}C]tyrosine were employed to test for incorporation of the β-carbon of these aromatic amino acids into the carbon-bound methyl group of ubiquinone, it was found, contrary to expectations, that all of the radioactivity was in the side chain (derived from the acetate pool) and none was in the ring fragment. This led to the novel conclusion that the whole side chain of tyrosine was lost in the metabolism leading to Q formation, and that *de novo* methylation of the ring occurred at a later stage (Olson *et al.*, 1963).

Gold and Olson (1966) observed in liver slices that the incorporation of [2-^{14}C]mevalonate into both cholesterol and ubiquinone-9 in rat liver slices obeyed saturation kinetics as measured by the ratio of specific activity of product to precursor. The apparent K_m for cholesterol biosynthesis was 1.0 mM, whereas that for ubiquinone-9 biosynthesis was 0.2 mM. It was also observed that when liver slices were incubated for various periods of time with [2-^{14}C]mevalonate, incorporation of radioactivity into cholesterol was linear with time, whereas that for ubiquinone-9 was observed to accumulate during the lag period. These results will be discussed in Section IV,B.

Mevalonic acid is converted by a series of enzymatic steps to isopentenyl pyrophosphate (Bloch *et al.*, 1959; Lynen *et al.*, 1958). Isopentenyl pyrophosphate when added to yeast extracts was found to be converted to farnesyl pyrophosphate (Lynen *et al.*, 1958). The mechanism by which this active isoprene is elongated has been described as a head-to-tail condensation (Lynen *et al.*, 1959) and this mechanism has been extensively reviewed (Lynen, 1959; Popjak *et al.*, 1964). Head-to-tail condensation of farnesyl pyrophosphate with isopentenyl pyrophosphate may lead to the formation of a series of higher isoprenoid pyrophosphates. Lynen (1961) proposed that polyprenyl pyrophosphates serve as immediate precursors for ubiquinone side chains. Condensation of given polyprenyl pyrophosphates with the ubiquinone precursor 4-hydroxybenzoate by the enzyme 4-hydroxylbenzoate:polyprenyltransferase has been demonstrated *in vitro* using preparations from *R. rubrum, E. coli, Saccharomyces carlsbergensis*, and the rat (Raman *et al.*, 1969; Cox *et al.*, 1969; Thomas and Threlfall, 1973; Momose and Rudney, 1972).

It is of interest to note that in all organisms examined, the polyprenyl pyrophospate transferase is a membrane-bound enzyme. In eukaryotes, this enzyme has been found to be associated with the inner membrane of the mitochondria (Momose and Rudney, 1972). Studies with rat mitochondria indicate an apparent lack of specificity of this enzyme for isoprene chain length. Similar results have been observed using *E. coli* (Young *et al.*, 1972), suggesting the length of the side chain of ubiquinone within a species is regulated at the level of polyprenyl pyrophosphate biosynthesis.

Recently it has been shown that compactin (ML236B), a competitive inhibitor of 3-hydroxy-3-methylglutaryl-CoA reductase, inhibits both cholesterol and ubiquinone-10 biosynthesis in human fibroblasts (Faust *et al.*, 1979; Nambudiri *et al.*, 1980; Ranganathan *et al.*, 1981).

B. BENZOQUINONE RING

Except for estrogenic compounds, most higher animals have lost their ability to synthesize aromatic rings from simple precursors, relying solely on dietary sources for aromatic compounds. In contrast, prototrophic microorganisms and many plants are able to synthesize a range of aromatic compounds from such simple precursors as acetate

(Busch, 1953), or glucose via chorismate (Davis, 1952). Olson *et al.* (1963) and Rudney and Parson (1963) simultaneously reported the identification of 4-hydroxybenzoate as the essential aromatic precursor of ubiquinone. In Rudney's laboratory 4-hydroxybenzaldehyde was found to be a trace contaminant of the [U-^{14}C]tyrosine. When added by itself, 40% of the mass was converted to ubiquinone. In Olson's laboratory the discovery that the whole side chain of tyrosine was lost in Q biosynthesis led them to test foreshortened products of phenylamino acid metabolism. They discovered that ^{14}C-ring-labeled benzoate was incorporated into the benzoquinone moiety of Q, but not [^{14}C]carboxyl-labeled benzoate. Acheson and Gibbard (1962) had shown that benzoate was converted to 4-hydroxybenzoate in rats and Olson (1965) showed that 4-hydroxybenzoate was a better precursor of Q than benzoate in liver slices by 2.5-fold. Aiyar and Olson (1964) demonstrated that 4-hydroxy[U-^{14}C]benzoate was a 2.5 times better precursor than the corresponding aldehyde. 4-Hydroxybenzoate, as well as the aldehyde, have been shown by Parson and Rudney (1964) to be incorporated into ubiquinone in *R. rubrum, Azotobacter vinelandii, Saccharomyces cerevisiae,* and rat kidney.

Proof that the common biosynthetic pathway for aromatic amino acids in microorganisms is utilized for Q synthesis was first demonstrated by Cox and Gibson (1964) who showed the incorporation of [U-^{14}C]shikimic acid into ubiquinone in *E. coli.* Furthermore, this incorporation could be "swamped" by exogenous 4-hydroxybenzoic acid. In animals that have lost this "shikimate pathway," tyrosine and/or phenylalanine serve as the source for the aromatic ring for its conversions to the benzoquinone moiety. [U-^{14}C]Tyrosine was found to be a 3-fold better precursor than phenylalanine in rat liver slices (Olson, 1965).

C. Ring Substituents

Uchida and Aida (1972) demonstrated with mass spectrometry that the quinone ring oxygen atoms are derived from $^{18}O_2$ and not $H_2^{18}O$. Rudney and Sugimura (1961) reported the incorporation of [^{14}C]formate and [*methyl*-^{14}C]methionine into ubiquinone in yeast. Similar results were obtained in the rat using formate and methionine (Wiss *et al.*, 1961b). Formate was shown to be a source of the benzoquinone rings methyl groups in the rat by Kuhn–Roth and Zeisel degradation of formate-labeled ubiquinone (Bentley *et al.*, 1968). Based on analogy with other well-studied C- and O-methylation reactions, *S*-adenosylmethionine was proposed to be the immediate methyl group donor. Jackman *et al.* (1967) demonstrated in bacteria that [*methyl*-^{14}C]methionine was incorporated into both the C- and O-methyl groups of ubiquinone.

Raman *et al.* (1969) showed that S-adenosylmethionine was the methyl group donor in *R. rubrum* cell extracts. In experiments with rat liver mitochondria, Trumpower and Olson (1971) demonstrated that the C-5 methoxy group of ubiquinone was labeled by S-adenosylmethionine. Similarly, 6-methoxy-2-nonaprenylphenol was found to be labeled by [*methyl*-^{3}H]methionine in rat liver slives (Nowicki *et al.*, 1972). It appears, therefore, that both prokaryotic and eukaryotic organisms draw from the same metabolic pools for their synthesis of methyl groups in ubiquinone as well as the other portions of the molecule.

IV. METABOLIC PATHWAY FOR BIOSYNTHESIS OF UBIQUINONES IN PROKARYOTIC AND EUKARYOTIC ORGANISMS

A. GENERATION OF 4-HYDROXYBENZOATE

The aromatic ring of ubiquinone can be synthesized from either glucose via shikimic acid or tyrosine. Both pathways generate 4-hydroxybenzoate, which is the pivotal precursor of the aromatic ring of ubiquinone. The intermediary metabolism leading to 4-hydroxybenzoate synthesis in various precursors has been reviewed by Cox and Gibson (1964), Rudney and Rana (1966), and Olson (1966).

A pathway from tyrosine to 4-hydroxybenzoate was originally proposed by Booth *et al.* (1960) as a result of urinary excretion studies of phenolic acids after administration of tyrosine metabolites. They concluded that the conversion of tyrosine to 4-hydroxybenzoate involved the β-oxidation of 4-hydroxyphenylpropionic acid. Zannoni and Weber (1966) isolated an aromatic α-keto acid reductase from sheep heart which is widely distributed in animal tissues and accounts for up to 80% of the phenyl lactate derived from phenyl pyruvate in the mammal. The conversion of *p*-hydroxycinnamic acid to 4-hydroxybenzoic acid follows the type reactions of β-oxidation and probably involves the appropriate coenzyme A derivative. The pathway involving benzoate as an intermediate could assume greater significance under conditions of impaired phenylalanine hydroxylase activity, such as in phenylketonuria (Napier *et al.*, 1964). Acheson and Gibbard (1962) demonstrated the conversion of benzoate to 4-hydroxybenzoate in the intact animal.

In studies of ubiquinone synthesis from various tyrosine metabolites

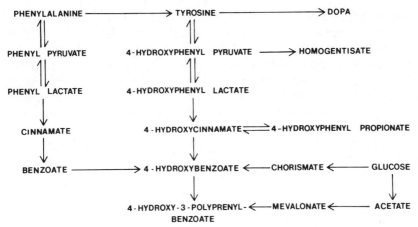

FIG. 3. Pathways from phenylalanine and tyrosine to 4-hydroxy-3-polyprenylbenzoate.

in the rat, Olson (1965) found the p-hydroxyphenyl pyruvate, p-hydroxycinnamate, p-hydroxyphenyl propionate, p-hydroxybenzyl alcohol, and p-hydroxybenzaldehyde greatly reduced the incorporation of isotopic tyrosine into Q-9, whereas homogentisate, orsellinic acid, and 3,4-dihydroxyphenylalanine did not. In a more direct approach, the phenolic acids were isolated from slices of liver incubated with [U-^{14}C]-tyrosine, radioactive p-hydroxyphenyl propionate and p-hydroxyphenyl lactate were isolated by chromatography and reincubated with freshly prepared liver slices. The rates of incorporation of label from these acids into Q-9 was somewhat greater than that obtained with [U-^{14}C]tyrosine. On the basis of these combined data, the scheme of biosynthesis presented in Fig. 3 was suggested for the pathway from phenylalanine to 4-hydroxybenzoate (Olson, 1965).

B. PATHWAY FROM 4-HYDROXYBENZOATE TO UBIQUINONE

Since 1965, the bulk of the work on the biosynthesis of ubiquinone in plants, animals, and microorganisms has been devoted to determination of the sequence of steps in the metabolic pathway between 4-hydroxybenzoate and ubiquinone. In 1965 Parsons and Rudney (1965) observed an unidentified lipophilic compound derived from p-[U-^{14}C]hydroxybenzoate, which accumulated in the cultures of $R.$ $rubrum$ incubated anaerobically in the dark, which could be converted into ubiquinone-10 by continued incubation in the light. It was less polar than ubiquinone on TLC and could be labeled by acetate, but not by methionine. At this point, Rudney joined forces with Karl Folkers, then at the Stanford Research Institute, and a large scale isolation of the new compound was achieved. It was identified as 2-de-caprenylphenol (Olsen *et al.*, 1965). Work in Olson's laboratory provided evidence that another lipophilic compound distinct from 2-non-aprenylphenol accumulated in the first hour of incubation of rat tissue slices incubated with [U-^{14}C]benzoate. It was more polar than ubiquinone-9 and more substituted than 2-nonaprenylphenol, although not totally substituted as indicated by retention of isotope when 4-[U-^{3}H]hydroxybenzoate was the substrate (Olson and Aiyar, 1966). It was finally identified as 5-demethoxyubiquinone-9 (Trumpower *et al.*, 1972).

Trumpower *et al.* (1972) then tested ^{14}C-ring-labeled nonaprenyl-phenol as a precursor of ubiquinone-9 in the rat and found it inactive. Furthermore, 2-nonaprenylphenol did not "swamp" the incorporation of 4-hydroxybenzoate into ubiquinone in rat liver slices. When 4-hy-droxy[G-^{3}H]benzoate was incubated with rat liver slices 6-methox-ynonaprenylphenol, a new intermediate, and 5-demethoxyubi-quinone-9 were highly labeled (each 50% of the total radioactivity), whereas nonaprenylphenol was unenriched (only 0.3% of the total radioactivity) (Nowicki *et al.*, 1972). These data led them to conclude that the pathway for the biosynthesis of ubiquinone in animals (and perhaps all eukaryotes) was different in certain respects from that in prokaryotes.

1. *The Pathway in Prokaryotes*

In 1965, Folkers and his group at Stanford reported in quick succession the identification of 2-decaprenylphenol, 2-decaprenyl-6-methoxy-phenol, 2-decaprenyl-6-methoxy-1,4-benzoquinone, and 2-de-caprenyl-3-methyl-6-methoxy-1,4-benzoquinone (5-demethoxyubi-quinone-10) in extracts of *R. rubrum* by molecular distillation and mass spectrometry. On the basis of characterization of these four compounds, Friis *et al.* (1966) postulated a complete sequence of hypothetical intermediates between 4-hydroxybenzoate and ubiquinone which included a number of basic steps. These were alkylation of *p*-hy-droxybenzoic acid to a prenylated derivative, decarboxylation of the product to a 2-polyprenylphenol, followed by ortho-hydroxylation and methylation to form 2-polyprenyl-6-methoxyphenol. Hydroxylation para to the phenolic group and oxidation led to the corresponding 1,4-benzoquinone. C-methylation in the position ortho to the polyprenyl group to form 5-demethoxyubiquinone was followed by hydroxylation and methylation of the remaining unsubstituted position to yield ubiquinone. Nilsson *et al.* (1968) showed that 3-decaprenyl-4-hydroxyben-zoate in *R. rubrum* was labeled *in vitro* by 4-hydroxybenzoate.

Studies in *E. coli* and selected *E. coli* mutants by Cox and his col-leagues in Australia (1968, 1969) more or less confirmed the Folkers hypothesis. Two mutants, which were unable to synthesize ubi-quinone, were found to accumulate either 3-octaprenyl-4-hy-droxybenzoate or 2-octaprenylphenol. The two genes, *ubiB* and *ubiD*, concerned with these two successive reactions were found to be closely linked. They also showed that cell extracts of the mutant strain carry-ing the *ubiD* ⁻ allele lacked 3-octaprenyl-4-hydroxybenzoic decarbox-ylase. It is of interest that the mutant having the gene *ubiD* ⁻, which accumulates 3-octaprenyl-4-hydroxybenzoate, still produces some ubiquinone-8 by an alternate pathway.

Young *et al.* (1971) reported the isolation of two more *E. coli* mutants which accumulated, respectively, 2-octaprenyl-6-methoxy-1,4-benzo-quinone and 5-demethoxyubiquinone-8. Stroobant *et al.* (1972) re-ported another *E. coli* mutant which accumulated sufficient amounts of 5-demethylubiquinone-8 for identification by mass spectrometry. Altogether this group has isolated eight mutants of *E. coli* defective in ubiquinone biosynthesis representing blocks in seven steps of the pro-karyotic metabolic pathway for ubiquinone synthesis and mapped the genes on the *E. coli* chromosome (Gibson, 1973). This pathway is shown in Fig. 4.

2. *The Pathway in Eukaryotes*

As already mentioned, 6-methoxy-2-nonaprenylphenol (Nowicki *et al.*, 1972), 5-demethoxyubiquinone-9 (Trumpower *et al.*, 1972), and 5-demethylubiquinone-9 (Houser and Olson, 1974) were shown to be bonafide intermediates in ubiquinone biosynthesis in the rat. The cor-responding intermediates in the ubiquinone-6 series have been demon-strated to be labeled by isotopic 4-hydroxybenzoate in yeast (Casey and Threlfall, 1978). On the other hand, nonaprenylphenol, an intermedi-ate in the biosynthesis of ubiquinone-9 by prokaryotes, was found not to be an intermediate in the rat (Trumpower *et al.*, 1974). Thus it appeared that although prokaryotes and eukaryotes share portions of this biosynthetic pathway, significant differences exist among them as shown in Fig. 4. An alternate pathway for 4-hydroxybenzoate metabo-lism in the rat was proposed by Nowicki *et al.* (1972).

Recent studies of mutants of the prototrophic strain of *S. cerevisiae*, deficient in ubiquinone-QH_2–cytochrome reductase activity, have re-vealed two new intermediates in ubiquinone synthesis which have been identified as, 3,4-dihydroxy-5-hexaprenylbenzoate (Goewert *et*

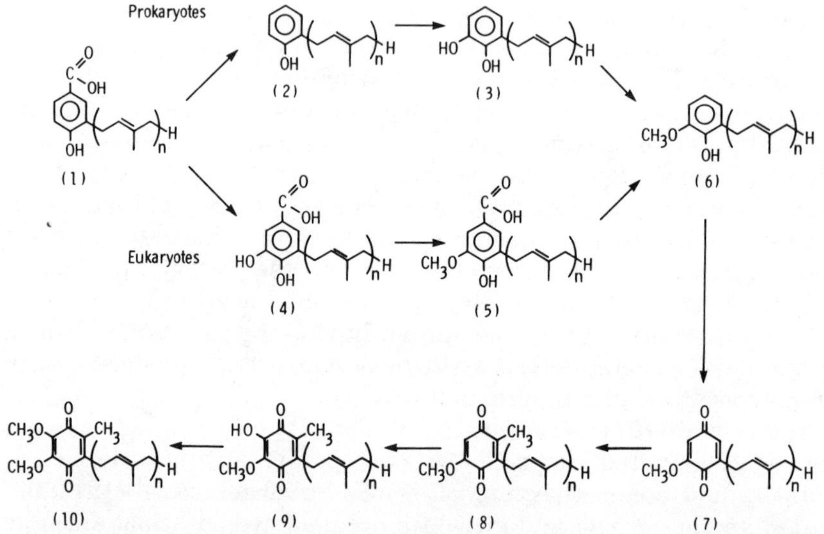

FIG. 4. The pathway of biosynthesis from 4-hydroxybenzoate to ubiquinone. The divergent and common pathways are indicated: (1) 4-hydroxy-3-polyprenylbenzoate; (2) 2-polyprenylphenol; (3) 6-hydroxy-2-polyprenylphenol; (4) 3,4-dihydroxy-5-polyprenylbenzoate; (5) 3-methoxy-4-hydroxy-5-polyprenylbenzoate; (6) 6-methyoxy-2-polyprenylphenol; (7) 6-methoxy-2-polyprenyl-1, 4-benzoquinone; (8) 6-methoxy-3-methyl-2-polyprenyl-1, 4-benzoquinone (5-demethoxyubiquinone-n); (9) 5-hydroxy-6-methoxy-3-methyl-2-polyprenyl-1, 4-benzoquinone (5-demethylubiquinone-n); (10) ubiquinone-n.

al., 1977, 1981a) and 3-methoxy-4-hydroxy-5-hexaprenylbenzoate (Goewert *et al.*, 1978, 1981b).

a. Identification of 3,4-Dihydroxy-5-hexaprenylbenzoate. The ubiquinone-deficient strain E3-24 (described by Tzagoloff *et al.*, 1975) grown in the presence of p-[U-^{14}C]hydroxybenzoate was found to incorporate 11–20% of the label into a novel polar metabolite. This metabolite, in the amount of 60 μg, was isolated from 32.9 g of lyophilized E3-24 and purified to a constant specific activity. The mass spectra for this natural product displayed a molecular ion at m/e 562 in addition to both the characteristic chromanylium and tropylium ions at m/e 207 and 167, respectively, suggesting this compound to be 3,4-dihydroxy-5-hexaprenyl benzoate (3,4-DHHB). The synthetic nonaprenyl homolog and phytyl analog were prepared and their mass spectra gave the appropriate ions, verifying the proposed structure. Nuclear magnetic resonance spectrum for 3,4-dihydroxy-5-nonaprenylbenzoate showed two singlets at 7.31δ and 6.58δ, corresponding to the two catecholic protons. The ultraviolet and infrared spectra exhibited absorption bands at 253 and 294 nm, and at 3.05, 3.68–4.60, 5.95, and 6.08 μm, respectively. These spectral data are consistent with the assigned structure.

3,4-Dihydroxy-5-hexaprenylbenzoate was also observed to accumulate in yeast strains blocked in methionine biosynthesis, e.g., in a met 2 mutant [blocked at homoserine O-transacetylase (EC 2.3.1.31)]. When 4-hydroxy[U-^{14}C]benzoate was washed out from these cultures and methionine restored in a pulse–chase experiment, radioactivity from 3,4-dihydroxy-5-hexaprenylbenzoate was observed to move into ubiquinone-6, demonstrating a precursor–product relationship (Goewert *et al.*, 1977, 1981a).

b. Identification of 3-Methoxy-4-hydroxy-5-hexaprenyl Benzoate. Another ubiquinone-deficient strain 26H, first described by deKok and Slater (1975), was found to accumulate a previously unidentified ubiquinone intermediate when grown in the presence of [U-^{14}C]- and p-[7-^{14}C]hydroxybenzoate. In addition, [*methyl*-^{3}H]methionine was also found to label this metabolite. This compound, in the amount of 31 μg, was isolated from 18.7 g of lyophilized 26H and purified to a constant specific activity. The mass spectra of the metabolite demonstrated a prominent molecular ion at *m/e* 576 and two key fragments, the chromenylium ion and tropylium ion at *m/e* 235 and 181, respectively. An intense peak at *m/e* 97, characteristic of vanillic acid, was also identified, suggesting this compound's structure to be 3-methoxy-4-hydroxy-5-hexaprenylbenzoate (3-MHHB). The methyl ester of this compound, prepared by treatment with diazomethane, gave a mass spectra with a molecular ion at *m/e* 590 which corresponds to an empirical formula of $C_{39}H_{58}O_4$. The molecular ion readily lost a methoxy group *m/e* 559 (M^+-OCH$_3$) and its ester group *m/e* 531 (M^+-COOCH$_3$). The methyl ester chromenylium ion and tropylium ion were present at *m/e* 250 and 195, respectively. A quantity, 18.2 mg, of 3-methoxy-4-hydroxy-5-hexaprenylbenzoate was isolated from a 100-liter batch culture and purified to a constant specific activity. The nuclear magnetic resonance spectrum of this material showed a predicted singlet at 3.88δ corresponding to the three methoxy protons. The remaining spectral data were consistent with the assigned structure. The ultraviolet and infrared spectra exhibited absorbances at 260 and 289 nm, and at 3.6, 6.0, 6.25, 6.8, and 7.0 μm, respectively, characteristic of the assigned structure.

In *in vitro* precursor–product experiments, isolated mitochondria from both wild-type yeast and rat liver were able to convert 10% of the labeled 3-methoxy-4-hydroxy-5-hexaprenylbenzoate to ubiquinone-6, demonstrating its role as an intermediate in eukaryotic ubiquinone biosynthesis (Goewert *et al.*, 1978, 1981a).

c. Alternate Pathways. There appears to be a considerable variation in the metabolism of 4-hydroxybenzoate (4-HBA) by animal cells. Although Momose and Rudney (1972) showed clearly that alkylation of 4-HBA to 4-hydroxy-3-polyprenylbenzoate was the first committed step in ubiquinone biosynthesis, Rudney's group has since shown that 4-HBA can be converted to 3,4-dihydroxybenzoate (protocatechuic acid) and to 3-methoxy-4-hydroxybenzoate (vanillic acid) in rat heart slices (Nambudiri *et al.*, 1977). These products then undergo prenyla-

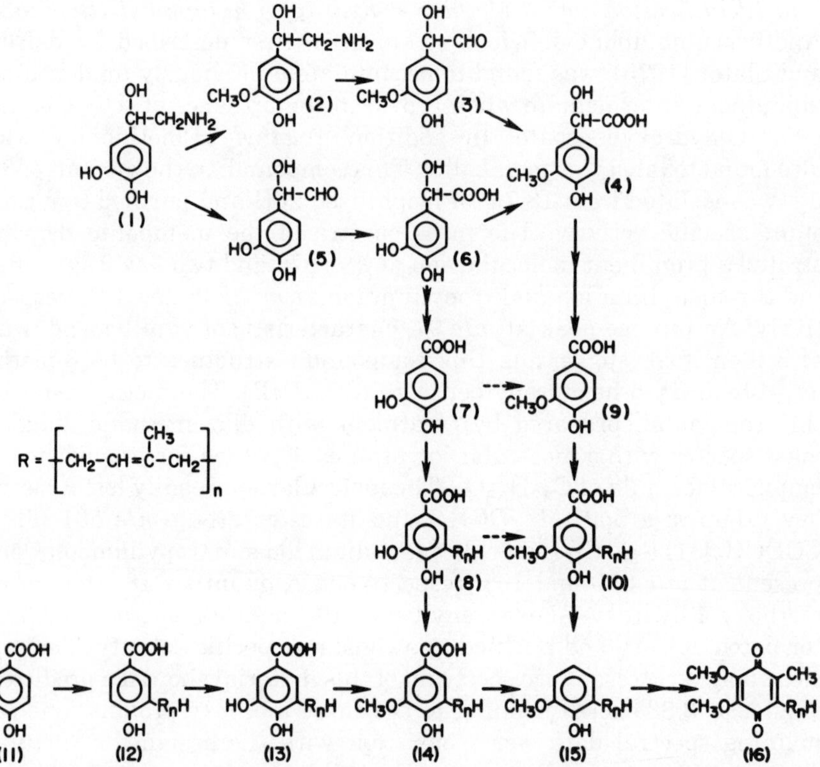

FIG. 5. Alternate pathways for ubiquinone synthesis in animal tissues involving norepinephrine metabolites. Tyrosine can be metabolized to norepinephrine and thence to intermediates in the established eukaryotic pathway for Q biosynthesis. The compounds shown are (1) norepinephrine; (2) 3-*O*-methylnorepinephrine; (3) 3-methoxy-4-hydroxymandelaldehyde; (4) 3-methoxy-4-hydroxymandelate; (5) 3,4-dihydroxymandelaldehyde; (6) 3,4-dihydroxymandelate; (7) 3,4-dihydroxybenzoate; (8),(13) 3,4-dihydroxy-5-polyprenylbenzoate; (9) 3-methoxy-4-hydroxybenzoate; (10),(14) 3-methoxy-4-hydroxy-5-polyprenylbenzoate; (11) 4-hydroxybenzoate; (12) 4-hydroxy-3-polyprenylbenzoate; (15) 6-methoxy-2-polyprenylphenol; (16) CoQ.

tion to intermediates analogous to those identified by Goewert *et al.* (1981a,b) in yeast (Nambudiri *et al.*, 1977) (see Fig. 5).

The observations that vanillic and protocatechuic acids can be prenylated by liver mitochondria raised the question of whether norepinephrine, which is metabolized to vanillic acid in man (Rosen and Goodall, 1962), could be converted to ubiquinone, and whether norepinephrine could directly generate these potential aromatic Q precursors. Rudney (1977) has shown that when norepinephrine is incubated with rat liver mitochondria, not only are vanillate and protocatechuate formed, but in addition they are also prenylated. Thus it seems possible that an alternate pathway from tyrosine to norepinephrine to protocatechuic acid and thence from 3,4-dihydroxy-5-polyprenylbenzoate to Q is possible, as shown in Fig. 5. The direct conversion of norepinephrine all the way to Q has not yet been demonstrated but is certainly possible. It may, in fact, be a "salvage pathway" for recycling tyrosine metabolites for Q synthesis.

V. CHARACTERIZATION OF ENZYMES IN THE PATHWAY FOR UBIQUINONE BIOSYNTHESIS

A. 4-HYDROXYBENZOATE:POLYPRENYLTRANSFERASE

The properties of 4-hydroxybenzoate:polyprenyltransferase and the system synthesizing polyprenyl pyrophosphate have been studied in mitochondria from rat and guinea pig livers. The assay system uses 1 μM 4-[7-^{14}C]HBA, 10 mM MgCl$_2$, 5 μM solanesyl PP, 0.01% Triton X-100, plus mitochondrial protein in 1.0 ml. The reactants are incubated for 30 minutes at 37°C and the hydrophobic prenylated product extracted into chloroform–methanol, 1:2. With solanesyl pyrophosphate and 4-hydroxybenzoate the reaction was linear with time, concentration of protein, and concentration of solanesyl pyrophosphate. Solanesyl monophosphate was inactive as a substrate and was noninhibitory. Detergents such as Triton X-100, Tween-80, and sodium deoxycholate activated the enzyme in mitochondria, which were aged by freezing at −20°C for periods ranging from 1 hour to several days. Maximum activation also required Mg^{2+}. In agreement with previous observations, the effect of Mg^{2+} and Triton X-100 on fresh mitochondria was quite variable. Activation with aged preparations, however, was very consistent. Treatment with Triton X-100 used an alteration in the biosynthetic pattern of rat liver mitochondria so that nonaprenyl rather than decaprenyl pyrophosphate was preferentially made in the presence of solanesyl pyrophosphate and isopentenyl pyrophosphate. In the case of guinea pig liver mitochondria a different pattern is observed with Triton X-100. The *de novo* formation of decaprenyl pyrophosphate from isopentenyl pyrophosphate appears to be inhibited by Triton X-100, but the synthesis of decaprenyl pyrophosphate from isopentenyl pyrophosphate and nonaprenyl pyrophosphate was not inhibited. The data also indicate that in guinea pig liver, in a system synthesizing decaprenyl pyrophosphate from isopentenyl pyrophosphate, there does not appear to be a detectable pool of nonaprenyl pyrophosphate. These results show that detergents can affect the specificity of the mitochondrial system synthesizing polyprenyl pyrophosphates (Nishino and Rudney, 1977).

B. 4-HYDROXY-5-POLYPRENYLBENZOATE HYDROXYLASE

The assay system for 4-hydroxy-5-nonaprenylbenzoate hydroxylase from rat kidney and liver mitochondria uses 50 mM NaH_2PO_4, 40 mM niacinamide, 3 mM ATP, 4 mM succinate, 0.2 mM NADP, 0.5 mM NADH, and 1 mM S-adenosylhomocysteine, pH 7.5, and mitochondrial protein in 1.0 ml. The substrate 4-hydroxy-5-nonaprenyl [*carboxy*-^{14}C]benzoate is added and the reaction carried out for 1 hour at 37°C. The reaction is stopped with methanol, the mixture extracted with diethyl ether, and the extract dried. A concentrated aliquot was then spotted on a silica G-25 TLC plate that had been pretreated with 0.1 M borate, pH 7.0, and developed in cyclohexane:diethyl ether:acetic acid (50:50:0.5). The areas corresponding to the product, 3,4-dihydroxy-5-nonaprenylbenzoate (R_f=0.20), and the substrate (R_f=0.27) were scraped and counted (Goewert *et al.*, 1981). Preliminary studies show levels of activity for the hydroxylase in the rat liver mitochondria of 5–7 pmol per hour per mg of protein and 9–12 pmol per hour per mg protein in rat kidney mitochondria. The inner membranes have a 6-fold enhancement of this specific activity. By applying the method of Ghazarian *et al.* (1974), it was possible to demonstrate the involvement of cytochrome P-450 in this reaction in rat kidney mitochondria.

C. S-ADENOSYLMETHIONINE:3,4-DIHYDROXY-5-POLYPRENYLBENZOATE O-METHYLTRANSFERASE

This enzyme is the first methylase in the eukaryotic pathway of Q biosynthesis and is located in the inner mitochondrial membrane. The enzyme is assayed in a phosphate buffer, 0.025 M, pH 6.3, containing 1 μM [7-^{14}C]3,4-dihydroxy-5-polyprenylbenzoate and 200 μM S-adenylosyl[*methyl*-³H]methionine, by incubation for 1 hour at 30°C. The product is extracted with diethyl ether and chromatographed on TLC using benzene:acetone (1:1). For the methylated product, which is nicely separated from the reactants, the yield is calculated from the $^3H/^{14}C$ ratio.

Partial purification of this methylase has been accomplished from yeast mitochondrial inner membranes by triton solubilization and chromatography on DEAE-cellulose in the presence of 5mM mercaptoethanol. A 20-fold purification of the enzyme from the initial mitochondrial-specific activity has been achieved.

D. S-ADENOSYLMETHIONINE:5-DEMETHYLUBIQUINONE-9-O-
   METHYLTRANFERASE

The methyltransferase responsible for the conversion of 6-de-methylubiquinone-9 to ubiquinone-9 in rat liver mitochondira has been shown to be localized in the inner membrane of rat liver mitochondria. NADH was required to generate the hydroquinone, which was the immediate substrate for methylation. The K_m for 5-de-methylubiquinone-9 was estimated to be in the range of 60 to 80 nM and the K_m for S-adenosylmethionine was found to be 22 μM. The methyltransferase was solubilized by Triton X-100, a procedure which inactiviated the 5-demethylubiquinone-9 reductase. Dithionite was found to partially substitute for NADH in both membranous and soluble systems. Inhibitors of catechol O-methyltransferase were not effective inhibitors of 5-demethylubiquinone-9-methyltransferase. In addition, catechol O-methyltransferase and 5-demethylubiquinone-9-methyltransferase were found to have reciprocal subcellular localizations. It is likely that the hydrophobic side chain of ubiquinone, added to 4-hydroxybenzoate in the first biosynthetic step, is required for attachment to the lipid bilayer. This permits subsequent metabolism of the ring system by membrane-bound enzymes, including the final methylation to form ubiquinone-9 (Houser and Olson, 1977).

VI. REGULATION OF UBIQUINONE BIOSYNTHESIS

A. ANIMAL STUDIES

1. *Effects of Starvation*

The effect of starvation is to greatly lower the activity of human menopausal gonadotropin (HMG)–CoA reductase in rat liver (Regen *et al.*, 1966; Hamprecht *et al.*, 1969). This decrease is associated with the early observations of a concomitant decrease in the rate of acetate incorporation into cholesterol (Tompkins and Chaikoff, 1952; Bucher *et al.*, 1959). Inamdar and Ramasarma (1971) also observed that tissue concentrations of ubiquinone were decreased in fasting and this was verified by Aiyar and Olson (1972) who observed that incorporation of [^{14}C]acetate into the side chain was greatly decreased.

Analogous studies with [^{14}C]mevalonic acid as the labeled precursor indicated that the specific radioactivity of the ubiquinone was unchanged (Aiyar and Olson, 1972) or even increased (Inamdar and Ramasarma, 1971). The increase was attributed to the elevated specific radioactivity of the mevalonic acid pool which was postulated to result from the diminished production of endogenous mevalonic acid. Inamdar and Ramasarma further reported that the degradation of ubiquinone was also decreased during starvation. Thus, their data indicated that fasting had a strong negative effect on ubiquinone biosynthesis by limiting the production of mevalonate.

2. *Effects of Cholesterol and Ubiquinone Feeding*

It has long been observed that cholesterol fed to rats decreased the incorporation of labeled acetate into endogenously formed cholesterol (Taylor and Gould, 1950; Tompkins and Chaikoff, 1952). This was shown to be primarily due to a depression of HMG–CoA reductase activity (Siperstein and Fagan, 1966; Linn, 1967; White and Rudney, 1970). The cholesterol effect, however, was not seen on ubiquinone synthesis. Rao and Olson (1967) found no effect of cholesterol on the pool size of ubiquinone or the incorporation of acetate into Q. The incorporation of mevalonic acid into sterols was also lowered by cholesterol feeding but the incorporation into ubiquinone was severalfold higher. Rao and Olson considered that the small amount of residual mevalonate synthesized in the livers of the cholesterol-fed rat was very efficiently used for the assembly of the side chain of ubiquinone. They further reasoned that the secondary block at the level of the cyclization of squalene would help to channel the isoprene precursors into the ubiquinone pathway. The presence of such a secondary site of regulation was first observed by Gould and Swyryd in 1966. Krishnaiah *et al.* (1967a) obtained similar results and they reported that feeding ubiquinone to rats seemed to decrease the synthesis of mevalonic acid and they suggested that ubiquinone might be a feedback regulator of reductase activity.

Later work (Aiyar and Olson, 1972) pointed to the biosynthesis of mevalonate as the limiting factor in the synthesis of ubiquinone. They observed mevalonate-enhanced incorporation of quinone ring precursors into ubiquinone in liver slices and that the enhancement was more pronounced in slices from fasted or cholesterol-fed rats. They also observed that the incorporation of ring precursors into ubiquinone was lowered in fasting and cholesterol feeding, thus confirming the earlier findings on [^{14}C]mevalonate incorporation into ubiquinone. This enhancement of the incorporation of ring precusors into ubiquinone by mevalonate has been observed in rat kidney minces (Momose and Rudney, 1972) and in isolated rat heart cells (Ranganathan et al., 1979). Ranganathan and Ramasarma (1975) observed that the incorporation of 4-hydroxybenzaldehyde into ubiquinone was decreased by starvation and cholesterol or folic acid feeding, but not by ubiquinone feeding. Thus, it seems that in general, ubiquinone plays a minimal role as a feedback regulator of its own synthesis.

3. Hormonal Effects

Hyperthyroidism, induced by administering thyroxin or thyroxin precursors, has been reported to increase the concentration of ubiquinone in rat liver (Aiyar et al., 1959; Edwin et al., 1960; Beyer et al., 1962). Inamdar and Ramasarma (1969) found that administration of thyroxin enhanced ubiquinone synthesis from mevalonic acid; in addition, it appeared to decrease the catabolism of ubiquinone. Hypothyroidism, induced by thiouracil, had a minimal effect on the concentration and synthesis of ubiquinone. It is unclear as to how these effects could influence the polyisoprenoid pathway. Administration of triiodothyronine to normal rats abolishes the circadian rhythm in reductase activity and maintains it at a peak level throughout the day (Dugan et al., 1974).

Epinephrine treatment is known to decrease the reductase activity in rats (Edwards, 1973). Inamdar (1968) has reported increases in the concentration and biogenesis of ubiquinone from mevalonate under similar conditions. On the other hand, the stimulation of reductase by catecholamines in rat liver or isolated rat hepatocytes (George and Ramasarma, 1977; Edwards, 1975) did not appear to be associated with any changes in the content or in the biosynthesis of ubiquinone (Inamdar, 1968). Other hormones, i.e., insulin, glucagon, glucocorticoids, and estrogens, have not as yet been examined for their effect on ubiquinone synthesis. These hormones do affect reductase activity and cholesterol synthesis (Lakshmanan et al., 1973; Ingebritsen et al., 1979; Cavanee and Melnykovich, 1977; Subbaiah, 1977).

4. Effects of Drugs

Many compounds and treatments are known which affect the biosynthesis of cholesterol and several of these were studied by Inamdar (1968). Other studies by a variety of authors are described in a review by Ramasarma (1972). This latter review lists, in tabular form, the substances and treatments and their effect on ubiquinone biosynthesis. α-Phenyl butyrate, an inhibitor of acetate activation (Steinberg and Frederickson, 1955), as well as of a postmevalonate step (Inamdar, 1968), inhibits both cholesterol and ubiquinone biosynthesis. SKF-525A (β-diethylaminoethylphenyl propylacetate hydrochloride), an inhibitor acting between isopentenyl pyrophosphate and squalene (Holmes and Benz, 1960), decreased the synthesis of ubiquinone from mevalonic acid.

Clofibrate (parachlorophenoxyisobutyrate, CPIB) has paradoxical effects. This drug markedly inhibits HMG–CoA reductase in rat liver (White, 1971; Cohen et al., 1974). Krishnaiah and Ramasarma (1970) observed that ubiquinone synthesis from labeled acetate was decreased by clofibrate treatment. However, the same treatment caused considerable enhancement of hepatic ubiquinone content. When labeled mevalonate was used as a tracer, ubiquinone synthesis was greater in controls than after a short-term drug treatment of 10 days. However, after longer treatment (25 days), the rate of ubiquinone synthesis was lower in the controls. This raised the possibility that the increase in ubiquinone synthesis was an apparent one since endogenous mevalonate production was blocked which could lead to an increased specific activity of the mevalonic acid pool. On the other hand, more recent work (Ranganathan and Ramasarma, 1975) showed that the incorporation of a ring precursor, 4-hydroxybenzaldehyde, was increased with clofibrate treatment, suggesting an actual enhancement of synthesis. It is suggested that the accumulation of ubiquinone in liver might be due in part to decreased catabolism.

Compactin (ML-236B), an analog of mevalonic acid, has been shown to be a powerful competitive inhibitor of HMG–CoA reductase in all systems that have been tested (Endo et al., 1976, 1977; Kaneko et al., 1978; Brown et al., 1978; Bensch et al., 1978). In whole animals, this compound inhibits the incorporation of [^{14}C]acetate into cholesterol and causes an acute reduction in plasma cholesterol after single, oral doses (Endo et al., 1976). It was observed by Brown et al. (1978) that this drug, when applied to the medium in fibroblast cultures, greatly reduced the activity of HMG–CoA reductase; however, the cells responded with a large increase in the synthesis of enzyme protein. This has also been observed in whole animals by Alberts et al. (1980) with an analog of compactin, mevinolin. Treatment of heterozygous familial hypercholesterolemic patients with compactin resulted in a lowered serum cholesterol (Mabuchi et al., 1981). Total serum ubiquinone content, however, remained the same even though the ubiquinone carried in the LDL fraction decreased by 50%. No studies on the effects of compactin or its analogs on the biosynthesis of ubiquinone in whole animals have been performed.

5. Effects of Radiation

X-Rays appear to have paradoxical effects on the synthesis of polyisoprene compounds. Whole body X-irradiation stimulated HMG–CoA reductase activity (Berndt and Gaumert, 1971; Aiyar et al., 1972) and the rate of cholesterol synthesis (Gould and Popjak, 1957; Gould et al., 1959; Berndt and Gaumert, 1970) in livers of rats and mice. Similar treatment of rats fed ad libitum had no stimulatory effect on ubiquinone synthesis (Aiyar et al., 1972). However, irradiation of fasted rats resulted in a 2- to 3-fold increase in the labeling of hepatic ubiquinone by [2-^{14}C]acetate, [U-^{14}C]benzoate, and [CH$_3$-^{14}C]methionine. There was no change in the incorporation of [2-^{14}C]mevalonate. Similar results were obtained in cholesterol-fed rats. The changes in incorporation of precursors into ubiquinone could be observed both in vivo and in vitro (Aiyar et al., 1972). These results suggest that HMG–CoA reductase is rate-limiting for ubiquinone synthesis in fasted or cholesterol-fed rats but not in Chow-fed animals.

B. Yeast Cells

1. Mechanism of "Catabolite Repression" of Ubiquinone Biosynthesis in Yeast

It is well known that respiration in yeast is inhibited by high external glucose concentrations. Lester and Crane (1969) observed that when yeast was grown anaerobically a significant reduction in the levels of ubiquinone-6 occurred. Sugimura and Rudney (1960) found that anaerobiosis depressed ubiquinone-6 levels in yeast from 180 to ca. 20 μg per g dry weight. These depressed levels were restored to normal when yeast cultures were incubated with 0.5% glucose and oxygen for 7 hours. In S. cerevisiae, the repressive effect of glucose on ubiquinone biosynthesis occurs in parallel with reduction in synthesis of cytochromes in the electron transport chain (Gordon and Stewart, 1969; Schatz and Mason, 1974). Gordon and Stewart (1969) found that high concentrations of glucose (i.e., 5.4%) and/or reduced oxygen tension inhibited ubiquinone biosynthesis, whereas similar concentrations of galactose inhibited ubiquinone biosynthesis to a lesser degree.

Preliminary experiments in Olson's laboratory (Sippel et al., 1979) confirmed the reciprocal relationship between the concentration of glucose in the medium and the levels of Q-6 in a wild-type strain (D273-10B) of *S. cerevisiae*. These same experiments demonstrated that the newly discovered intermediate 3,4-dihydroxy-5-hexaprenyl-benzoate (3,4-DHHB) accumulated as Q-6 levels fell. In more recent experiments, in the chemostat, in which these yeast cells were grown at constant pH, cell density, oxygen tension, and temperature in the presence of [U-^{14}C]4-hydroxybenzoate and various glucose concentrations, it was found that levels of 3,4-dihydroxy-5-hexaprenylbenzoate varied inversely with the diminished levels of Q-6 as shown in Fig. 6. These data suggest that O-methylation of 3,4-DHHB, the first methylation in ubiquinone synthesis, is a regulated step in "catabolite repression."

Fang and Butow (1970) observed that the inhibitory effect of high levels of glucose on mitochondrial respiration could be reversed in protoplasts if they were incubated with 1.2 mM cAMP. Sippel *et al.* (1983) showed that the inhibition of ubiquinone biosynthesis, in protoplasts of yeast cells incubated with 10% glucose, could be reversed by

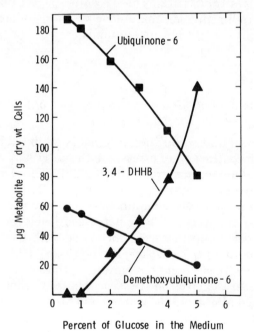

FIG. 6. Relationship between exogenous glucose concentrations and levels of Q-6, DMQ-6, and 3,4-DHHB in yeast cells. The triangles denote 3,4-dihydroxy-5-hexaprenylbenzoate concentrations, the squares ubiquinone-6 concentrations, and the circles 5-demethoxyubiquinone-6 concentrations.

1.2 μM cAMP or 10^{-4} M theophylline with a $t_{1/2}$ of 2.5 hours. Cycloheximide at 100 $\mu g/ml$ inhibited protein synthesis in yeast but did not affect the reversal of glucose repression by protoplast cAMP. Q-6 biosynthesis could not be restored by cAMP, in isolated mitochondria from yeast grown in the presence of 10% glucose, unless a cytosolic fraction was present. This evidence suggests that control of Q-6 biosynthesis is mediated through cAMP and that a cytosolic component, possibly a protein kinase, may be responsible for the phosphorylation and consequent activation of the 3,4-DHHB methylase. Since glucose is known to lower cAMP levels in cells, the "catabolite repression" of Q-6 synthesis in yeast cells may be due to the presence of an unphosphorylated and thus inactive methylase which permits the accumulation of 3,4-DHHB.

2. Regulation of 4-Hydroxybenzoate Synthesis from Tyrosine and Shikimate

Goewert (1979) found by using [U-^{14}C]shikimate and [U-^{14}C]tyrosine in yeast mutants blocked at various points in the aromatic amino acid biosynthetic pathway, that both shikimate and tyrosine can serve as precursors to ubiquinone-6. In general, aromatic pathway mutants blocked prior to chorismate rely on tyrosine as a source of 4-hydroxybenzoate, while mutants blocked after chorismate utilize the normal biosynthetic route via chorismate to 4-hydroxybenzoate. It was found that wild-type strains, employing the normal synthetic pathway, have elevated levels of 4-hydroxyphenylpyruvate with relatively low levels of p-hydroxyphenyl lactate. Mutants blocked prior to chorismate, which derive 4-hydroxybenzoate from tyrosine, contain a reduced level of 4-hydroxyphenyl pyruvate with elevated levels of 4-hydroxyphenyl lactate, indicating a possible point of regulation.

When shikimate (50 $\mu g/ml$) was added to a culture of aro 1c cells (blocked prior to shikimate) and allowed to grow 1 cell doubling time, the relative levels of 4-hydroxyphenyl pyruvate and 4-hydroxyphenyl lactate attained wild-type levels. This reversion was cycloheximide-independent, indicating regulation was at the level of substrate and did not involve new enzyme synthesis. A K_m of 0.27 mM was determined for the enzyme, 4-hydroxyphenyl pyruvate reductase (HPPR).

Various aromatic amino acid pathway intermediates were tested as possible effectors of this reaction. Only prephenate was found to significantly affect the activity of HPPR acting in a noncompetitive manner. These results indicate that the pathway from tyrosine to 4-hydroxybenzoate is negatively controlled at the substrate level by prephenate as shown in Fig. 7.

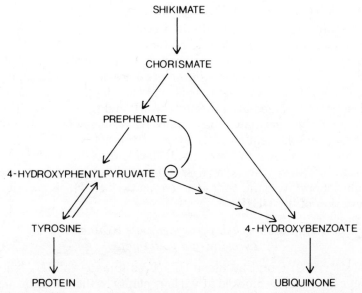

FIG. 7. The regulation of 4-hydroxybenzoate formation from tyrosine by prephenate in *S. cerevisiae.*

C. CULTURED CELLS

It is now well established that mammalian cells in culture respond to an absence of an exogenous supply of cholesterol with a large increase in the rate of cholesterol synthesis (Rothblat, 1972; Bailey, 1973; Goldstein and Brown, 1976, 1977). The increased cholesterol synthesis is also reflected in a stimulation of HMG–CoA reductase protein. Detailed studies on the effects of oxygenated sterols (Kandutsch *et al.*, 1978), of inhibitors of the reductase (Brown and Goldstein, 1980; Nambudiri *et al.*, 1980), and of growth and cell density (Chen, 1981; Sexton *et al.*, 1982; Panini *et al.*, 1982) on isoprenoid biosynthesis have utilized cultured cells.

1. *Effects of Lipoproteins and Inhibitors of HMG–CoA Reductase*

The uptake of cholesterol is regulated by the number of receptors which are generated in response to the level of cholesterol carried in low-density lipoproteins. The addition of LDL to a culture medium results in suppression of reductase and, thereby, an increase in endogenous sterol synthesis (Brown *et al.*, 1973; Brown and Goldstein, 1979).

The interrelationship of cholesterol and ubiquinone syntheses, under conditions where the activity of HMG–CoA reductase is altered severalfold, has recently been examined in cultured human fibroblasts (Faust et al., 1979; Nambudiri et al., 1980; Ranganathan et al., 1981; Rudney et al., 1981). When endogenous mevalonate production was inhibited by compactin or LDL, the incorporation of exogenous mevalonate into ubiquinone was increased two to three times faster than into cholesterol (Faust et al., 1979). In the absence of LDL, the reverse was true and a large increase of mevalonate into cholesterol was observed compared to that into ubiquinone. These results were interpreted to indicate that when the synthesis of cholesterol was inhibited at a postmevalonate step, the isopentenyl pyrophosphate units resulting from mevalonate were shifted into the ubiquinone pathway to form more ubiquinone. They also agreed with the earlier conclusions reached by Rao and Olson (1967) and Krishnaiah et al. (1967a) on the effect of cholesterol feeding on sterol and ubiquinone synthesis in rat liver, that the ubiquinone pathway could be saturated at much lower levels of mevalonate than the cholesterol pathway.

Nambudiri et al. (1980), on the other hand, interpreted the increased incorporation of [^{3}H]mevalonate into ubiquinone in the presence of compactin and LDL as due to the higher specific radioactivity of the intracellular pool of mevalonate resulting from the inhibition of HMG–CoA reductase. They observed that the incorporation of 4-hydroxybenzoate into ubiquinone under similar conditions was greatly inhibited. The inhibition could be overcome by the addition of mevalonic acid to the medium which indicated that HMG–CoA reductase was rate-limiting under these conditions. This was a different conclusion from that of Faust et al. (1979) who had made similar observations with labeled methionine. They found the synthesis of ubiquinone as measured by the incorporation of [$methyl$-^{3}H]methionine decreased by 76% in the presence of compactin and LDL. Ranganathan et al. (1981) also showed that compactin inhibited the incorporation of 2-[^{14}C]acetate and 4-hydroxybenzoate into ubiquinone to the same extent.

Nambudiri et al. (1980) and Ranganathan et al. (1981) observed that the incorporation of labeled acetate or 4-hydroxybenzoate into ubiquinone appeared to be higher in cells grown in medium supplemented with whole human serum as compared to cells in a medium supplemented with lipoprotein-deficient serum. This occurred despite the fact that there was a 20-fold increase in the activity of HMG–CoA reductase in lipoprotein-deficient serum. Addition of LDL to these cells caused a further reduction in the incorporation of these precursors into ubiquinone. These authors suggested that whole human serum may contain a stimulatory factor for ubiquinone biosynthesis which is removed when lipoproteins are separated from the serum. Recent work (Sexton *et al.*, 1982) shows, however, that this effect is observed only in cells that have reached the stationary phase of growth. In cells growing logarithmically, the treatment produced a two- to threefold increase in the incorporation of 4-hydroxybenzoate into ubiquinone.

Another class of inhibitors which is being used to study the regulation of HMG–CoA reductase are the oxygenated sterols. The inhibitory effect of oxygenated sterols on HMG–CoA reductase activity was first observed by Kandutsch and Chen (1973, 1974). Kandutsch *et al.* (1978) suggested that oxygenated sterols may represent the physiological feedback regulator of reductase. This suggestion comes from the observation that highly purified cholesterol caused little inhibition of reductase activity. The addition of 8-ketocholesterol or 25-hydroxycholesterol to human fibroblasts, grown in the presence or absence of lipoproteins, inhibited both the reductase activity and the incorporation of 4-hydroxybenzoate into ubiquinone (Nambudiri *et al.*, 1980). As in the previous observations of Nambudiri *et al.* (1980) and Rudney *et al.* (1981), this inhibition could be reversed by the addition of mevalonate to the culture medium.

2. *Effects of Changes in Cell Density*

The effect of cell density on the activity of the sterol biosynthetic pathway has been examined in several cell lines (Chen, 1981; Sexton *et al.*, 1982; Panini *et al.*, 1982). Chen observed that the activity of HMG–CoA reductase decreased linearly with increasing cell density. There was a parallel decrease in the incorporation of [^{14}C]acetate into cholesterol and fatty acids, and of [^{3}H]thymidine into DNA. Similar observations were made with cultured human fibroblasts (Sexton *et al.*, 1982). In cultures of rat intestinal epithelial cells (IEC-6), Panini *et al.* (1982) observed that reductase specific activity increased during logarithmic growth and decreased after confluency. They measured the incorporation of [^{3}H]acetate and [U-^{14}C]4-hydroxybenzoate into ubiquinone and observed a progressive decrease with growth in both cell lines to approximately 50% of the rates observed in the log phase. These results suggested that cell growth was coordinately regulating the pathway for isoprenoid biosynthesis at some stage that was common to both sterols and ubiquinone.

3. *Regulation at Points beyond HMG–CoA Reductase*

The differential effect of rates of inhibitors of the synthesis of the ubiquinone and sterol pathways has generally led to the acceptance of a view stated by Gold and Olson (1966) that an enzyme in the pathway for ubiquinone formation is more readily saturated with isoprenoid substrates than are the enzymes in the pathway for cholesterol biosynthesis. It seemed reasonable to expect that if the cholesterol pathway was inhibited, an increase might be expected in the ubiquinone pathway, or at least there would be no decrease. The differing interpretations of similar experiments by Faust et al. (1979) and Nambudiri et al. (1980) have already been alluded to. In a recent study, Volpe and Obert (1982) studied the effects of 3β-[2-diethylaminoethoxy]androst-5-en-17-one [U-1866A] on the biosynthesis of cholesterol and ubiquinone in cultured C-6 glial cells. Treatment of these cells with U-1866A resulted in an inhibition of [^{14}C]acetate incorporation to cholesterol and a corresponding increase into ubiquinone. There was no corresponding effect of this compound on HMG–CoA reductase activity. Volpe and Obert interpreted these results in support of the observations of Faust et al. (1979) that there was a tight link between sterol and ubiquinone synthesis in neural tissue. Recent work from our laboratory (Panini et al., 1983) on the effects of U-1866A on human fibroblasts and IEC-6 cells indicated that there was little or no stimulation of 4-hydroxybenzoate incorporation into ubiquinone under these conditions. However, in agreement with Volpe and Obert (1982), the increase of acetate and mevalonate incorporation into ubiquinone was also observed. Further studies show that this large enhancement of the incorporation of acetate was into a compound which contaminated the ubiquinone fraction. Panini et al. (1982) have indicated that this is a derivative of squalene, namely the 2,3:22,22-dioxide, which results from the inhibition of the 2,3-oxidosqualene cyclase by U-1866A.

D. Overview of the Regulation of Isoprenoid Biosynthesis

The current understanding of the factors regulating isoprenoid synthesis is summarized in Fig. 8. Many of these have been discussed in previous sections of this article. While HMG–CoA reductase appears to be the primary regulatory point, other steps in the pathway are also susceptible to regulation. Hormonal factors may not only affect the content of HMG–CoA reductase, but also regulate interconversion of active and inactive forms of the enzyme (Dugan, 1981; Beg and Brewer, 1981). Inhibition of HMG–CoA synthetase, squalene oxidocyclase, and methylsterol oxidase by LDL cholesterol and oxysterols in cultured cells and by cholesterol feeding of intact animals has been noted (Brown and Goldstein, 1980; Chang and Limanek, 1980; Quereshi and Porter, 1981; Gaylor, 1981). Regulation of membrane-bound

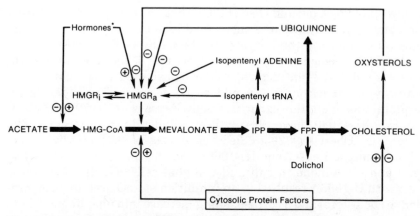

F $_{\text{IG}}$. 8. Factors regulating isoprenoid compound biosynthesis. Bold arrows are used to indicate the formation of intermediates and products. Thin arrows indicate probable sites of action of effectors. Positive and negative signs indicate activation or inhibition of the indicated step(s) in the pathway. IPP, Isopentenyl pyrophosphate; FPP, farnesyl pyrophosphate; HMGR$_i$ and HMGR$_a$, inactive and active forms of HMG–CoA reductase. The cytosolic factors include sterol carrier protein, supernatant protein factor, and fatty acid binding protein. Hormones include thyroxine, catecholamines, insulin, glucocorticoids, and estrogens.

enzymes of sterol synthesis in concert by various cytosolic protein factors has been proposed (Gaylor, 1981).

The subcellular localization of various enzymes of isoprenoid synthesis could also play a role in regulation. While HMG–CoA reductase in mammalian systems is associated with endoplasmic reticulum, enzymes leading to the formation of HMG–CoA from acetyl-CoA and those between mevalonate and farnesyl pyrophosphate are chiefly cytosolic (Quereshi and Porter, 1981; Dugan, 1981; Poulter and Rilling, 1981). HMG–CoA synthase has been observed in both cytoplasmic and mitochondrial compartments in chicken liver and kidney (Clinkenbeard *et al.*, 1975). The cytoplasmic enzyme may play a regulatory role in isoprenoid synthesis because of its response to cholesterol feeding (White and Rudney, 1970), oxysterols (Chang and Limanek, 1980), and glucocorticoids (Ramachandran *et al.*, 1978). Mitochondrial acetoacetyl-CoA thiolase and HMG–CoA synthase do not respond to dietary cholesterol and are therefore considered to be involved only in ketogenesis and not in isoprenoid synthesis (Quereshi and Porter, 1981). Since the syntheses of 2,3-dihydrodolichyl pyrophosphate (Daleo *et al.*, 1977) and solanesyl pyrophosphate (Momose and Rudney, 1972) are reported to be associated with the mitochondria, the possibility exists that these organelles may possess a complete prenyl biosynthetic pathway leading to the production of dolichols and the sidechain of ubiquinone. Wong and Lennarz (1982b) and Adair and Keller (1982) have found that the microsomal fraction from rat liver is capable of the complete synthesis of dolichol from farnesyl pyrophosphate. When isopentenyl pyrophosphate was used as the precursor, supplementation of microsomes with cytosol fraction was necessary for the synthesis of dolichol (Wong and Lennarz, 1982b). Total ubiquinone biosynthesis can be accomplished in rat liver mitochondria (Trumpower and Olson, 1971; Trumpower et al., 1974).

VII. Ubiquinone–Ubichromenol–α-Tocopherol Interrelationships

When this issue was reviewed in 1966 (Olson, 1966) there was a controversy about the biosynthesis of ubichromenol, a cyclic isomer of ubiquinone, from ubiquinone. At that time Joshi et al. (1963) raised the question of whether ubiquinone or ubichromenol was the primary synthetic product from [2-^{14}C]mevalonate in kidney and liver tissue from the rat. They claimed that in their experiments a higher specific activity was found in ubichromenol than in ubiquinone. Olson et al. (1965) carried out two kinds of experiments to check this rather remarkable conclusion and could not confirm the conversion of ubichromenol to ubiquinone. In their first experiments Olson et al. (1965) incubated [U-^{14}C]benzoate with liver slices and isolated ubiquinone-9 and ubichromenol-9 by standard procedures. The total activity incorporated into ubiquinone-9 was 200 times that of ubichromenol-9. The specific radioactivity of ubiquinone-9 was 20 times that of ubichromenol-9.

In another study ubiquinone-9 was labeled biologically in the side chain with [2-C^{14}]mevalonate and purified to radiochemical purity. A portion of this product was converted to ubichromenol-9 by refluxing with pyridine and was isolated by chromatography. These two metabolites were separately complexed with albumin and incubated with liver slices for 5 hours at 37°C. The washed tissue slices were extracted with alcohol–ether (3:1) and the Q-9 and ubichromenol-9 were isolated and purified by chromatography. When ubiquinone-9 was labeled, the ubiquinone-9 of the tissues became richly labeled and the specific activity of the tissue ubichromenol-9 attained half the specific activity of its precursor. This represented an appreciable transformation of ubiquinone to ubichromenol. On the other hand, when ubichromenol was the substrate, tissue ubichromenol became labeled but the tissue ubiquinone-9 was essentially unlabeled. It was suggested that although ubiquinone-9 can be metabolized to ubichromenol-9, the reverse transformation occurs in an extraordinarily slow and most likely insigificant rate.

The turnover of Q is relatively slow in the animal body so that its rate of synthesis clearly meets the needs of the tissues. On the other hand, α-tocopherol has been established as a vitamin in animals and man. The range of deficiency diseases, reported in a large number of species, is impressive.

More recently it has been claimed that α-tocopherol quinone, which is a homolog of ubiquinone, is synthesized in rats (Hughes and Tove 1980), but the report has been questioned (Bieri and Tolliver, 1982; Plack and Bieri, 1964). The levels of tocopherol quinone reported to be found in rat tissues of Hughes and Tove (1980) are 10 times higher than those found by other workers. Tyrosine is known to be a precursor of tocopherol in plants by way of the homogentisate pathway which contrasts with the pathway for tyrosine to 4-hydroxybenzoate in ubiquinone biosynthesis. More work is necessary before this claim can be evaluated.

VIII. Summary

Ubiquinone is an essential component of electron transport systems in mitochondria in most prokaryotic and all eukaryotic cells. Ubiquinone is biosynthesized from a number of precursor molecules in the inner membrane of mitochondria. The isoprenyl side chain is derived from mevalonate, the ring from tyrosine (or chorismate), the hydroxyl groups from molecular oxygen, and the methyl groups from S-adenosylmethionine. 4-Hydroxybenzoate is the pivotal aromatic precursor.

The first committed step in ubiquinone biosynthesis is the alkylation of 4-hydroxybenzoate by polyprenyl pyrophosphate. The initial stages of the biosynthesis of polyprenyl pyrophosphate are accomplished in the cytosol and the product is transported through the external mitochondrial membrane to the internal membrane where the alkylation reaction occurs. It is possible that some chain elongation occurs in the mitochondria. The rate of alkylation is driven by the concentration of isoprenyl pyrophosphate in proximity to the enzyme. The transferase is quite nonspecific with respect to chain length of the polyprenyl pyrophosphate so that length of the side chain is regulated by the isoprenyl phosphate polymerase(s).

Detailed metabolic pathways for the biosynthesis of ubiquinone in both prokaryotic and eukaryotic cells have now been established. Most interesting is the fact that the pathway from 4-hydroxypolyprenyl benzoate (4-HPB) to 6-methoxypolyprenyl phenol is different in pro- and eukaryotic organisms. The process in prokaryotic organisms involves decarboxylation, hydroxylation, and methylation in that order. In eukaryotic organisms, the order is hydroxylation, methylation, and carboxylation. It is not clear why this difference occurs, but it may serve regulatory purposes in eukaryotic cells.

The regulation of the biosynthesis of ubiquinone occurs at different points. HMG–CoA reductase appears to be the primary regulatory site for isopentenyl pyrophosphate biosynthesis. It appears, furthermore, that hormonal factors may not only affect the content of HMG–CoA reductase but also regulate interconversion of active and inactive forms of the enzyme. The inhibition of HMG–CoA synthase, CoA synthetase, squalene oxidocyclase, and methylsterol oxidase by LDL-cholesterol and oxysterols in cultured cells and by cholesterol feedings in studies with intact animals has been noted. In yeast cells the first methylase in the eukaryotic metabolic sequence, namely SAM;4-hydroxy-5-polyprenyl benzoate-O-methyltransferase, appears to be regulated by the concentration of cAMP. This methylase appears to require phosphorylation for activity and explains "catabolite repression" of Q-6 synthesis in yeast. When glucose levels in the medium are high and cAMP levels low, biosynthesis of ubiquinone is interrupted and 3,4-dihydroxy-5-polyprenyl benzoate accumulates. Reduction of glucose levels by the addition of cAMP to protoplasts will restore Q-6 synthesis. In rats, vitamin A deficiency increases ubiquinone biosynthesis by diverting more polyprenyl phosphate to ubiquinone biosynthesis at the squalene oxidocyclase stage.

Several of the enzymes in the sequence leading to the biosynthesis of Q have been partially purified. Since these are all membrane bound enzymes, progress has been modest in purifying them and describing their properties. It is expected that this field will continue to be an interesting one for researchers in the future.

Acknowledgments

The authors wish to acknowledge support by grants which aided in the conduct of some of the work reported here and in the preparation of this manuscript. REO acknowledges the support of the National Institutes of Health, AM-10004 and HR acknowledges the support of the National Science Foundation, PCM-820-4817 and the National Institutes of Health, AM-12402.

REFERENCES

Acheson, R. M., and Gibbard, S. (1962). The hydroxylation of benzoic acid by rats and guinea pigs. *Biochim. Biophys. Acta* **59**, 320–325.

Adair, W. L., Jr., and Keller, R. K. (1982). Dolichol metabolism in rat liver. *J. Biol. Chem.* **257**, 8990–8996.

Aiyar, A. S., and Olson, R. E. (1964). Biosynthesis of the benzoquinone ring of coenzyme Q_9 in the rat. *Fed. Proc., Fed. Am. Soc. Exp. Biol.* **23**, 425.

Aiyar, A. S., and Olson, R. E. (1972). Enhancement of ubiquinone-9 biosynthesis in rat liver slices by exogenous mevalonate. *Eur. J. Biochem.* **27**, 60–64.

Aiyar, A. S., Sulebele, G. A., Rege, D. V., and Sreenivasan, A. (1959). Pantothenic acid deficiency and ubiquinone levels in rat liver mitochondria. *Nature (London)* **184**, 1867–1868.

Aiyar, A. S., Gopalaswamy, U. V., and Sreenivasan, A. (1972). Stimulation of ubiquinone biosynthesis in irradiated rats. *Environ. Physiol. Biochem.* **2**, 86–95.

Albers-Schonberg, G., Joshua, H., Lopez, M., Hensens, O., Springer, J., Chen, J., Ostrove, S., Hoffman, C., Alberts, A., and Patchett, A. (1981). Dihydromevinolin, a potent hypocholesterolemic metabolite produced by *Aspergillus terreus. J. Antibiot.* **34**, 507–512.

Alberts, A. W., Chen, G., Kuron, G., Hunt, V., Huff, J., Hoffman, C., Rothrock, J., Lopez, M., Josua, H., Harris, E., Patchett, A., Monaghan, R., Currie, S., Stapley, E., Albers-Schonberg, G., Hensens, O., Hirshfield, J., Hoogsteen, K., Liesch, J., and Springer, J. (1980). Mevinolin: A highly potent competitive inhibitor of hydroxymethylglutaryl-coenzyme A reductase and a cholesterol-lowering agent. *Proc. Natl. Acad. Sci. U.S.A.* **77**, 3957–3961.

Avoy, D. R., Swyryd, E. A., and Gould, R. G. (1965). Effects of α-p-chlorophenoxypybutyryl ethyl ester (cPIB) with and without androsterone on cholesterol biosynthesis in rat liver. *J. Lipid Res.* **6**, 369–376.

Bailey, J. M. (1973). Regulation of cell cholesterol content. *Ciba Found. Symp.* **12**, 63–92.

Bakke, J. E., and Olson, R. E. (1982). Detection of 4-hydroxy-5-nonaprenyl benzoate hydroxylase in rat liver and kidney mitochondria. *Fed. Proc. Fed. Am. Soc. Exp. Biol.* **41**, 668.

Beg, Z. H., and Brewer, H. B., Jr. (1981). Regulation of liver 3-hydroxy-3-methylglutaryl-CoA. *Curr. Top. Cell Regul.* **20**, 139–184.

Beirne, O. R., Heller, R., and Watson, J. A. (1977). Regulation of 3-hydroxy-3-methylglutaryl coenzyme A reductase in minimal hepatoma 7288C. *J. Biol. Chem.* **252**, 950–954.

Bell, J. J., Sargeant, T. E., and Watson, J. A. (1976). Inhibition of 3-hydroxy-3-methylglutaryl coenzyme A reductase activity in hepatoma tissue culture cells by pure cholesterol and several cholesterol derivatives. Evidence supporting two distinct mechanisms. *J. Biol. Chem.* **251**, 1745–1758.

Bensch, W. R., Ingrebritsen, T. S., and Diller, E. R. (1978). Lack of correlation between the rate of cholesterol biosynthesis and the activity of 3-hydroxy-3-methylglutaryl coenzyme A reductase in rats and in fibroblasts treated with ML-236B. *Biochem. Biophys. Res. Commun.* **82**, 247–254.

Bentley, R., Ramsey, V. G., Springer, C. M., Dialameh, G. H., and Olson, R. E. (1961). The origin of the benzoquinone ring of coenzyme Q in the rat. *Biochem. Biophys. Res. Commun.* **5**, 443–446.

Bentley, R., Springer, C. M., Ramsey, V., Dialameh, G. H., and Olson, R. E. (1968). The origin of the carbon methyl group and its point of attachment. *J. Biol. Chem.* **243,** 174–177.

Berndt, J., and Gaumert, R. (1970). The in vitro biosynthesis of cholesterol and the cholesterol content in the liver of X-irradiated mice. *Radiat. Res.* **42,** 292–304.

Berndt, J., and Gaumert, R. (1971). Stimulation of hydroxymethylglutaryl coenzyme A reductase in mouse liver by X-rays. *FEBS Lett.* **13,** 49–52.

Beyer, R. E., Noble, W. M., and Hirschfeld, T. J. (1962). Alterations of rat tissue coenzyme Q (ubiquinone) levels by various treatments. *Biochim. Biophys. Acta* **57,** 376–379.

Bieri, J., and Tolliver, T. J. (1982). On the occurrence of α-tocopherol-quinone in rat tissue. *Lipids* **16,** 777–779.

Bloch, K., Chaykin, S., Phillips, A. H., and DeWaard, A. (1959). Mevalonic acid pyrophosphate and isopentenylpyrophosphate. *J. Biol. Chem.* **234,** 2595–2604.

Booth, A. N., Masri, M. S., Robbins, D. J., Emerson, O. H., Jones, F. T., and DeEds, F. (1960). Urinary phenolic acid metabolites of tyrosine. *J. Biol. Chem.* **235,** 2649–2652.

Brown, M. S., and Goldstein, J. L. (1974). Suppression of 3-hydroxy-3-methylglutaryl coenzyme A reductase activity and inhibition of growth of human fibroblasts by 7-ketocholesterol. *J. Biol. Chem.* **249,** 7306–7314.

Brown, M. S., and Goldstein, J. L. (1979). Receptor-mediated endocytosis: Insights from the lipoprotein receptor system. *Proc. Natl. Acad. Sci. U.S.A.* **76,** 3330–3337.

Brown, M. S., and Goldstein, J. L. (1980). Multivalent feedback regulation of HMG-CoA reductase, a control mechanism coordinating isoprenoid synthesis and cell growth. *J. Lipid Res.* **21,** 505–517.

Brown, M. S., Dana, S. E., and Goldstein, J. L. (1973). Regulation of 3-hydroxy-3-methylglutaryl coenzyme A reductase activity in human fibroblasts by lipoproteins. *Proc. Natl. Acad. Sci. U.S.A.* **70,** 2162–2166.

Brown, M. S., Dana, S. E., and Goldstein, J. L. (1974). Regulation of 3-hydroxy-3-methylglutaryl coenzyme A reductase activity in cultured human fibroblasts. *J. Biol. Chem.* **249,** 789–796.

Brown, M. S., Fausy, J. R., and Goldstein, J. L. (1978). Induction of 3-hydroxy-3-methylglutaryl coenzyme A reductase activity in human fibroblasts incubated with compaction (ML-236B), a competitive inhibitor of the reductase. *J. Biol. Chem.* **253,** 1121–1128.

Bucher, N. L. R., McGarrahan, K., Gould, E., and Loud, A. V. (1959). Cholesterol biosynthesis in preparations of liver from normal, fasting, X-irradiated, cholesterol-fed, Triton, or Δ^4-cholesten-3-one-treated rats. *J. Biol. Chem.* **234,** 262–267.

Bucher, N. L. R., Overath, P., and Lynen, F. (1960). β-hydroxy-β-methylglutaryl coenzyme A reductase, cleavage and condensing enzymes in relation to cholesterol formation in rat liver. *Biochim. Biophys. Acta* **40,** 491–501.

Busch, H. (1953). Studies on metabolism of acetate-1-C^{14} in tissues of tumor-bearing rats. *Cancer Res.* **13,** 789–794.

Casey, J., and Threlfall, D. R. (1978). Synthesis of 5-demethoxyubiquinone-6 and ubiquinone-6 from 3-hexaprenyl-4-hydroxybenzoate in yeast mitochondria. *FEBS Lett.* **85,** 249–253.

Cavenee, W. K., and Melnykovych, G. (1977). Induction of 3-hydroxy-3-methylglutaryl coenzyme A reductase in HeLa cells by glucocorticoids.*J. Biol. Chem.* **252,** 3272–3276.

Chang, T. Y., and Limanek, J. S. (1980). Regulation of cytosolic acetoacetyl coenzyme A thiolase, 3-hydroxy-3-methylglutaryl coenzyme A synthase, 3-hydroxy-3-methylglutaryl coenzyme A reductase, and mevalonate kinase by low density lipoprotein and by 25-hydroxycholesterol in Chinese hamster ovary cells. *J. Biol. Chem.* **255,** 7787–7795.

Chen, H. W. (1981). The activity of 3-hydroxy-3-methylglutaryl coenzyme A reductase and the rate of sterol synthesis diminish in cultures with high cell density. *J. Cell Physiol.* **108,** 91–97.

Clinkenbeard, K. D., Sugiyama, T., Reed, W. D., and Lane, M. P. (1975). Cytoplasmic 3-hydroxy-3-methylglutaryl coenzyme A synthase from liver. *J. Biol. Chem.* **250,** 3124–3135.

Cohen, B. I., Raicht, R. F., Shefer, S., and Mosbach, E. H. (1974). Effects of clofibrate on sterol metabolism in the rat. *Biochim. Biophys. Acta* **369,** 79–85.

Collins, M. D., and Jones, D. (1981). Lipid composition of the entomopathogen *Corynebacterium okanaganae* (Luthy). *FEMS Microbiol. Lett.* **10,** 157–159.

Cox, G. B., and Gibson, F. (1964). Biosynthesis of vitamin K and ubiquinone. Relation to the shikimic acid pathway in *Escherichia coli. Biochim. Biophys. Acta* **93,** 204–206.

Cox, G. B., Gibson, F., and Pittard, J. (1968). Mutant strains of *Escherichia coli* K-12 unable to form ubiquinone. *J. Bacteriol.* **95,** 1591–1598.

Cox, G. B., Young, I. G., McCann, L. M., and Gibson, F. (1969). Biosynthesis of ubiquinone in *Escherichia coli* K-12: Location of genes affecting the metabolism of 3-octaprenyl-4-hydroxybenzoic acid and 2-octaprenylphenol. *J. Bacteriol.* **99,** 450–458.

Crane, F. L. (1965). Distribution of ubiquinones. *In:* "Biochemistry of Quinones" (R. A. Morton, ed.), pp. 183–206. Academic Press, New York.

Crane, F. L., Hatefi, Y., Lester, R. L., and Widmer, C. (1957). Isolation of quinone from beef heart and beef heart mitochondria. *Biochim. Biophys. Acta* **25,** 220–221.

Daleo, G. R., Hopp, H. E., Romero, P. A., and Pont-Lezica, R. (1977). Biosynthesis of dolichol phosphate by subcellular fractions from liver. *FEBS Lett.* **81,** 411–414.

Daves, G. D., Jr., Moore, H. W., Schwab, D. E., Olsen, R. K., Wilczynsk, J. J., and Folkers, K. (1967). Synthesis of 2-multiprenylphenols and 2-multiprenyl-6-methoxyphenols, biosynthetic precursors of the ubiquinones. *J. Org. Chem.* **32,** 1414–1417.

Davis, B. D. (1952). Aromatic biosynthesis. IV. Preferential conversion, in incompletely blocked mutants, of a common precursor of several metabolites. *J. Bacteriol.* **64,** 729–748.

DeKok, J., and Slater, E. C. (1975). Ubiquinone redox potential in *Saccharomyces cerevisiae. Biochim. Biophys. Acta* **376,** 27–41.

DeLuca, H. F. (1979). The vitamin D system in the regulation of calcium and phosphorus metabolism. *Nutr. Rev.* **37,** 161–193.

Dialameh, G. H., and Olson, R. E. (1959). Incorporation of acetate-1-C^{14} into coenzyme Q. *Fed. Proc. Fed. Am. Soc. Exp. Biol.* **18,** 214.

Dialameh, G. H., Nowicki, H. G., Yekundi, K. G., and Olson, R. E. (1970). Involvement of p-OH-benzoyl-coenzyme A in the biosynthesis of ubiquinone-9 in the rat. *Biochem. Biophys. Res. Commun.* **40,** 1063–1069.

Dugan, R. E. (1981). Regulation of HMG-CoA reductase. *In:* "Biosynthesis of Isoprenoid Compounds" (J. W. Porter and S. L. Spurgeon, eds.), pp. 95–160. Wiley, New York.

Dugan, R. E., Ness, G. C., Lakshmanan, M. R., Nepokroeff, C. M., and Porter, J. W. (1974). Regulation of hepatic β-hydroxy-β-methylglutaryl coenzyme A reductase by the interplay of hormones. *Arch. Biochem. Biophys.* **151,** 499–504.

Edelhoch, H. (1967). Spectroscopic determination of tryptophan and tyrosine in proteins. *Biochemistry* **6,** 1948–1954.

Edwards, P. A. (1973). Effect of adrenalectomy and hypophysectomy on the circadian rhythm of β-hydroxy-β-methylglutaryl coenzyme A reductase activity in rat liver. *J. Biol. Chem.* **248,** 2912–2917.

Edwards, P. A. (1975). The influence of catecholamines and cyclic AMP on 3-hydroxy-3-methylglutaryl coenzyme A reductase activity and lipid biosynthesis in isolated rat hepatocytes. *Arch. Biochem. Biophys.* **170,** 188–203.

Edwin, B. E., and Green, J. (1960a). Reversal by α-tocopherol and other substances of succinoxidase inhibition produced by a *Tetrahymena pyriformis* preparation. *Arch. Biochem. Biophys.* **87,** 337–338.

Edwin, B. E., Green, J., Diplock, A. T., and Bunyan, J. (1960b). The effect of thyroxine and 2,4-dinitrophenol on levels of ubiquinone and ubichromenol in the rat. *Nature,(London)* **186,** 725.

Endo, A. (1979). Monocolin K, a new hypocholesterolemic agent produced by a *Monabcus* species. *J. Antibiot.* **32,** 852–854.

Endo, A., Kuroda, M., and Tsujita, Y. (1976a). Presence of isomers in quinomycin E. *J. Antibiot.* **29,** 1346–1348.

Endo, A., Kuroda, M., and Tanzawa, K. (1976b). Hormonal regulation of liver mitochondrial pyruvate carrier in relation to gluconeogenesis and lipogenesis. *FEBS Lett.* **72,** 323–326.

Endo, A., Tsujita, Y., Kuroda, M., and Tanzawa, K. (1977). Inhibition of cholesterol synthesis in vitro and in vivo by ML-236A and ML-236B, competitive inhibitors of 3-hydroxy-3-methylglutaryl coenzyme A reductase. *Eur. J. Biochem.* **77,** 31–36.

Endo, A., Tsujita, Y., Kuroda, M., and Tanzawa, K. (1979). Effects of ML-236B on cholesterol metabolism in mice and rats: Lack of hypocholesterolemic activity in normal animals. *Biochim. Biophys. Acta* **575,** 266–276.

Ephrussi, B., and Slonimski, P. P. (1950). La synthese adaptative des cytochromes chez la levure de boulangerie. *Biochim. Biophys. Acta* **6,** 256–267.

Erickson, S. K., Matsui, S. M., Shrewsbury, M. A., Cooper, A. D., and Gould, R. G. (1978). Effects of 2,5-hydroxycholesterol on rat hepatic 3-hydroxy-3-methylglutaryl coenzyme A reductase activity in vivo, in perfused liver, and in hepatocytes. *J. Biol. Chem.* **253,** 4159–4164.

Fang, M., and Butow, R. (1970). Nucleotide reversal of mitochondrial repression in *Saccharomyces cerevisiae. Biochem. Biophys. Res. Commun.* **41,** 1579–1583.

Faust, J. R., Goldstein, J. L., and Brown, M. S. (1979). Synthesis of ubiquinone and cholesterol in human fibroblasts: Regulation of branched pathway. *Arch. Biochem. Biophys.* **192,** 86–99.

Fears, R., Richards, D. H., and Ferres, H. (1980). The effect of compactin, a potent inhibitor of hydroxy-3-methylglutaryl coenzyme-A reductase activity, on cholesterolgenesis and serum cholesterol levels in rats and chicks. *Atherosclerosis* **35,** 439–449.

Festenstein, G. N., Heaton, F. W., Lowe, J. S., and Morton, R. A. (1955). A constituent of the unsaponifiable portion of animal tissue lipids. *Biochem. J.* **59,** 558–566.

Friis, P., Daves, G. D., Jr., and Folkers, K. (1966). Complete sequence of biosynthesis from p-hydroxybenzoic acid to ubiquinone. *J. Am. Chem. Soc.* **88,** 4754–4756.

Friis, P., Daves, G. D., and Folkers, K. (1967). New epoxyubiquinones.*Biochemistry* **6,** 3618–3624.

Gale, P. H., Arison, B. H., Trenner, N. R., Page, A. C., Jr., and Folkers, K. (1963a). Coenzyme Q. XXXVI. Isolation and characterization of coenzyme Q10 (H-10). *Biochemistry* **2,** 196–206.

Gale, P. H., Trenner, N. R., Arison, B. H., Page, A. C., Jr., and Folkers, K. (1963b).

Coenzyme Q. XLXI. Characterization of coenzyme Q10 (H-10) from *Pennicillium stipitatum. Biochem. Biophys. Res. Commun.* **12,** 414–417.

Gaylor, J. L. (1981). Formation of sterols in animals. *In* "Biosynthesis of Isoprenoid Compounds" (J. W. Porter and S. L. Spurgeon, eds.), Vol. 1, pp. 481–543. Wiley, New York.

George, R., and Ramasarma, T. (1977). Nature of the stimulation of biogenesis of cholesterol in the liver by noradrenaline. *Biochem. J.* **162,** 493–499.

Ghazarian, J. G., Jefcoate, C. R., Knutson, J. C., Orme-Johnson, W. H., and DeLuca, H. F. (1974). Mitochondrial cytochrome P_{450}—a component of chick kidney 25-hydroxycholecalciferol-1α-hydroxylase. *J. Biol. Chem.* **249,** 3026–3033.

Gibson, F. (1956). Chorismic acid: Purification and some chemical and physical studies. *Biochem. J.* **90,** 256–261.

Gibson, F. (1973). Chemical and genetic studies on the biosynthesis of ubiquinone by *Escherichia coli. Biochem. Soc. Trans.* **1,** 317–326.

Gloor, U., and Wiss, O. (1959). On the biosynthesis of ubiquinone (50). *Arch. Biochem. Biophys.* **83,** 216–222.

Goewert, R. R. (1979). Studies of the biosynthesis of ubiquinone in *Saccharomyces cerevisiae.* Ph.D. Dissertation, St. Louis University.

Goewert, R. R., Sippel, C. J., and Olson, R. E. (1977). The isolation and identification of a novel intermediate in ubiquinone-6 biosynthesis by *Saccharomyces cerevisiae. Biochem. Biophys. Res. Commun.* **77,** 599–605.

Goewert, R. R., Sippel, C. J., Grimm, M. F., and Olson, R. E. (1978). Identification of 3-methoxy-4-hydroxy-5-hexaprenylbenzoic acid as a new intermediate in ubiquinone biosynthesis by *Saccharomyces cerevisiae. FEBS Lett.* **87,** 219–221.

Goewert, R. E., Sippel, C. J., Grimm, M. F., and Olson, R. E. (1981a). Identification of 3-methoxy-4-hydroxy-5-hexaprenyl-benzoic acid as a new intermediate in ubiquinone biosynthesis by *Saccharomyces cerevisiae. Biochemistry* **20,** 5611–5616.

Goewert, R. R., Sippel, C. J., and Olson, R. E. (1981b). Identification of 3,4-dihydroxy-5-hexaprenyl-benzoic acid as an intermediate in the biosynthesis of ubiquinone-6 by *Saccharomyces cerevisiae. Biochemistry* **20,** 217–4223.

Gold, P. H., and Olson, R. E. (1966). Studies on coenzyme Q. The biosynthesis of coenzyme Q_9 in rat tissue slices. *J. Biol. Chem.* **241,** 3507–3516.

Goldstein, J. L., and Brown, M. S. (1976). The LDL pathway in human fibroblasts: A receptor-mediated mechanism for the regulation of cholesterol metabolism. *Curr. Top. Cell Regul.* **11,** 147–181.

Goldstein, J. L., and Brown, M. S. (1977). The low-density lipoprotein pathway and its relation to atherosclerosis. *Annu. Rev. Biochem.* **46,** 897–930.

Gordon, P. A., and Stewart, P. R. (1969). Ubiquinone formation in wild type and petite yeast: The effect of catabolite repression. *Biochim. Biophys. Acta* **177,** 358–360.

Gould, R. G., and Popjak, G. (1957). Biosynthesis of cholesterol in vivo and in vitro from DL-β-hydroxy-β-methyl-δ-[2-^{14}C]valerolactone. *Biochem. J.* **66,** 51P.

Gould, R. G., and Swyryd, E. A. (1966). Sites of control of hepatic cholesterol biosynthesis. *J. Lipid Res.* **7,** 698–707.

Gould, R. G., Bell, V. L., Lilly, E. H., Keegan, P., Riper, J. V., and Jonnard, M. L. (1959). Stimulation of cholesterol. Biosynthesis from acetate in rat liver and adrenals by whole body X-irradiation. *Am. J. Physiol.* **196,** 1231–1237.

Green, D. E., and Fleischer, S. (1968). Role of lipids in mitochondrial function. *In* "Metabolism, Physiology and Significance of Lipids" Cambridge, England

Green, D. E., and Lester, R. L. (1959). Role of lipids in the mitochondrial electron transport system. *Fed. Proc. Fed. Am. Soc. Exp. Biol.* **18,** 987–1000.

Hamprecht, B., Nussler, C., and Lynen, F. (1969). Rhythmic changes of hydroxymethylglutaryl coenzyme A reductase activity in livers of fed and fasted rats. *FEBS Lett.* **4,** 117–124.

Hatefi, Y., and Quiros-Perez, F. (1959). Studies on the electron transport system. XVII. Effects of adenosine on the steady-state oxidoreduction level of coenzyme Q. *Biochim. Biophys. Acta* **31,** 502–512.

Ho, L., Nilsson, J. L. G., Skelton, F. S., and Folkers, K. (1973). Preparation of uniformly ^{14}C-labeled p-hydroxybenzoic acid. *J. Org. Chem.* **38,** 1059–1060.

Holmes, W. L., and Benz, J. D. (1960). Inhibition of cholesterol biosynthesis in vitro by β-diethylaminoethyl diphenylpropylacetate hydrochloride (SKF 525-A). *J. Biol. Chem.* **235,** 3118–3122.

Houser, R. M., and Olson, R. E. (1974). 5-Desmethylubiquinone-9 methyltransferase from rat liver mitochondria. I. Characterization, localization and solubilization. *Life Sci.* **14,** 1211–1219.

Houser, R. M., and Olson, R. E. (1977). 5-Desmethylubiquinone-9 methyltransferase from rat liver mitochondria. I. Characterization, localization and solubilization. *J. Biol. Chem.* **252,** 4017–4021.

Hughes, P. E., and Tove, S. B. (1980). Synthesis of α-tocopherolquinone by the rat and its reduction by mitochondria. *J. Biol. Chem.* **255,** 7095–7097.

Inamdar, A. R. (1968). Metabolism of ubiquinone in relation to nutritional status. Ph.D. Thesis, Indian Institute of Science, Bagalore, India.

Inamdar, A. R., and Ramasarma, T. (1969). Metabolism of ubiquinone in relation to thyroxine status. *Biochem. J.* **111,** 479–486.

Inamdar, A. R., and Ramasarma, T. (1971). Influence of starvation on the metabolism of ubiquinone in the rat. *Indian J. Biochem. Biophys.* **8,** 271–274.

Ingebritsen, T. S., Geelan, M. J. H., Parker, R. A., Evenson, K. J., and Gibson, D. M. (1979). A high molecular weight DNA polymerase from Drosophila melanogaster embryos. *J. Biol. Chem.* **254,** 9986–9989.

Jackman, L., O'Brien, I. G., Cox, G. B., and Gibson, F. (1967). Methionine as the source of the methyl groups in ubiquinone and vitamin K. *Biochim. Biophys. Acta* **141,** 1–7.

Joshi, V. C., Jayaraman, J., and Ramasarma, T. (1963). Tissue concentrations of coenzyme Q ubichomenol and tocopherol in relation to protein status in the rat. *Biochem. J.* **88,** 25–31.

Kandutsch, A. A., and Chen, H. W. (1973). Inhibition of sterol synthesis in cultured mouse cells by 7α-hydroxycholesterol, 7β-hydroxycholesterol, and 7-ketocholesterol. *J. Biol. Chem.* **248,** 8408–8417.

Kandutsch, A. A., and Chen, H. W. (1974). Inhibition of sterol synthesis in cultured mouse cells by cholesterol derivatives oxygenated in the side chain. *J. Biol. Chem.* **249,** 6057–6061.

Kandutsch, A. A., Chen, H. W., and Heiniger, H.-J. (1978). Biological activity of some oxygenated sterols. *Science* **201,** 498–501.

Kaneko, I., Hazama-Shimada, Y., and Endo, A. (1978). Inhibitory effects on lipid metabolism in cultured cells of ML-236B, a potent inhibitor of 3-hydroxy-3-methylglutaryl-coenzyme A reductase. *Eur. J. Biochem.* **87,** 313–321.

Krishnaiah, K. V., and Ramasarma, T. (1970). Effect of α-p-chlorophenoxy isobutyrate on the metabolism of isoprenoid compounds in the cat. *Biochem. J.* **116,** 321–327.

Krishnaiah, K. V., Joshi, V. C., and Ramasarma, T. (1967a). Effect of dietary cholesterol and ubiquinone on isoprene synthesis in rat liver. *Arch. Biochem. Biophys.* **121,** 147–153.

Krishnaiah, K. V., Inamdar, A. R., and Ramasarma, T. (1967b). Regulation of steroido-genesis by ubiquinone. *Biochem. Biophys. Res. Commun.* **27**, 474–478.

Kuroda, M., Tsujita, Y., Tanzawa, K., and Endo, A. (1979). Hypolipidemic effects in monkeys of ML-236B, a competitive inhibitor of 3-hydroxy-3-methylglutaryl co-enzyme A reductase. *Lipids* **14**, 585–589.

Lakshmanan, M. R., Phillips, W. E.J., and Brien, R. L. (1968). Effect of p-chlorophenoxy-isobutyrate (CPIB) fed to rats on hepatic biosynthesis and catabolism of ubiquinone. *J. Lipid Res.* **9**, 353–356.

Lakshmanan, M. R., Nepokoreff, C. M., Nes, G. C., Dugan, R. E., and Porter, J. W. (1973). Stimulation by insulin of rat liver β-hydroxy-β-methylglutaryl coenzyme A reductase and cholesterol-synthesizing activities. *Biochem. Biophys. Res. Commun.* **50**, 704–710.

Langdon, R., El-Masry, S., and Counsell, R. E. (1977). Induction of HMG-CoA reductase by the administration of 20,25-diazocholesterol. *J. Lipid Res.* **18**, 24–31.

Lavate, W. V., Dyer, J. R., Springer, C. M., and Bentley, R. (1962). The new naturally occurring member of the coenzyme Q group: Tetrahydrocoenzyme Q10. *J. Biol. Chem.* **237**, PC2715-PC2716.

Lavate, W. V., Dyer, J. R., Springer, C. M., and Bentley, R. (1965). Studies of coenzyme Q. The isolation, characterization, and general properties of a partly reduced co-enzyme Q10 *Penicillium stipitatum. J. Biol. Chem.* **240**, 524–531.

Leppik, R. A., Stroobant, P., Shineberg, B., Young, I. G., and Gibson, F. (1976). Mem-brane-associated reactions in ubiquinone biosynthesis. 2-Octaprenyl-3-methyl-5-hy-droxy-6-methoxy-1,4-benzoquinone methyltransferase. *Biochim. Biophys. Acta* **428**, 146–156.

Lester, R. L., and Crane, F. L. (1959). The natural occurrence of coenzyme Q and related compounds. *J. Biol. Chem.* **234**, 2169–2175.

Lester, R. L., and Fleischer, S. (1959). The specific restoration of succinoxidase activity by coenzyme Q compounds in acetone-extracted mitochondria. *Arch. Biochem. Bi-ophys.* **80**, 470–473.

Lester, R. L., and Fleischer, S. (1961). Studies on the electron transport system. XXVII. The respiratory activity of acetone-extracted beef heart mitochondria. Role of co-enzyme Q and other lipids. *Biochim. Biophys. Acta* **47**, 358–377.

Linn, T. C. (1967). The effect of cholesterol feeding and fasting upon β-hydroxy-β-meth-ylglutaryl coenzyme A reductase. *J. Biol. Chem.* **242**, 990–993.

Linnane, W., and Lukins, H. B. (1975). Isolation of mitochondria and techniques for studying mitochondrial biogenesis in yeasts. *In* "Methods in Cell Biology" (D. M. Prescott, ed.), Vol. XII, pp. 293–307, Academic Press, New York.

Lipmann, F., and Tuttle, L. C. (1945). A specific micromethod for the determination of acyl phosphates. *J. Biol. Chem.* **159**, 21–28.

Lynen, F. (1961). Studies on the biosynthesis of terpenoid side chains of quinones. In "Ciba Foundation Symposium on Quinones in Electron Transport" (G. Wolsten-holme and C. O'Connor, eds.), pp. 244–263. Little, Brown, Boston, Massachusetts.

Lynen, F., Eggerer, H., Henning, U., and Kessel, I. (1958). Farnesyl-pyrophosphat und 3-methy-butenyl-1-pyrophosphate, die biologischen voistufendes squalens. *Angew. Chem.* **70**, 738.

Lynen, F., Agranoff, B. W., Eggerer, H., Henning, U., and Maslein, E. M. (1959). Die-methyl-allyl-pyrophosphat biologische vorstufen des squalens. *Angew. Chem.* **71**, 657.

Mabuchi, H., Haba, T., Tatami, R., Miyamoto, S., Sakai, Y., Wakasurgi, T., Watanabe, A., Koizumi, J., and Takeda, R. (1981). Effects of an inhibitor of 3-hydroxy-3-methylglutaryl coenzyme A reductase on serum lipoproteins and ubiquinone-10 levels in patients with familial hypercholesterolemia. *New Engl. J. Med.* **305**, 478–482.

Mitchell, P. (1961). Coupling of phosphorylation to electron and hydrogen transfer of a chemi-osmotic type of mechanism. *Nature (London)* **91**, 144–148.

Mitchell, P. (1966). "*Chemiosmotic Coupling in Oxidative and Photosynthetic Phosphorylation.*" Glynn Research, Ltd., Bodmin, Cornwall, England.

Mitchell, P. (1967). Possible molecular mechanisms of the protonmotive function of cytochrome system. *J. Theor. Biol.* **62**, 327–367.

Momose, K., and Rudney, H. (1972). 3-Polyprenyl-4-hydroxybenzoate synthesis in the inner membrane of mitochondria from p-hydroxybenzoate and isopentenyl pyrophosphate. *J. Biol. Chem.* **247**, 3930–3940.

Morton, R. A., Gloor, U., Schindler, O., Wilson, G. M., Copard-dit-Jean, L. H., Hemming, F. W., Isler, O., Leat, W. M. F., Pennock, J. F., Ruegg, R., Schwieter, U., and Wiss, O. (1958). Die Struktur des Ubichinons aus Schweineherzen. *Helv. Chim. Acta* **41**, 2343–2357.

Nambudiri, A. M. D., Brockman, D., Alam, S. S., and Rudney, H. (1977). Alternate routes for ubiquinone biosynthesis in rats. *Biochem. Biophys. Res. Commun.* **786**, 282–288.

Nambudiri, A. M. D., Ranganathan, S., and Rudney, H. (1980). The role of 3-hydroxy-3-methylglutaryl coenzyme A reductase activity in the regulation of ubiquinone synthesis in human fibroblasts. *J. Biol. Chem.* **255**, 5894–5899.

Napier, E. A., Jr., Kreyden, R. W., Henley, K. S., and Pollard, H. M. (1964). Coenzyme Q and phenylketonuria. *Nature (London)* **202**, 806–807.

Nilsson, J. L. G., Farley, T. M., and Folkers, K. (1968). Determination of biosynthetic precursors from p-hydroxybenzoic acid-U-^{14}C to ubiquinone. *Anal. Biochem.* **23**, 422–428.

Nishino, T., and Rudney, H. (1977). Effects of detergents on the properties of 4-hydroxybenzoate. Polyprenyl transferase and the specificity of the polyprenyl pyrophosphate synthetic system in mitochondria. *Biochemistry* **16**, 605–609.

Nowicki, H. G., Dialameh, G. H., and Olson, R. E. (1972). Isolation and identification of 6-methoxy-2-nonaprenylphenol as an intermediate in the biosynthesis of ubiquinone-9 in the rat. *Biochemistry* **11**, 896–904.

Olsen, R. K., Smith, J. L., Daves, G. D., Jr., Moore, H. W., Folkers, K., Parson, W. W., and Rudney, H. (1965). 2-Decaprenylphenol, biosynthetic precursor of ubiquinone-10. *J. Am. Chem. Soc.* **87**, 2298–2300.

Olson, R. E. (1965). Anabolism of the coenzyme Q family and their biological activities. *Fed. Proc. Fed. Am. Soc. Exp. Biol. Symp.* **24**, 85–92.

Olson, R. E. (1966). Biosynthesis of ubiquinones in animals. *Vitam. Horm.* **24**, 551–574.

Olson, R. E., and Aiyar, A. S. (1966). Evidence for a new aromatic intermediate in the biosynthesis of coenzyme Q_9 in the rat. *Fed. Proc. Fed. Am. Soc. Exp. Biol.* **25**, 217.

Olson, R. E., and Dialameh, G. H. (1960). On the biosynthesis of coenzyme Q_9 in the rat. *Biochem. Biophys. Res. Commun,* **2**, 198–202.

Olson, R. E., Dialameh, G. H., and Bentley, R. (1961). The biosynthesis of coenzyme Q in the rat. *In* "Ciba Foundation Symposium on Quinones in Electron Transport" (G. E. W. Wolstenholme and C. M. O'Connor, eds.), pp. 284–302. Churchill, London.

Olson, R. E., Bentley, R., Dialameh, G. H., and Gold, P. H. (1962). On phenylalanine as a source of the benzoquinone moiety of coenzyme Q_9. *Biochem. J.* **82**, 14P-15P.

Olson, R. E., Bentley, R., Aiyar, A. S., Dialameh, G. H., Gold, P. H., Ramsey, V. G., and Springer, C. M. (1963). Benzoate derivative as intermediate in the biosynthesis of coenzyme Q_9 in the rat. *J. Biol. Chem.,* **238**, PC3146-PC3148.

Olson, R. E., Dialameh, G. H., Bentley, R., Springer, C. M., and Ramsey, V. G. (1965). Studies on coenzyme Q. Pattern of labeling in coenzyme Q_9 after administration of isotopic acetate and aromatic amino acids to rats. Studies on coenzyme Q. *J. Biol. Chem.* **240**, 514–523.

Panini, S. R., Sexton, R. C., and Rudney, H. (1982). Regulation of 3-hydroxy-3-methylglutaryl coenzyme A reductase (HMGR) activity and cholesterol (CH) synthesis in cultured rat intestinal epithelial cells. *Fed. Proc. Fed. Am. Soc. Exp. Biol.* **41**, 1215.

Parson, W. W., and Rudney, H. (1964). The biosynthesis of the benzoquinone ring of ubiquinone from p-hydroxybenzaldehyde and p-hydroxybenzoic acid in rat kidney, *Azobacter vinelandii,* and baker's yeast. *Proc. Natl. Acad. Sci. U.S.A.* **51**, 444–450.

Parson, W., and Rudney, H. (1965). An intermediate in the conversion of p-hydroxybenzoate-U-C-14 to ubiquinone in *Rhodospirillum rubrum. Proc. Natl. Acad. Sci. U.S.A.* **53**, 599–606.

Pennock, J. F. (1966). Occurrence of vitamin K and related quinones. *Vitam. Horm.* **24**, 307–329.

Phillips, W. E. J. (1960). *In vitro* studies on the biosynthesis of ubiquinone. *Can. J. Biochem. Physiol.* **38**, 1105–1115.

Plack, P. A., and Bieri, J. G. (1964). Metabolic products of α-tocopherol with livers of rats given intraperitoneal injections of [^{14}C]-α-tocopherol. *Biochim. Biophys. Acta* **84**, 729–738.

Popjak, G., Goodman, D., Cornforth, J. W., Cornforth, R. H., and Ryhafe, R. J. (1964). Studies on the biosynthesis from farnesylpyrophosphate and from mevalonate. *J. Biol. Chem.* **236**, 1934–1947.

Poulter, C. D., and Rilling, H. C. (1981). Prenyl transferases and isomerase. *In* "Biosynthesis of Isoprenoid Compounds" (J. W. Porter and S. L. Spurgeon, eds.), Vol. 1, pp. 161–224. Wiley, New York.

Pumphrey, A. M., and Redfearn, E. R. (1959). The rate of reduction of the endogenous ubiquinone in a heart muscle preparation. *Biochem. J.* **72**, 2P.

Quereshi, N. and Porter, J. W. (1981). Conversion of acetyl-coenzyme A to isopentenyl pyrophosphate. *In* "Biosynthesis of Isoprenoid Compounds" (J. W. Porter and S. L. Spurgeon, eds.), Vol. 1, pp. 47–94. Wiley, New York.

Ramachandran, C. K., Gray, S. L., and Melnykovych, G. (1978). Coordinate repression of cholesterol biosynthesis and cytoplasmic 3-hydroxy-3-methylglutaryl coenzyme A synthase by glucocorticoids in HeLa cells. *Arch. Biochem. Biophys.* **189**, 205–211.

Raman, T. S., Rudney, H., and Buzzelli, N. K. (1969). The incorporation of p-hydroxybenzoate and isopentenyl pyrophosphate into polyprenylphenol precursors of ubiquinone by broken cell preparations of *Rhodospirillum rubrum. Arch. Biochem. Biophys.* **130**, 164–174.

Ramasarma, T. (1972). Control of biogenesis of isopenoid compounds. *Curr. Top. Cell. Regul.* **6**, 169–207.

Ranganathan, S., and Ramasarma, T. (1975). The regulation of the biosynthesis of ubiquinone in the rat. *Biochem. J.* **148**, 35–39.

Ranganathan, S., Nambudiri, A. M. D., and Rudney, H. (1979). The biosynthesis of ubiquinone in isolated rat heart cells. *Arch. Biochem. Biophys.* **198**, 506–511.

Ranganathan, S., Nambudiri, A. M. D., and Rudney, H. (1981). The regulation of ubiquinone synthesis in fibroblasts: The effect of modulators of hydroxymethylglutaryl-coenzyme A reductase activity. *Arch. Biochem. Biophys.* **210**, 592–597.

Rao, K. S., and Olson, R. E. (1967). The effect of exogenous cholesterol on the synthesis in vivo of cholesterol, ubiquinone, and squalene in rat liver. *Biochem. Biophys. Res. Commun.* **26**, 668–673.

Regen, D., Piepertinger, C., Hamprecht, B., and Lynen, F. (1966). The measurement of β-hydroxy-β-methylglutaryl-CoA reductase in rat liver. Effects of fasting and refeeding. *Biochem. Z.* **346**, 78–84.

Rosen, L., and Goodall, M. (1962). Identification of vanillic acid as a catabolite of non-adrenaline metabolism in the human. *Proc. Soc. Exp. Biol. Med.* **110**, 767–769.

Rothblat, G. H. (1972). Cellular sterol metabolism. *In* "Growth, Nutrition, and Metabolism of Cells in Culture" (G. H. Rothblat and V. J. Cristofalo, eds.), Vol. 1, pp. 297–325. Academic Press, New York.

Rudney, H. (1977). The biosynthesis of coenzyme Q and its relation to cellular metabolism and function. *In* "Biomedical and Clinical Aspects of Coenzyme Q" (K. Folkers and Y. Yamamura, eds.), pp. 29–46. Elsevier, Amsterdam.

Rudney, H., and Parson, W. W. (1963). The conversion of p-hydroxybenzaldehyde to the benzoquinone ring of ubiquinone in *Rhodospirillum rubrum. J. Biol. Chem.* **238**, PC3137–PC3138.

Rudney, H., and Raman, T. S. (1966). Biosynthesis of ubiquinones and vitamin K in microorganisms. *Vitam. Horm.* **24**, 531–549.

Rudney, H., and Sugimura, T. (1961). Studies on the biosynthesis of the ubiquinone (coenzyme Q) series in animals and microorganisms. *In* "Ciba Foundation Symposium on Quinones in Electron Transport" (G. E. W. Wolstenholme and C. M. O'Connor, eds.), p. 211–232. Churchill, London.

Rudney, H., Nambudiri, A. M. D., and Ranganathan, S. (1981). Regulation of the synthesis of coenzyme Q in fibroblasts and in heart muscle. *In* "Biomedical and Clinical Aspects of Coenzyme Q" (K. Folkers and Y. Yamamura, eds.), Vol. 3, pp. 279–290. Elsevier, Amsterdam.

Ruegg, R., Gloor, U., Goel, R. N., Ryser, G., Wiss, O., and Isler, O. (1959). Synthese von ubichinon (45) and ubichinon (50). *Helv. Chim. Acta* **42**, 2616–2621.

Sanghvi, A., and Parikh, B. (1978). Stimulation of hydroxymethylglutaryl-CoA reductase activity after a single dose of the porphyrogenic chemical, allylisopropylacetamide. *Biochim. Biophys. Acta* **531**, 79–85.

Schatz, G., and Mason, T. L. (1974). The biosynthesis of mitochondrial proteins. *Annu. Rev. Biochem.* **43**, 51–87.

Schnaitman, C., and Grenawalt, J. W. (1968). Enzymatic properties of the inner and outer membranes of rat liver mitochondria. *J. Cell Biol.* **38**, 158–175.

Schneider, W. C. (1948). Intracellular distribution of enzymes. III. The oxidation of octanoic acid by rat liver fractions. *J. Biol. Chem.* **176**, 259–266.

Schroepfer, G. J., Jr., Parish, E. J., Chen, H. W., and Kandutsch, A. A. (1977). Inhibition of sterol biosynthesis in L cells and mouse liver cells by 15-oxygenated sterols. *J. Biol. Chem.* **252**, 8975–8980.

Schroepfer, G. J., Jr., Pascal, R. A., Shaw, R., and Kandutsch, A. A. (1978). Inhibition of sterol biosynthesis by 14α-hydroxymethyl sterols. *Biochem. Biophys. Res. Commun.* **83**, 1024–1031.

Sexton, R. C., Panini, S. R., and Rudney, H. (1982). Factors regulating cholesterol (CH) and ubiquinone (UQ) synthesis in fibroblasts: Cell density serum lipoproteins and 3-hydroxy-methylglutaryl coenzyme A reductase (HMGR). *Fed. Proc. Fed. Am. Soc. Exp. Biol.* **41**, 1388.

Siperstein, M. D., and Fagan, V. M. (1966). Feedback control of mevalonate synthesis by dietary cholesterol. *J. Biol. Chem.* **241**, 602–609.

Sippel, C. J., Goewert, R. R., and Slachman, F. N. (1979). The regulation of ubiquinone-6 biosynthesis in *Saccharomyces cerevisiae. Fed. Proc. Fed. Am. Soc. Exp. Biol.* **38**, 1475.

Sippel, C. J., Goewert, R. R., Slachman, F. N., and Olson, R. E. (1983). The regulation of ubiquinone-6 biosynthesis by *Saccharomyces cerevisiae*. *J. Biol. Chem.* **258**, 1057–1061.

Steinberg, D., and Frederickson, D. S. (1955). Inhibition of lipid synthesis by alpha-phenyl-N-butyrate and related compounds. *Proc. Soc. Exp. Biol. Med.* **90**, 232–236.

Stroobant, P., Young, I. G., and Gibson, F. (1972). Mutants of *Escherichia coli* K-12 blocked in the final reaction of ubiquinone biosynthesis: Characterization and genetic analysis. *J. Bacteriol.* **109**, 134–139.

Subbaiah, M. T. R. (1977). Effect of long-term administration of estrogens on the subcellular distribution of cholesterol and the activity of rate-limiting enzymes of cholesterol biosynthesis and degradation in pigeon liver. *Endokrinologie* **70**, 257–262.

Sugimura, T., and Rudney, H. (1960). The adaptive form of ubiquinone 30 (coenzyme Q_6) in yeast. *Biochim. Biophys. Acta* **37**, 560–561.

Taylor, C. B., and Gould, R. C. (1950). Effect of dietary cholesterol on rate of cholesterol synthesis in the intact animal measured by means of radioactive carbon. *Circulation* **2**, 467–468.

Thomas, G., and Threlfall, D. R. (1973). Polyprenyl pyrophosphate-p-hydroxybenzoate polyprenyltransferase activity in mitochondria of broad-bean seeds and yeast. *Biochem. J.* **134**, 811–814.

Tomkins, G. M., and Chaikoff, I. L. (1952). Cholesterol synthesis by liver. I. Influence of fasting and of diet. *J. Biol. Chem.* **196**, 569–573.

Tony Lam, Y. K., Gullo, V. P., Goegelman, R. T., Jorn, D., Huang, L., DeRiso, C., Monaghan, R. L., and Putter, I. (1981). Dihydrocompactin, a new potent inhibitor of 3-hydroxy-3-methylglutaryl coenzyme A reductase from *Penicillium citrinum*. *J. Antibiot.* **34**, 614–616.

Trumpower, B. L. (1981). New concepts on the role of ubiquinone in the mitochondrial respiratory chain. *J. Bioenerg. Biomembr.* **13**, 1–24.

Trumpower, B. L., and Olson, R. E. (1971). Biosynthesis of ubiquinone-9 from p-hydroxybenzoate by a cell-free system from rat liver. *Biochem. Biophys. Res. Commun.* **45**, 1323–1330.

Trumpower, B. L., Palkar, V. S., Ramasarma, T., and Olson, R. E. (1968). Noninvolvement of 2-nonaprenyl phenol in the biosynthesis of ubiquinone-9 in the rat. *Fed. Proc. Fed. Am. Soc. Exp. Biol.* **27**, 524.

Trumpower, B. L., Aiyar, A. S., Opliger, C. E., and Olson, R. E. (1972). Studies on ubiquinone. The isolation and identification of 5-demethoxyubiquinone-9 as an intermediate in biosynthesis of ubiquinone-9 in the rat. *J. Biol. Chem.* **247**, 2499–2511.

Trumpower, B. L., Houser, R. M., and Olson, R. E. (1974a). Studies on ubiquinone. Demonstration of the total biosynthesis of ubiquinone-9 in rat liver mitochondria. *J. Biol. Chem.* **249**, 3041–3047.

Trumpower, B. L., Opliger, C. E., and Olson, R. E. (1974b). Synthesis and stability of ^{3}H-5-demethoxyubiquinone-9. *Chem. Phys. Lipids* **13**, 123–132.

Tsujita, Y., Kuroda, M., Tanzawa, K., Kitano, N., and Endo, A. (1979). Hypolipidemic effects in dogs of ML-236B, a competitive inhibitor of 3-hydroxy-methylglutaryl coenzyme A reductase. *Atherosclerosis* **32**, 307–313.

Tzagoloff, A. (1969). Assembly of the mitochondrial membrane system. II. Synthesis of the mitochondrial adenosine triphosphatase. *J. Biol. Chem.* **244**, 5027–5033.

Tzagoloff, A., Akai, A., and Needleman, R. B. (1975). Assembly of mitochondrial membrane system. Characterization of nuclear mutants of *Saccharomyces cerevisiae* with defects in mitochondrial ATPase and respiratory enzymes. *J. Biol. Chem.* **250,** 8228–8235.

Uchida, K., and Aida, K. (1972). Incorporation of molecular oxygen during the biosynthesis of ubiquinone in an aerobic bacteria, *Pseudomonas desmolytica. Biochem. Biophys. Res. Commun.* **46,** 130–135.

Volpe, J. J., and Obert, K. A. (1982). Interrelationships of ubiquinone and sterol synthesis in cultured cells of neural origin. *J. Neurochem.* **38,** 931–938.

Weis, H. J., and Dietschy, J. M. (1975). The interaction of various control mechanisms in determining the rate of hepatic cholesterolgenesis in the rat. *Biochim. Biophys. Acta* **398,** 315–324.

Whistance, G. R., and Threlfall, D. R. (1970). Biosynthesis of phytoquinones. Homogentisic acid: A precursor of plastoquinones, tocopherols and α-tocopherolquinone in higher plants, green algae and blue-green algae. *Biochem. J.* **117,** 593–600.

White, L. W. (1971). Regulation of hepatic cholesterol biosynthesis by clofibrate administration. *J. Pharmacol. Exp. Ther.* **178,** 361–370.

White, L. W. (1972). Feedback regulation of cholesterol biosynthesis: Studies with cholestyramine. *Circ. Res.* **31,** 899–907.

White, L. W., and Rudney, H. (1970). Regulation of 3-hydroxy-3-methylglutarate and mevalonate biosynthesis by rat liver homogenates. Effects of fasting, cholesterol feeding, and triton administration. *Biochemistry* **9,** 2725–2731.

Winrow, M. J., and Rudney, H. (1969). Incorporation of p-hydroxybenzoic acid and isopentenylpyrophosphate into ubiquinone precursors by cell-free preparations of rat tissues. *Biochem. Biophys. Res. Commun.* **37,** 833–840.

Wiss, O., Gloor, V., and Weber, F. (1961a). Biosynthesis of ubiquinones. *In* "Ciba Foundation Symposium on Quinones in Electron Transport" (G. Wolstenholme and C. M. O'Connor, eds.), pp. 264–283. Churchill, London.

Wiss, O., Gloor, V., and Weber, F. (1961b). Vitamin A function in ubiquinone and cholesterol biosynthesis. *Am. J. Clin. Nutr.* **9,** 27–35.

Wolf, D. E., Hoffman, C. H., Trenner, N. R., Arison, B. H., Shunk, C. H., Linn, B. O., McPherson, J. F., and Folkers, K. (1958). Coenzyme Q. Structure studies on the coenzyme Q group. *J. Am. Chem. Soc.* **80,** 4752.

Wong, T. K., and Lennarz, W. J. (1982). Biosynthesis of dolichol and cholesterol during embryonic development of the chicken. *Biochim. Biophys. Acta* **710,** 32–38.

Yamamoto, A., Sudo, H., and Endo, A. (1980). Therapeutic effects of ML-236B in primary hypercholesterolemia. *Atherosclerosis* **35,** 259–266.

Young, I. G., Leppik, R. A., Hamilton, J. A., and Gibson, F. (1972). Studies on ubiquinone biosynthesis in *Escherichia coli* K-12: 4-Hydroxybenzoate octaprenyl transferase. *J. Bacteriol.* **11,** 18–25.

Young, I. G., McCann, L. M., Stroobant, P., and Gibson, F. (1971). Characterization and genetic analysis of a mutant strain of *Escherichia coli* K-12 accumulating the ubiquinone precursors 2-octaprenyl-6-methoxy-1,4-benzoquinone and 2-octaprenyl-3-methyl-6-methoxy-1,4-benzoquinone. *J. Bacteriol.* **105,** 769–779.

Zannoni, V. G., and Weber, W. W. (1966). Isolation and properties of aromatic α-keto acid reductase. *J. Biol. Chem.* **241,** 1340–1345.

Synthesis and Analysis of the Pteroylpolyglutamates

CARLOS L. KRUMDIECK, TSUNENOBU TAMURA, AND ISAO ETO

Department of Nutrition Sciences, University of Alabama, Birmingham, Alabama

I. INTRODUCTION

Although the discovery of poly-γ-glutamyl derivatives of folic acid dates back to the mid 1940s, it is only during the last 10 or 12 years that these forms of the folates have become the subject of intensive study. The main reason for this prior lack of attention to what many investigators recognized as the naturally occurring forms of the folate coenzymes was methodological limitations. The nonavailability of synthetic pteroylpolyglutamates, other than "teropterin," the pteroyltriglutamate synthesized by the Lederle group in the late 1940s, made the study of the biological role of these compounds extremely difficult. Nevertheless, the biological importance of the polyglutamyl chain was recognized on the basis of its universal occurrence and by the fact that, during evolution, the ability to synthesize the peptide chain has been retained, even by organisms that have lost the pathways for folic acid synthesis. That loss of the polyglutamate-synthesizing system represents a very serious survival handicap was clearly demonstrated by McBurney and Whitmore (1974a,b), they showed that artificial mu-

45

tants of Chinese hamster ovary cells, incapable of making polyglutamates, could not survive unless supplied with purines, glycine, and
thymidine. It is now believed by most investigators in the field, that
the polyglutamyl chain of the folates plays a role in the regulation of
one-carbon metabolism. A large body of literature has accumulated
supporting the idea that polyglutamates are the best cosubstrates of
the folate-requiring enzymes, and that some of these enzymes show a
clear preference for certain specific polyglutamyl chain lengths. The
part played by the poly-γ-glutamyl chain in affecting the translocation
of folates across cellular and subcellular membranes is well established. This role acquires special practical significance when considering the pharmacodynamics of polyglutamyl derivatives of folic acid
analogs possessing antitumor activity. Changes in the patterns of distribution of polyglutamates of different chain lengths have been shown
to occur under conditions which alter the steady-state of one-carbon
metabolism, a necessary effect if the polyglutamyl chain is indeed
involved in regulation. Finally, the properties of the enzymes of polyglutamate biosynthesis and degradation are now being defined. The
accumulation of much of this impressive body of knowledge depended
on the development of methods of synthesis and analysis of the biologically active forms of the pteroylpolyglutamates. It is to the review of
these methods that we have addressed ourselves. The reader interested
in the biochemistry and biology of the polyglutamates should refer to
the excellent reviews of Kisliuk (1981), McGuire and Bertino (1981),
Cichowicz *et al.* (1981), Covey (1980), and Goldwin *et al.* (1983).

II. History

The isolation and characterization of a previously unknown micronutrient require a biological assay system to follow the progress of the
purification procedures. It is apparent that the chemical entity isolated
in the end will be one to which the chosen assay system is capable of
responding, and that closely related molecules which the assay system
fails to "see" will be excluded from the final isolate. The history of the
folates illustrates this very clearly, particularly with regard to the
discovery of the longer chain pteroylpolyglutamates. Shortly after
Wills (1931) demonstrated the curative effect of yeast and yeast extracts, as well as crude liver, in cases of "pernicious anemia of prenan-
cy," an animal model of the disease using monkeys was developed by
Wills and Bilimoria (1932). The use of a monkey assay proved, howev-

er, too difficult to permit any significant progress in the purification of the antianemic factor (Day, 1944). This situation changed when a number of independent investigators, attacking the seemingly unrelated problems of purification of a bacterial growth factor required by certain strains of lactobacilli and streptococci, and an antianemic factor for chicks, developed the first two practical bioassay procedures. These procedures were to guide all subsequent work of isolation and purification of the folates. Hogan *et al.* (1935) had succeeded in formulating a simplified ration for the chick which, for many months, seemed to be entirely adequate. Their initial success could not, however, be consistently duplicated. The problems were traced to variability of the commercial liver extracts used in the preparation of their diet. Investigating this problem further, Hogan and Parrot (1940) discovered that extracting autolyzed hog liver with 95% alcohol at 70°C removed an unknown factor, different from any of the vitamins then recognized, in whose absence the chicks developed a severe macrocytic anemia. They named the new factor "the B_c vitamin [because] it belongs to the old vitamin B complex . . . the small c is added because this substance is essential for the chick." A new chick assay for the study of the antianemia factors of liver and yeast was later perfected by O'Dell and Hogan (1943). In 1940, Snell and Peterson, studying the growth requirements of lactic acid bacteria, described a factor present in yeast and liver, easily adsorbed by Norite (a brand of activated charcoal), which was essential for the growth of *Lactobacillus casei*. This study proved to be a very important contribution which provided two valuable procedures, a rapid microbiological assay and a potent means of concentrating the active principle by adsorption and elution from charcoal. Progress in the purification and characterization of the bacterial growth factor by two independent groups followed rapidly. Mitchell *et al.* (1941) reported the isolation, from four tons of spinach leafs, of an acid which supported the growth of *Streptococcus lactis R* and of *L. casei* in a fashion indistinguishable from the "Norite eluate factor" of Snell and Peterson (1940). Mitchell and co-workers named the new substance "folic acid" because of its abundance in green leafs (Latin, folium—leaf). They recognized that "this acid, or one with similar chemical and physiological properties, occurs in a number of animal tissues of which liver and kidney are best sources." Scarcely 2 months after the publication of the letter by Mitchell *et al.*, Hutchings *et al.* (1941a) submitted a paper describing the purification of the *L. casei* growth factor from liver. Both of these early purifications of folic acid were based on the adsorption of the acid onto charcoal and its subsequent desorption at alkaline pH values, and both made use of microbiological assays to monitor the purification procedures. The major contribution to these successful attempts by the prior work of Snell and Peterson (1940) deserves to be noted.

A better understanding of the properties of the factor led Hutchings and his collaborators (1941b) to recognize that the bacterial factor had many properties in common with the chick antianemia factor and with other chick growth factors described before by Stokstad and Manning (1938) and Schumacher *et al.* (1940). Hutchings *et al.* (1941b) published a note showing that a concentrated *L. casei* factor obtained from liver promoted the growth of deficient chicks. The close relationship between the *L. casei* factor and the antianemia factor of Hogan and Parrot (1940) was firmly demonstrated a year later by Mills *et al.* (1942), who successfully prevented the anemia by feeding the "Norite eluate factor" to deficient chicks. The converse experiment, showing growth stimulation of *L. casei* by crystalline preparations of the hog liver antianemia factor purified using the chick assay, was reported by Pfiffner *et al.* in 1943. The identity of the "Norite eluate factor" with the chick antianemia factor "vitamin B_c" and with "folic acid" was thus established.

It is of interest to note that since all isolation attempts had to start from very large amounts of homogenates which took many hours to process, degradation of the naturally occurring polyglutamates by intrinsic pteroylpolyglutamate hydrolases (conjugases) must have always taken place. This, together with the lack of response of the microbiological assays to the polyglutamates, and the lack of protection from oxidation, led to the isolation of a fully oxidized molecule, pteroylglutamic acid, which we now know occurs in minimal quantities, if at all, in biological materials and which must therefore be recognized as an artifact of isolation.

Interest in the constituents of yeast which cured the macrocytic anemia of pregnancy stimulated the group of Pfiffner and collaborators (Binkley *et al.*, 1944), at Parke Davis, to isolate and characterize the active principle. These investigators used both the *L. casei* growth-stimulating acivity and the chick antianemia activity to monitor their purification attempts. They soon realized that yeast extracts, highly active as measured in the anemic chick, were essentially inactive in stimulating the growth of *L. casei*. Similar observations had been reported by Totter *et al.* (1944) who compared the antianemic effect of yeast, measured by a monkey assay, with its *S. lactis R* growth-supporting activity. It became evident that the yeast antianemia factor differed chemically from the "vitamin B_c" which these investigators had previoulsy isolated from liver and shown to be identical with folic acid. The possibility that the antianemia factor of yeast was actually a *biosynthetic precursor* of folic acid which the animal liver, but not the assay bacteria, was capable of converting to the vitamin was apparently supported by the work of Wright and Welch (1943). These authors reported experiments which seemed to indicate the synthesis of folic acid by fresh rat liver homogenates incubated with a variety of substances. After incubation there was always a considerable increase in folic acid as measured by the *S. lactis R* assay. Control incubations of liver homogenates *without* any additions were apparently not done. When yeast or yeast extracts were incubated with liver homogenates or with homogenates from other tissues (Mims *et al.*, 1944; Laskowski *et al.*, 1945; Mims and Laskowski, 1945; Bird *et al.*, 1945), there was indeed a marked increase in the *S. lactis R* activity of the preparation. Understanding the true nature of the enzyme-mediated activation of yeast extracts required the isolation of the active principle and the demonstration that it was a high-molecular-weight derivative of folic acid (Binkley *et al.*, 1944; Pfiffner *et al.*, 1945). It is interesting to note that yeast is among the few biological sources of folates which contain no conjugase activity (Bird *et al.*, 1945) and was therefore a uniquely appropriate starting material for isolation of the pteroylpolyglutamates. The peptide nature of the yeast antianemia factor, or the "B$_c$ conjugate" as it was called, was described a year later by Pfiffner *et al.* (1946). Furthermore, these authors demonstrated that folic acid was liberated from the "conjugate" by the enzyme-mediated activation. This clearly demonstrated that the process of activation was degradative rather than biosynthetic, and that the conjugases were in effect peptidases. Also in 1946, Angier *et al.* published evidence indicating that a previously isolated *L. casei* growth factor (Hutchings *et al.*, 1944), the source of which was not divulged, yielded on degradation three molecules of glutamic acid per mole of *p*-aminobenzoic acid. This substance, later described as the "fermentation *L. casei* factor" (Hutchings *et al.*, 1948a,b; Stokstad *et al.*, 1948) and given the trivial name of "teropterin," was finally assigned the structure pteroyl-γ-glutamyl-γ-glutamylglutamic acid after the synthesis of pteroylglutamic acid was carried out by Waller *et al.* (1948), and after the exact configuration of the peptide chain had been determined by comparison with synthetic isomeric peptides. The synthesis of teropterin was accomplished by two methods (Boothe *et al.*, 1948, 1949) briefly discussed in Section IV,A. It marks the culmination of the early work of isolation, structural elucidation, and synthesis of the folates. No other pteroyl-γ-glutamates were synthesized until the development of the solid-phase synthesis procedure of Krumdieck and Baugh in 1969.

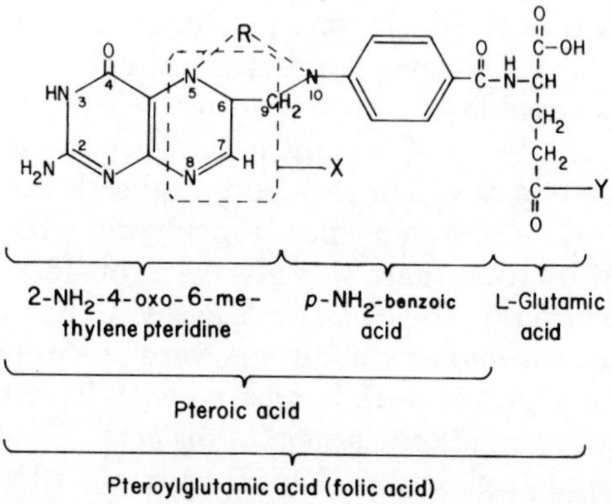

X	R	Name of Compound
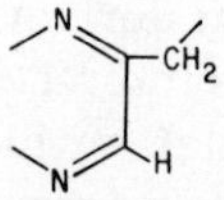 (pyrazine N, –CH₂)	–H at N-10	Pteroyl glutamic acid (folic acid)
	–CHO at N-10	10-formyl folic acid
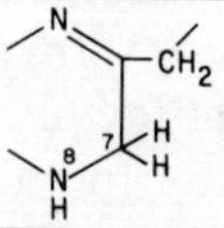 (7,8-dihydro)	–H at N-10	7,8-dihydrofolic acid
	–CH₃ at N-5	5-methyl " " "
	–CHO at N-10	10-formyl " " "
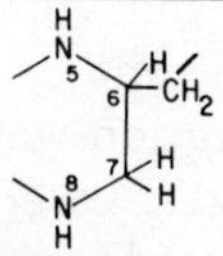 (5,6,7,8-tetrahydro)	–H at N-10	5,6,7,8-tetrahydrofolic acid
	–CH₃ at N-5	5-methyl " " "
	–CHO at N-5	5-formyl " " "
	–CHNH at N-5	5-formimino " " "
	–CHO at N-10	10-formyl " " "
Note: asymmetric C at position 6, ∴ optical isomers d, l.	≡CH≡ at N-5–N-10	5,10-methenyl or (methylidyne) " " "
	–CH₂– at N-5–N-10	5,10-methylene " " "

Y		Name of Compound
	– OH	Pteroyl - mono glutamate
	(glutamate chain, n)	n ≥ 0 = Pteroyl-poly-γ-glutamates
		n + 2 = number of glutamic acid residues attached to pteroic acid.

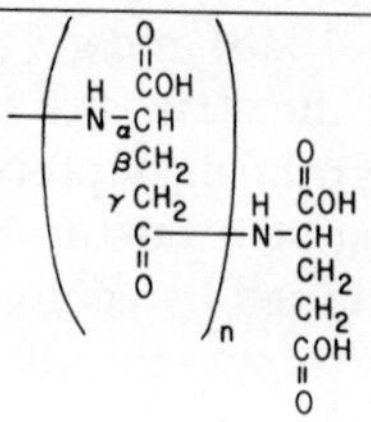

Fig. 1. Structure and nomenclature of the naturally occurring folates.

III. Structure and Nomenclature

The naturally occurring pteroylpolyglutamates constitute a large family of closely related compounds arising from modifications of three parts of the parent compound pteroylglutamic acid. Changes in the state of reduction of the pteridine moiety, addition of various kinds of one-carbon substituents, and addition of glutamic acid residues lead to a wide array of compounds. Baugh and Krumdieck (1971), based on the three known states of reduction of the pyrazine ring, the six different one-carbon substituents that may occur at N-5 and/or N-10, and assuming that the polyglutamyl chain would have no more than seven glutamyl residues, calculated that the theoretical number of folates approached 150. This often-quoted figure includes compounds which have never been identified in natural materials. If only those folates known to occur in nature are included, the family of folates can be depicted as in Fig. 1. Since it is clear now that the polyglutamyl chain reaches at least 8 residues in animal tissues (and as many as 12 in bacterial cells), the number of folates that might be expected to occur in animal tissues still approaches 100 compounds. It becomes important, therefore, to adopt, from the onset, a systematic nomenclature to refer to this large family of compounds. The trivial name "polyglutamates" will be used only to refer to pteroyl-(γ-glutamyl)$_n$-glutamic acids where the chain lengths, the one-carbon substituent, and the state of reduction of the pyrazine ring are not specified. The abbreviations used for the various folates are based on the tentative IUPAC–IUB rules as set forth in *Biochem. J.* **102**, 19 (1967). Thus, PteGlu refers to pteroylglutamic acid (folic acid), H_2PteGlu and H_4PteGlu to the 7,8-dihydro- and 5,6,7,8-tetrahydro-PteGlu, respectively. The term folic acid may, as in Fig. 1, be used instead of pteroylglutamic acid. 5-CH_3, 5-CHO, 5-CHNH, 10-CHO, etc., preceding the abbreviation, refer to the nature and position of the one-carbon substituent and a subscript, i.e., PteGlu$_n$, denotes the number of glutamic acid residues in γ-peptide linkage.

IV. Synthesis of the Fully Oxidized, Unsubstituted Pteroylpolyglutamates

A. Synthesis of Pteroyl-γ-glutamyl-γ-glutamylglutamic Acid (Teropterin)

The degradation of the fermentation *L. casei* factor showed that it contained three molecules of glutamic acid which could occur in the

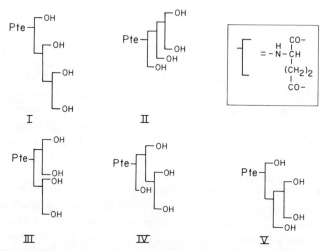

FIG. 2. Isomeric configurations of pteroyltriglutamate. **I**, Pteroyl-γ-glutamyl-γ-glutamylglutamic acid; **II**, pteroyl-α-glutamyl-α-glutamylglutamic acid; **III**, pteroyl-α,γ-glutamyl-di-glutamic acid; **IV**, pteroyl-α-glutamyl-γ-glutamylglutamic acid; **V**, pteroyl-γ-glutamyl-α-glutamylglutamic acid.

five different isomeric configurations shown in Fig. 2. All five isomeric compounds were synthesized by the Lederle group (Boothe *et al.*, 1948, 1949; Mowat *et al.*, 1948, 1949; Semb *et al.*, 1949) and only one, pteroyl-γ-glutamyl-γ-glutamylglutamic acid, had biological activity. The first reported synthesis of this compound (Boothe *et al.*, 1948; Fig. 3, First synthesis) started with α-ethyl carbobenzoxyglutamate which was converted to the acid chloride (**I**) and treated with diethyl glutamate to form the corresponding carbobenzoxy (CBX) dipeptide. After reductively removing the CBX group, the resulting triethyl-γ-glutamylglutamate was condensed once again with the acid chloride (**I**) to form tetraethylcarbobenzoxy-γ-glutamyl-γ-glutamylglutamate (**II**). After removing the carbobenzoxy group the tetraethyl-γ-glutamyl-γ-glutamylglutamate hydrochloride (**III**) was *p*-nitrobenzoxylated. The *p*-nitrobenzoyl tripeptide (**IV**) was reduced to the corresponding *p*-aminobenzoyl derivative (**V**) and condensed with α,β-dibromopropionaldehyde (**VI**) and with 2,4,5-triamino-6-hydroxypyrimidine (**VII**) to complete the pteroyl ring system and obtain the desired pteroyl-γ-glutamyl-γ-glutamylglutamic acid (**VIII**). This synthesis was not practical since it resulted in very low yields. It is however of great historical significance since it served to demonstrate the poly-γ-glutamyl peptide structure of the fermentation *L. casei* factor.

A year later Boothe *et al.* (1949) described a new synthesis (Fig. 3, Second synthesis) suitable as a preparative method for large-scale

First synthesis

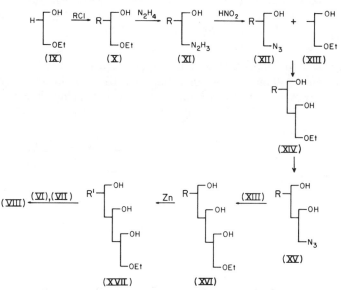

Fig. 3. First and second synthesis of pteroyl-γ-glutamyl-γ-glutamylglutamic acid (teropterin). For explanation see text.

work. This synthesis started from γ-ethyl glutamate (**IX**) which was *p*-nitrobenzoylated by treating with *p*-nitrobenzoyl chloride. The γ-ethyl *p*-nitrobenzoylglutamate (**X**) was converted to the hydrazide (**XI**) by hydrazine hydrate and to the azide (**XII**) by nitrous acid. The azide was reacted with γ-ethyl glutamate (**XIII**) to yield the *p*-nitrobenzoyl dipeptide as the γ-ethyl monoester (**XIV**). After preparing successively the disodium salt, the hydrazide, and the azide (**XV**), the latter was treated with γ-ethyl glutamate to yield the *p*-nitrobenzoyl-γ-glutamyl-γ-glutamyl-γ-ethyl glutamate (**XVI**). This compound was subsequently reduced with zinc dust to the corresponding *p*-aminobenzoyl tripeptide (**XVII**) and condensed directly with 2,3-dibromopropionaldehyde (**VI**) and 2,4,5-triamino-6-hydroxypyrimidine (**VII**) to yield, after removal of the ester group, the desired pteroyl-γ-glutamyl-γ-glutamylglutamic acid (**VIII**).

B. Solid Phase Synthesis

Krumdieck and Baugh (1969) reported a method of synthesis of the pteroylpoly-γ-glutamates based on a modification of Merrifield's solid-phase peptide synthesis. Details of the procedure are given in Krumdieck and Baugh (1980) and Baugh *et al.* (1970).

The starting material is t-butyloxycarbonyl-L-glutamic acid α-benzyl ester (Fig. 4, **I**) which is commercially available. This compound is esterified through its unprotected γ-carboxyl group to the chloromethylated Merrifield's resin (**II**). The yield of the esterification step following the original method (Krumdieck and Baugh, 1969) seldom exceeds 35%. This low yield is of concern when the synthesis of a radioactively labeled polyglutamate, bearing the tracer in the C-terminal glutamic acid, is attempted. A modified esterification based on the use of the cesium salt of the amino acid has been developed (Krumdieck and Baugh, 1980). The yield increases to more than 70% of the capacity of the resin.

The poly-γ-glutamyl chain is built going through cycles of deprotection of the amine group of the resin-bound moiety and peptide formation. An additional molecule of (**I**) (Fig. 4) is added per cycle. Since the resin−ester linkage via the γ-carboxyl group of glutamic acid is weaker than the usual α-carboxy resin−ester bonds formed in conventional solid-phase peptide synthesis, the deprotection step had to be modified

---

FIG. 4. Solid-phase synthesis of pteroylpoly-γ-glutamates. For explanation see text. Abbreviations: *t*Boc, tertiary butyloxycarbonyl; Bz, benzyl; R, resin; F$_3$AC, trifluoroacetyl.

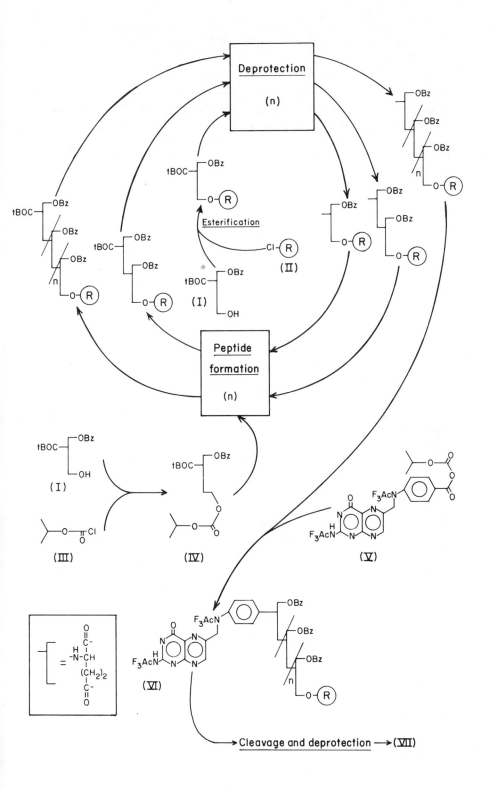

to avoid cleavage of the product from the resin. Twenty percent tri-fluoroacetic acid in methylene chloride effects complete removal of the tBoc group with negligible loss of resin-bound product. The activation of the entering amino acid through the use of a carbodiimide, as in the original procedure of Marshall and Merrifield (1965), was ineffective in promoting formation of the γ-peptide linkages. On the other hand, activation of the γ-carboxyl of (I) by formation of a mixed anhydride (IV) with isobutylchloroformate (III) resulted in nearly quantitative yields of the peptide-forming steps (Krumdieck and Baugh, 1969). After going through the necessary cycles of deprotection and peptide formation to achieve the desired poly-γ-glutamyl chain length, the pteroyl moiety is coupled in the form of a ditrifluoroacetylated deriva-tive (N-2,N-10-ditrifluoroacetylpteroic acid) which is readily soluble in dimethylformamide. Pteroic acid can be conveniently obtained from folic acid by removal of the glutamic acid, using a pteroylglutamic acid-degrading pseudomonad (Levy and Goldman, 1967; Houlihan et al., 1972; Scott, 1980). The pteroic acid precipitates from the culture medium and is recovered by centrifugation together with the bacterial cells. These are separated after dissolving the pteroic acid in alkaline sodium carbonate. The crude pteroic acid thus obtained is purified by column chromatography (Houlihan et al., 1972; Scott, 1980). Recently a chemical procedure to prepare pteroic acid from folic acid has been described (Temple et al., 1981). This method still requires column pu-rification of the final product. Since this is the most laborious step in obtaining pure pteroic acid, the chemical method does not seem to offer a substantial advantage over the microbiological degradation proce-dure.

The coupling of the trifluoroacetylated derivative of pteroic acid to the poly-γ-glutamyl-resin complex is carried out, preparing the mixed anhydride (V) with isobutylchloroformate (III). The yield of the cou-pling of pteroic acid is usually about 75%.

Cleavage of the final product from the resin can be done in several ways. The original method made use of gaseous HBr in trifluoroacetic acid with removal of the base-labile-protecting groups as the last step of the synthesis. Cleavage of the resin−ester bond and final deprotec-tion can be carried out in one single operation treating with nitrogen-saturated base in acetone (Krumdieck and Baugh, 1980). After neu-tralization and concentration of the final solution, the products can be precipitated at an acidic pH. The salt-free precipitates are easily col-lected and redissolved at neutral pH prior to column purification. The products obtained are purified by chromatography on a column of DEAE-cellulose.

The solid-phase synthesis of pteroylpoly-γ-glutamates is simple enough to be carried out by persons with limited expertise in organic chemistry. Its main shortcomings are that it is not suited to large-scale preparations and that small quantities of intermediate-length polyglutamates contaminate the final products. These contaminants arise whenever the yield of the peptide-forming steps is less than quantitative. Acetylating the growing peptide immediately after the coupling of each entering amino acid terminates the elongation of the unreacted chains and minimizes the problem of contamination in the end. Because of the ease of purification of the final products, this problem has not limited the usefulness of the method.

Pteroylpoly-γ-glutamates and p-aminobenzoylpoly-γ-glutamates of up to 12 glutamyl residues have been prepared. In addition, the synthesis of a number of analogs bearing different amino acid residues in the carboxyl end (Baugh et al., 1970) and of polyglutamyl derivatives of methotrexate (Baugh et al., 1973; Nair and Baugh, 1973) has been accomplished. The synthesis lends itself easily to the introduction of radioactively labeled glutamyl residues at any position in the poly-γ-glutamyl chain. Radioactive pteroylpolyglutamates have proven useful in studies of folate absorption (Butterworth et al., 1969; Baugh et al., 1971; Rosenberg, 1976; Halsted et al., 1981) and in the preparation of substrates for conjugase assay (Krumdieck and Baugh, 1970).

In spite of its shortcomings, this procedure is the most commonly used for the preparation of pteroylpolyglutamates (PteGlu$_n$) which, after conversion to reduced and one-carbon substituted forms, have been extensively used in the study of the enzymology of the folate-requiring reactions (Kisliuk, 1981; Covey, 1980; McGuire and Bertino, 1981) and the biosynthesis and biological role of the polyglutamates (Mcguire and Bertino, 1981; Cichowicz et al., 1981).

C. Synthesis in Solution

Meienhofer et al. (1970) described a method to synthesize, in solution, oligo-γ-glutamylglutamic acid peptides having two to seven glutamyl residues. They verified the previously reported observation (Krumdieck and Baugh, 1969) that the standard procedures for solid-phase peptide synthesis of Marshall and Merrifield (1965) using dicyclohexylcarbodiimide were not suitable for the synthesis of γ-glutamyl polypeptides. The yield at each peptide-forming step was less than quantitative, resulting in contamination of the final poly-γ-glutamyl peptide with small but significant quantities of peptides of intermediate lengths which, prior to the coupling of pteroic acid, were difficult to separate in preparative quantities. Their approach to synthesis in solution is shown schematically in Fig. 5. The starting material is N-carbobenzoxy-L-glutamic acid di-t-butyl ester (**I**). After removal of the N-carbobenzoxy group by catalytic hydrogenation, the formation of the peptide chain is initiated by coupling N-carbobenzoxy-L-glutamic acid α-t-butyl ester (**II**) activated as the carbonic acid–carboxylic acid-mixed anhydride (**IV**) of isobutylchloroformate (**III**) as described before by Krumdieck and Baugh (1969). Following each peptide-forming step the products have to be purified either by recrystallization or, for the heptapeptide, by chromatography on a large (190 × 5 cm) Sephadex LH-20 column and subsequent crystallization. Attempts to elongate the peptide chain by the use of pentachlorophenyl and N-hydroxysuccinimide γ-esters of the entering N-carbobenzoxy-L-glutamic acid α-t-butyl ester proved unsatisfactory. In a subsequent paper Godwin *et al.* (1972) described the coupling of N-10-trifluoroacetylpteroic acid as the mixed anhydride formed with isobutylchloroformate (**V**). The still protected products are purified by Sephadex LH-20 column chromatography, deprotected, and repurified by gel filtration. This synthesis has the advantage of being applicable to larger scale preparation of the polyglutamates and of yielding products of high purity. It is, however, considerably more involved and time consuming than the preceding solid-phase procedures.

Drey and Priestley (1978, 1979) described a number of improvements in the synthesis of the γ-L-glutamic acid peptides required for the preparation of the pteroylpolyglutamates. These authors selected C-terminal elongation as the mode of peptide synthesis, primarily because purification of intermediate acid peptides as quaternary ammonium salts was seen as a definite advantage. Furthermore, rather than elongating the peptide by the addition of one glutamyl residue at a time, they adopted the "block coupling" approach in which key intermediate peptides are linked to one another.

In their first communication, Drey and Priestley (1978) focused their efforts on the development of γ-glutamyl peptide intermediates which would be readily crystallizable and easily purified. To this end these authors introduced the basic picolyl ester group, in conjunction with 4-nitrobenzyl and t-butyl esters, for protection of the glutamyl–carboxyl groups. The use of these various carboxyl-protecting groups was, however, abandoned in their more recent work (Drey and Priestley, 1979) in order to simplify the final deprotection step. They selected N-carbobenzoxy-L-glutamic acid-α-t-butyl ester (**II** in Fig. 5) as their starting material. This compound is coupled, via its mixed anhydride with isobutylchloroformate (**IV** in Fig. 5), to L-glutamic acid-α-t-butyl ester.

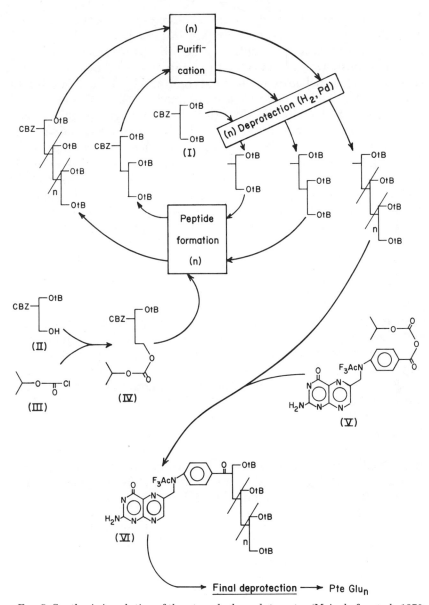

Fig. 5. Synthesis in solution of the pteroylpoly-γ-glutamates (Meienhofer *et al.*, 1970; Godwin *et al.*, 1972). For explanation see text. CBZ, Carbobenzoxy; *t*B, tertiary butyl; F₃AC, trifluoroacetyl.

The resulting acid dipeptide, N-carbobenzoxy-γ-[α-t-butylglutamyl]-t-butylglutamic acid (A), is one of two key intermediates in the synthesis of higher poly-γ-glutamyl peptides. The other is obtained by coupling (A) to the diester α,γ-di-t-butyl-L-glutamate to yield the fully protected tripeptide N-carbobenzoxy-γ-[α-t-butylglutamyl]$_2$-α,γ-di-t-butylglutamate (B). The higher peptides are obtained by "2 + 3" and "2 + 5" block coupling reactions. To this effect, the amino group of the tripeptide (B) is selectively deprotected by catalytic hydrogenation and the free-amino product coupled in γ-peptide linkage to a residue of (A), following the usual activation of the latter as the carbonic–carboxylic acid-mixed anhydride with isobutylchloroformate. The resulting fully protected pentapeptide provides, after catalytic hydrogenation, the free-amino peptide to which an additional "block" of the dipeptide (A) is added as before to obtain the fully protected heptaglutamate.

The desired pteroylpolyglutamates are obtained by coupling the mixed anhydride of N-10-trifluoroacetylpteroic acid and iso-butylchloroformate (V in Fig. 5) to the free-amino–carboxyl-protected peptides as described in the discussion of Godwin et al. (1972). Deprotection of the final products is obtained by trifluoroacetic acid treatment to remove the t-butyl groups, followed by aqueous piperidine to hydrolyze the trifluoroacetyl residue from N-10 of the pteroyl moiety.

An important contribution of these authors is the improved purification procedures of both the intermediate peptides and the final products. Their procedure is readily applicable to large-scale synthesis and results in high yields of products of very good quality.

Recently Piper and Montgomery (1983) and Piper et al. (1982) have described a synthetic approach to poly-γ-glutamyl analogs of methotrexate that, in principle, is also applicable to the synthesis of pteroyl-poly-γ-glutamates. Their method is based on earlier work of Piper and Montgomery (1977) that led to the synthesis of 6-(bromomethyl)-2,4-pteridinediamine hydrobromide (Fig. 6, I) which, when coupled to compounds of the general structure N-[4-(methylamino)-benzoyl]-L-α- and -γ-glutamyl-R$_{1,2}$ (II), resulted in the synthesis of methotrexate and substituted amides, peptides, and esters therof (III). To prepare poly-γ-glutamyl derivatives the appropriate oligo-γ-glutamate benzyl esters were synthesized in solution starting from L-glutamic acid dibenzyl ester and coupling t-butyloxycarbonyl-L-glutamic acid α-benzyl ester using diphenylphosphorylazide (Shioiri et al. 1972) as the coupling agent. Following deprotection of the amine the peptide was elongated by the addition of subsequent t-Boc-L-glutamyl-α-benzyl ester residues to the desired chain length. Deprotection of the peptide and coupling of (II) protected in the α-carboxyl by a benzyl group and in the amine by a

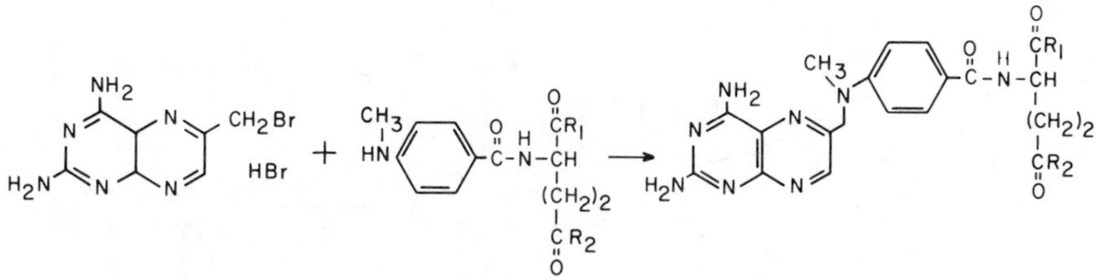

Fig. 6. Synthesis of poly-γ-glutamyl derivatives of methotrexate (Piper *et al.*, 1982; Piper and Montgomery, 1983). For explanation see text. R_1, OH; R_2, $-(\gamma$-glutamyl$)_n$-glutamic acid; Other peptides made include α-glutamyl peptides where R_1 = Glu, Asp, or Gly; R_2, = OH; and γ-glutamyl peptides where R_1 = OH; R_2, = Asp or Gly.

carbobenzoxy group yielded the final peptide which, following removal of the benzyl-and benzyloxycarbonyl-blocking groups, was smoothly coupled to (**I**) to give the desired poly-γ-glutamate of methotrexate. This elegant approach which results in products of excellent purity at very good yields has not yet been applied to the synthesis of polyglutamyl derivatives of folic acid. Difficulties in preparing the necessary 6-(bromomethyl)-2-amino-4-oxopteridine hydrobromide, which precluded the synthesis of the folypolyglutamates, have now been resolved by selective deamination of the 4 position of (**I**) (Montgomery, personal communication). When concluded, this approach will probably be the best yet devised to the large-scale synthesis of the pteroylpoly-γ-glutamates.

V. REDUCTION AND ONE-CARBON SUBSTITUTION OF THE PTEROYLPOLYGLUTAMATES

Figure 7 summarizes the most important chemical reactions used to prepare the reduced, one-carbon substituted pteroylpoly-γ-glutamates. The figure also shows a number of important degradation reactions, several of which form the basis of currently used analytical procedures for the quantitation and chain length determination of the pteroylpoly-γ-glutamates. The bold arrows indicate synthetic routes and the light arrows degradative reactions. The folates for which a cosubstrate role is known appear in rectangles drawn with bold lines.

Starting from a fully oxidized, unsubstituted pteroylpoly- (or mono-) glutamate the preparation of the various reduced, one-carbon substituted forms usually requires first their reduction to the tetrahydro derivatives. The recently described electrochemical reduction of Salem

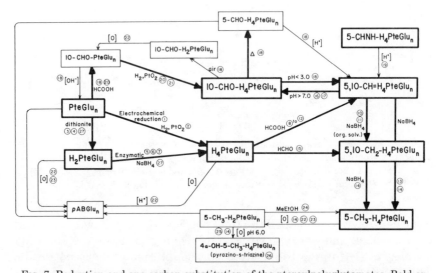

FIG. 7. Reduction and one-carbon substitution of the pteroylpolyglutamates. Bold arrows, synthetic routes to convert fully oxidized $PteGlu_n$ to the reduced one-carbon substituted cosubstrates (bold rectangles); light arrows, degradative reactions. References: 1. Salem *et al.* (1979); 2. Hatefi *et al.* (1960); 3. Futterman (1957); 4. Coward *et al.* (1975); 5. Mathews and Huennekens (1960); 6. MacKenzie and Baugh (1980); 7. Matthews and Baugh (1980); 8. Rowe (1968); 9. Baggott and Krumdieck (1979); 10. Farina *et al.* (1973); 11. Tatum *et al.* (1977); 12. Tatum *et al.* (1980); 13. Chanarin and Perry (1967); 14. Eto and Krumdieck (1980); 15. Osborn *et al.* (1960); 16. Kay *et al.* (1960); 17. Robinson and Jencks (1967); 18. May *et al.* (1951); 19. Uyeda and Rabinowitz (1965); 20. Huennekens *et al.* (1963); 21. Brody *et al.* (1979); 22. Maruyama *et al.* (1978); 23. Lewis and Rowe (1979b); 24. Donaldson and Keresztesy (1962); 25. Gapski *et al.* (1971); 26. Jongejan *et al.* (1979); 27. Hillcoat and Blakley (1964).

et al. (1979) is the best of the nonenzymatic methods available for this purpose. The yields obtained are essentially quantitative and since no reagents other than the volatile solvents triethylammonium bicarbonate (pH 9.25) and mercaptoethanol are used, the reduced folate is obtained, after lyophilization, as an essentially pure product. The compounds can be sealed in glass ampules under argon and stored indefinitely. An important advantage of this method is that the course of the reaction can be monitored spectrally. The operator can thus proceed for as long as necessary to effect complete conversion to the tetrahydro form. The method was designed to handle the small amounts of the expensive $PteGlu_n$ usually available. Depending on the power limitations of the available potentiostat, it can be applied to large-scale preparations.

The time-honored catalytic hydrogenation in glacial acetic acid

(Hatefi *et al.*, 1960) has been used for the reduction of poly-γ-gluta-mates. The method is, however, difficult and often results in disappointingly low yields. The very rapid decomposition of the reduced folates that follows exposure of the glacial acetic acid solution to air at the time of filtration of the catalyst is a problem familiar to all that have used this procedure. Also, as noted by Salem *et al.* (1979), the completeness of the reaction is seldom ascertained and, as a result, a mixture of products is usually obtained.

A major drawback of the chemical or electrochemical reductive procedures is that a *dl* mixture of the diastereoisomers formed by the introduction of the second asymmetric center at carbon 6 is always obtained. For biochemical work this represents, at best, a 50% drop in the yield of the biologically active product and at worst its contamination with an inhibitory isomer which cannot be removed. To obviate these difficulties the enzymatic preparation of the *l,L*-diastereoisomer, as first described by Mathews and Huennekens (1960), has been applied successfully to the polyglutamates (MacKenzie and Baugh, 1980; Matthews and Baugh, 1980). The fully oxidized compounds are first reduced by dithionite to the 7,8-dihydro derivatives as described originally by Futterman (1957) and modified by Coward *et al.* (1975). The $H_2PteGlu_n$ are then incubated with a dihydrofolate reductase preparation usually of bacterial origin (Poe *et al.*, 1972; Liu and Dunlap, 1974) in the presence of excess $NADPH + H^+$ or an $NADPH + H^+$ regenerating system. The l,L-$H_4PteGlu_n$ thus obtained can be purified by anion exchange or gel filtration chromatography in the presence of mercaptoethanol. Yields of 60–80% can be expected.

The preparation of the one-carbon substituted folates found in nature is conveniently carried out starting from $5,10$-$CH{=}H_4PteGlu_n$. These derivatives, as solids, are the most stable of the reduced folates and efficient ways for converting them to the other one-carbon substituted forms are available. A notable exception are the 5-formimino-tetrahydropteroylpoly-γ-glutamates for which no appropriate synthesis has been described. Baggott and Krumdieck (1979) applied, without modification, the method of Rowe (1968) to the synthesis of $5,10$-$CH{=}H_4PteGlu_n$ of chain lengths one through seven. A more recent procedure (Farina *et al.*, 1973; Tatum *et al.*, 1977) uses a mixture of formic acid (7.0 ml) and mercaptoethanol (3.2 ml) in glacial acetic acid (160 ml) instead of the 98% formic acid plus 2% mercaptoethanol (v/v) employed by Rowe. The small amount of formic acid used in the newer procedure permits the synthesis of one-carbon substituted tetrahydrofolates labeled with ^{14}C, ^{3}H, or ^{2}H in the one-carbon moiety with minimal dilution of the label present in the formic acid. Tatum *et al.* (1980) have described a useful purification of 5,10-CH=H_4 PteGlu using a phosphocellulose column eluted with a gradient of formic acid. Operating at acidic pH values prevents conversion of 5,10-CH=H_4Pte-Glu to the less stable 10-CHO—H_4PteGlu and lyophilization of the volatile eluant yields a salt-free preparation of the final product.

Reduction of 5,10-CH=H_4PteGlu$_n$ to 5-CH_3—H_4PteGlu$_n$ proceeds quantitatively by treatment with $NaBH_4$ in an acidic environment (Eto and Krumdieck, 1980). This method is based on the original communication of Chanarin and Perry (1967) which used 5-CHO—H_4Pte-Glu as the starting material. Probably because of incomplete conversion of 5-CHO—H_4PteGlu to 5,10-CH=H_4PteGlu their method resulted in low yields of the desired 5-CH_3—H_4PteGlu. In the procedure of Eto and Krumdieck (1980) the reduction to 5-CH_3—H_4Pte-Glu$_n$ proceeds very smoothly in spite of the rapid decomposition of the borohydride in the acidic solution. Evidently, the rate of the reduction must far exceed the rate of decomposition of the hydride.

The preparation of 5,10-CH_2—H_4PteGlu$_n$ is accomplished treating the tetrahydrofolates with dilute formaldehyde as originally described by Osborn *et al.* (1960). To our knowledge the separation of the diastereoisomers of *dl*, L-5,10-CH_2—PteGlu$_n$, in a way similar to that described by Kaufman *et al.* (1963) for the separation of the monoglutamyl diastereoisomers, has not been reported. Farina *et al.* (1973) described a stereoselective chemical reduction of 5,10-CH=H_4PteGlu to 5,10-CH_2—H_4PteGlu employing sodium borohydride, borodeuteride, or borotritide (Tatum *et al.,* 1977) in dimethyl sulfoxide:pyridine. Contrary to the borohydride reduction of 5,10-CH=H_4PteGlu$_n$ in acid which proceeds to the quantitative formation of the 5-CH_3 derivatives, the reduction in DMSO:pyridine stops at the intermediate 5,10-CH_2—H_4PteGlu form. It is worth noting that the stereospecificity of the latter reaction applies to the hydrogen atoms of the 5,10 methylene bridge and has nothing to do with the chirality of carbon 6.

10-CHO—H_4PteGlu$_n$ is obtained from 5,10-CH=H_4PteGlu$_n$ by simply raising the pH above neutrality. The reaction is fully reversible with an equilibrium constant for the monoglutamates [5,10-CH=H_4-PteGlu]/[10-CHO—H_4PteGlu] [H^+] equal to 9.0 × 10^5 M^{-1} (Kay *et al.,* 1960). Using this constant the equilibrium proportion of 10-CHO—H_4PteGlu at pH 7.0 is 92%, at pH 6.0 is 52.2%, and at pH 5.0 is 10.0%, dropping to insignificant proportions below pH 3.0. The marked susceptibility of 10-CHO—H_4PteGlu to air oxidation, with formation of 10-CHO—H_2PteGlu would, however, invalidate the above ratios unless precautions are taken to avoid this oxidation. The rate of hydrolysis of 5,10-CH=H_4PteGlu is very dependent on the nature and concentration of the buffer used (Robinson and Jencks, 1967). As a rule, the higher the pK_a, the pH, and the concentration of the buffer used, the faster the rate of hydrolysis.

VI. BIOLOGICAL SYNTHESIS

Certain yeast and bacteria have been used successfully for the biological synthesis of a number of one-carbon substituted and unsubstituted $H_4PteGlu_n$. These procedures, involving the isolation of a natural $H_4PteGlu_n$ in the form of a stable derivative which can be readily converted to various coenzyme forms, have two main advantages: they yield the biologically active l,L diastereoisomer and can be readily applied to the preparation of radioactively labeled polyglutamates of high specific activity.

Curthoys et al. (1972) used the purine-fermenting anaerobe *Clostridium acidiurici* as their biological source. This organism contains on a dry weight basis from 100 to 200 times more folates than found in rat liver, presumably all as triglutamate derivatives. These authors described the isolation of l 5,10-CH=$H_4PteGlu_3$ by two DEAE-cellulose column purifications and an acid-precipitation step. From this material l $H_4PteGlu_3$ was obtained by enzymatic arsenolysis using formyltetrahydrofolate synthetase. The l 5,10-CH=$H_4PteGlu_3$ was also converted to l 10-[^{14}C]CHO—$H_4PteGlu_3$ by incubating in the presence of [^{14}C]formate and formyltetrahydrofolate synthetase. In a preincubation step with ADP, the direction of the synthetase reaction is reversed and the nonradioactive starting triglutamate undergoes deformylation. Adding ATP shifts the equilibrium toward synthesis and promotes incorporation of the radioactive formate. In the same paper the synthesis of l [^{3}H]$H_4PteGlu_3$ from chemically prepared $PteGlu_3$ is described. Three steps were involved: (1) a [^{3}H]$NaBH_4$ reduction to obtain dl [^{3}H]$H_4PteGlu_3$; (2) conversion of the l isomer to the l 10-CHO—[^{3}H]$H_4PteGlu_3$ by formyltetrahydrofolate synthetase and its separation from the d [^{3}H]$H_4PteGlu_3$; and (3) the enzymatic arsenolysis of the l 10-CHO—[^{3}H]$H_4PteGlu_3$ to the desired [^{3}H]$H_4PteGlu_3$. The main limitation of the procedures described by Curthoys et al. (1972) is that the most interesting and difficult to obtain higher polyglutamates are apparently not synthesized by *Clostridium acidiurici*. This limitation does not apply to the work of Buehring et al. (1974) who used the common assay organisms *L. casei* and *Streptococcus faecium* to effect the biological synthesis of radioactive polyglutamates of up to nine glutamyl residues. Since these organisms lack the ability to synthesize folic acid, the biological conversion of [^{3}H]folic acid to the reduced polyglutamates present in the cells proceeds without dilution of the label. These authors were the first to report that the folic acid concentration of the medium influences the chain length of the polyglutamates synthesized by the cell. Longer forms appear at low (1.0–10.0 ng/ml) folic acid concentrations.

The approach of Buehring *et al.* (1974) to the isolation of the [^{3}H]Pte-Glu was based on the conversion of the cell's folates to the stable 5,10-CH=H$_4$PteGlu$_n$ by treatment of the extracts with concentrated formic acid. Reduction with NaBH$_4$ converted the 5,10-CH=H$_4$PteGlu$_n$ to the 5-CH$_3$—H$_4$PteGlu$_n$ which were resolved by QAE-Sephadex A-25 chromatography into four major peaks. The two major components were identified as 5-CH$_3$—H$_4$PteGlu$_8$ (42%) and 5-CH$_3$—H$_4$PteGlu$_9$ (19%) by cochromatography of their products of incomplete digestion with hog kidney conjugase, which yielded the complete homologous series of 5-CH$_3$—H$_4$PteGlu$_{1-9}$, with 5-CH$_3$—H$_4$PteGlu$_3$ and 5-CH$_3$—H$_4$PteGlu$_5$ synthetic markers used for reference.

Rao and Noronha (1978) have also described the isolation of 5-CH$_3$—H$_4$PteGlu$_{1,3,\text{ and }5}$, from bulk cultures of Torula yeast (*Candida utilis*). These authors established the chain length of their purified 5-CH$_3$—H$_4$PteGlu$_n$ by degradation and quantitative amino acid analysis.

VII. ANALYTICAL METHODS

The multiplicity of natural folates, the very low concentrations at which they are found in biological samples, their instability and the ubiquitous presence of enzymes that interconvert the one-carbon substituted forms and degrade the polyglutamyl chain, all combine to present a formidable obstacle to the separation, quantitation, and identification of these important coenzymes.

Taking the figure of 200 ng/g as the concentration of total folates in most biological samples and assuming that some of the folates in that sample may represent 5% or less of the total, the necessary sensitivity of the analytical procedures must extend down to 2–10 ng of folate, or 2–10 pmol, based on an average molecular weight of 1000 for the polyglutamates. Until recently only microbiologic and radioisotopic methods provided the needed sensitivity, however, several promising, highly sensitive, spectrophotometric (Eto and Krumdieck, 1982a; Shane, 1982), fluorometric (Furness and Loewen, 1981), and electrochemical (Lankelma *et al.*, 1980) procedures are being developed.

Compounding the difficulties of detection is the abnormal chromatographic behavior exhibited by the intact polyglutamates. These abnormalities, attributable mainly to adsorption artifacts, preclude the direct estimation of chain length based on the elution position of the reduced, one-carbon substituted pteroylpolyglutamates from molecular sieve (Kozloff *et al.*, 1970; Shin *et al.*, 1972a; Gawthorne and Smith, 1973; Buehring *et al.*, 1974) or from ion exchange columns (Baugh *et al.*, 1974; Kisliuk *et al.*, 1974; Moran *et al.*, 1976). In general, two approaches have been taken to develop analytical procedures for the study of the natural folates: (1) the first, directly attempting to resolve the mixture of intact folates, seeks to maintain the cofactors as they occur in nature and aims for a maximum of information, i.e., the quantitation of each of the one-carbon substituted, reduced, and oxidized forms, and determination of their corresponding polyglutamyl chain lengths; (2) the less ambitious approach, focuses primarily on the determination of the chain length of the polyglutamates, ignoring in most instances the nature of the one-carbon substituent or the state of reduction of the ring system. It must be said at the outset that no entirely satisfactory analytical procedure has yet been developed for the study of the natural folates.

A. MICROBIOLOGICAL ASSAYS

Table I summarizes the response of the three most commonly used assay organisms to a number of folic acid and pteroic acid derivatives. An increase in growth-supporting activity after treatment of the sample with a poly-γ-glutamyl hydrolase (conjugase) indicates the presence of pteroylpolyglutamates with more than three glutamyl residues if *L. casei* is the assay organism used. If *S. faecium* is employed, an increase in activity after conjugase treatment indicates the presence of polyglutamates greater than $PteGlu_2$ and bearing one-carbon substituents other than $5\text{-}CH_3$. Increased activity after conjugase for *Pediococcus cerevisiae* indicates the presence of tetrahydropolyglutamates longer than $H_4PteGlu_2$ and, as for *S. faecium*, bearing one-carbon substituents other than $5\text{-}CH_3$.

Tamura *et al.* (1972a) demonstrated that *L. casei* exhibits a significant growth response to $PteGlu_n$ having more than three glutamyl residues. These compounds were previously believed to be completely devoid of activity for this organism (see Table I). The response curves with polyglutamates having more than three glutamic acid residues showed progressively steeper slopes. The consequence of this is that samples containing significant amounts of the longer polyglutamates

TABLE I

GROWTH-SUPPORTING ACTIVITY OF FOLIC ACID AND PTEROIC ACID DERIVATIVES FOR *Lactobacillus casei* (ATCC 7469), *Streptococcus faecium*[a] (ATCC 8043), AND *Pediococcus cerevisiae*[b] (ATCC 8081)

Compound	L. casei		S. faecium	P. cerevisiae	Reference[c]
PteGlu	+	(100%)	+	−	1,2
H_2PteGlu	+		+	−	2
H_4PteGlu	+		+	+	2,3
10-CHO—PteGlu	+		+	−	2
10-CHO—H_2PteGlu	+		+	−	1,2
10-CHO—H_4PteGlu	+		+	+	2
5-CHO—H_4PteGlu	+		+	+	1,2,4
5-CH_3—H_4PteGlu	+		−	−	1,2,5,6
5,10-CH=H_4PteGlu	+		+	−	7
5-CH_3—H_4PteGlu$_2$	+		−	−	8
5-CHO—H_4PteGlu$_3$	+		−	+	9,10,11,12
PteGlu$_2$	+	(100%)	+	−	13,14
PteGlu$_3$	+	(100%)	−	−	2,14
PteGlu$_4$	+	(65%)	−	−	14
PteGlu$_5$	+	(20%)	−	−	14
PteGlu$_6$	+	(3.5%)	−	−	14
PteGlu$_7$	+	(2.4%)	−	−	14
5-CHO—H_4PteGlu$_n$[d]	−		−	−	8,9
5-CH_3—H_4PteGlu$_n$[d]	−		−	−	8,15
10-CHO—H_4PteGlu$_n$[d]	−		−	−	9
Pteroic acid	−		+	−	7
10-CHO—Pteroic acid	−		+	−	7
5-CHO—Pteroic acid	−		+	−	7

[a] Previously known as *Streptococcus lactis R* and *Streptococcus faecalis*.
[b] Previously known as *Leuconostoc citrovorum*.
[c] 1, Bird *et al.* (1965); 2, Silverman *et al.* (1961); 3, Bakerman (1961); 4, Sauberlich and Baumann (1948); 5, Keresztesy and Donaldson (1961); 6, Larrabee and Buchanan (1961); 7, Stokstad and Koch (1967); 8, Noronha and Silverman (1962); 9, Wittenberg *et al.* (1962); 10, Silverman and Wright (1956); 11, Usdin (1959); 12, Hakala and Welch (1957); 13, Rao and Noronha (1978); 14, Tamura *et al.* (1972a); 15, Noronha and Aboobaker (1963).
[d] The *n* unspecified; probably > 5.

read against a calibration curve prepared with a monoglutamate standard never give the same results when assayed at various dilutions. At low concentrations falsely low results are obtained, while the more concentrated solutions result in falsely high values. Furthermore, these authors showed that the *L. casei* activity of the longer chain

PteGlu$_n$ was sensitive to the length of incubation of the assay. Thus, the relative percentage of L. casei activity (with the response to PteGlu taken as 100%) to PteGlu$_5$ increased from 20 to 58% by merely extending the incubation time from 21 to 44 hours. Similarly, the responses to PteGlu$_6$ and PteGlu$_7$ increased from 3.6 to 7.9% and from 2.4 to 3.6%, respectively, prolonging the incubation time. It is clear that microbiological assays before and after conjugase treatment can provide some limited information regarding the chain length of the polyglutamates present in a sample. If there is a greater than 10-fold increase in L. casei activity after conjugase treatment, it is safe to conclude that the polyglutamates in the sample must be equal to or longer than PteGlu$_6$. On the other hand, if no increase in activity follows the conjugase treatment, the folates in the sample should be equal to or smaller than PteGlu$_3$.

Much effort has been invested in developing differential assays, using all three microorganisms, to identify and quantitate reduced and oxidized folates bearing different one-carbon substituents. Bird and McGlohon (1972) published an excellent review on this subject. The two most successful approaches are the use of P. cerevisae, which responds solely to tetrahydro forms of folic acid (with the exception of 5-CH$_3$—H$_4$PteGlu), for the determination of reduced derivatives, and the differential assay with L. casei and S. faecium for the quantitation of 5-CH$_3$ folates. A number of important sources of error involving chemical and enzymatic interconversions, as well as destruction of labile forms occurring during the extraction procedures and/or during the incubation period, must be avoided if accurate results are to be obtained. The polyglutamyl chain is particularly susceptible to rapid degradation by tissue conjugases liberated during homogenization of the sample. The need for instantaneous inactivation of these enzymes during sample preparation has been documented repeatedly (Bird and McGlohon, 1972; Tamura et al., 1972b; Krumdieck et al., 1976) and various strategies have been developed to achieve this, while at the same time avoiding the introduction of other modifications of the tissue folates. Autolytic changes begin to occur in homogenates, even at low temperatures, and accelerate rapidly when the homogenates are heated to inactivate the enzymes. Bird and McGlohon (1972) recommend the use of tissue slices to avoid the release of conjugases from disrupted subcellular organelles. Enzyme inactivation is achieved by dropping the slices into ascorbate buffers preheated to 95°C and heating for 5 minutes. Rat liver samples extracted in this fashion and assayed with L. casei after hog kidney conjugase treatment gave a total folate content of about 21 µg/g with only 2.18 µg/g assayable before conjugase treatment. Heating to 75°C, on the other hand, doubled the folates assayable prior to conjugase treatment indicating autolytic degradation of the polyglutamates before the conjugases were inactivated at this lower temperature. Alternative approaches involve homogenization in acid (Eto and Krumdieck, 1980; Foo et al., 1980; Shane, 1982) in 8 M urea:chloroform:mercaptoethanol mixtures (Francis et al., 1977), or in acetone:mercaptoethanol mixtures (Buehring et al., 1974). Although all of these procedures achieve instantaneous enzyme inactivation, chemical interconversions of the one-carbon substituents brought about by heat or by acidic pH values, and the apparent derivation of tetrahydrofolates by cyanate present in the high molarity urea solutions (Francis et al., 1977) do occur and complicate the interpretation of microbiological assays of the extracts thus prepared.

Another difficulty inherent in the use of microbiological assays is that a variety of reduced and oxidized one-carbon substituted and unsubstituted folates are quantitated against calibration curves prepared as a rule with PteGlu or 5-CHO—H_4PteGlu as standards. The basic assumption introduced here is that all active folate forms have identical equimolar growth-supporting activities for the assay organism used. This assumption is, however, a subject of controversy. For example, Bakerman (1961) clearly demonstrated that the activity of H_4PteGlu, relative to the standard 5-CHO—H_4PteGlu for P. cerevisiae, varies with concentration, temperature of incubation, and initial pH of the medium. A similar observation was reported by Bird et al. (1969) and Ruddick et al. (1978). More recently, Phillips and Wright (1982) have shown that the response of L. casei to 5-CH_3—H_4PteGlu could be as little as half that obtained with PteGlu. The response depended largely on the pH and on the buffer capacity of the medium. Contrary to these reports, Shane et al. (1980) could not demonstrate any difference in the growth response of L. casei to PteGlu, 5-CH_3—H_4PteGlu, 10-CHO—PteGlu, or 10-CHO—H_4PteGlu. It is difficult to estimate the extent of the errors in quantitation that may arise from assay conditions leading to unequal responses to the standard and to the sample's folates. This is particularly true when these different responses are complicated by the phenomenon of "positive drift," where a folate has less relative activity with respect to the standard at lower levels than at higher concentrations.

B. RADIOASSAYS

Any substance that can be labeled with a radioactive isotope and for which a specific high affinity binder exists can be quantitated by some form of radioisotope dilution assay. The first enunciation of the concept of a radioisotopic competitive binding assay was published by Herbert (1959) describing, very briefly, some preliminary work on the development of a vitamin B_{12} assay using intrinsic factor as a specific binder. The general principle has since been successfully applied to the determination of a large number of compounds (hormones, neurotransmitters, etc.) present in minute quantities in biological samples. Not surprisingly the discovery of folate binders in milk (Ghitis, 1967) and other sources prompted the development of numerous procedures for folate radioassays. The multiplicity of tissue folates was recognized early as a major obstacle to the successful application of these methods to the analysis of tissue samples. Ideally, the assay of a given molecule by means of a binder and a radiolabeled competitor requires that the molecule to be measured and its radioactive counterpart be either identical, or if not, that they bind to the binder with identical affinities. The chances that folates differing in state of reduction, one-carbon substitution, and length of the polyglutamyl chain would have equal affinities for the binder when compared to each other and to the radiolabeled competitor used (for example, an ^{125}I derivative of pteroylmonoglutamate) are rather low. Unless conversion of the multiple naturally occurring folates to a single compound is accomplished on a preliminary step, the requirements imposed on the binder are staggering and even contradictory. While required to be specific for folates, it would have to be, at the same time, nonspecific enough to ignore major structural differences in both the pteroyl and glutamyl parts of the molecules. Attempting to satisfy these requirements, many modifications of radioassays have been published including changes in pH (Givas and Gutcho, 1975), in the protein binders (Waxman and Schreiber, 1980), in the nature of the folate compounds used as radiolabeled competitors (Mitchell *et al.*, 1976; Johnson *et al.*, 1977), and in the order of addition of the sample and the labeled folate compounds, i.e., sequential vs simultaneous assays (Rothenberg *et al.*, 1974; Waxman and Schreiber, 1973). Four such different procedures, available commercially as radioassay kits, have been compared among themselves and against a standard *L. casei* assay (Shane *et al.*, 1980). A number of synthetic mono- and polyglutamyl derivatives of PteGlu, *l* 5-CH$_3$—H$_4$PteGlu, *dl* 5-CH$_3$—H$_4$PteGlu, and *l* 10-CHO—H$_4$PteGlu were assayed. Folate monoglutamates exhibited different responses in all the radioassay procedures depending on the one-carbon substituent and the oxidation state of the pyrazine ring. Folate polyglutamates exhibited an increased response indicative of a greater affinity of the binders used for the polyglutamates. Colman and Herbert (1979) observed the same phenomenon noting that folate triglutamate and heptaglutamate displaced more [³H]PteGlu from high-affinity folate binding proteins of human serum than did the monoglutamates. They warned against the possibility of errors in folate radioassays resulting from these differences in binder affinity. The study of Shane *et al.* (1980) also showed that the relative response of the polyglutamates increased with higher concentrations, precluding the normalization of the polyglutamate response curves to those of the monoglutamates. Because of this, these authors concluded that radioassays cannot be used for the direct determination of pteroylpolyglutamates. Furthermore, because of the variable response to different monoglutamyl derivatives, they found the radioassays unsuitable for the determination of a mixture of monoglutamates such as would be encountered in a natural sample after folate conjugase treatment. Of particular concern is the much lower affinity of the protein binders for folates with substituents at the formyl oxidation level, which are known to constitute a major fraction of total folates in tissues such as liver.

Similar discrepancies between radioassay kits and microbiological assays have also been reported by Baril and Carmel (1978), Longo and Herbert (1976), Jones *et al.* (1979), and McGown *et al.* (1978). In view of these discrepancies, the high correlation between total folate content of rat liver determined by *L. casei* assay after 5 hours of autolysis and by a radioassay procedure using a milk binder reported by Tigner and Roe (1979), is difficult to explain.

C. CHROMATOGRAPHIC METHODS

1. *Intact Folates*

Attempts to separate, identify, and quantitate the folate derivatives present in tissue extracts date back at least 30 years, when Winsten and Eigen (1950) and Wieland *et al.* (1952) applied paper chromatography and detection by bioautography to the study of folates in liver, yeast extracts, and some pharmaceutical preparations. Because of the limited resolutions achieved and the difficulties involved in hydrolyzing the polyglutamyl derivatives, either on the paper or in the bioautography plates, these early approaches were abandoned in favor of newer methods. Usdin and Porath (1957) reported the separation of PteGlu, 5-CHO—H₄PteGlu, and PteGlu₃, by column electrophoresis and by anion-exchange chromatography through Dowex-2 and triethylaminoethyl cellulose (TEAE-cellulose) columns. The latter anion exchanger was similar in properties to the then recently described diethylaminoethyl cellulose (DEAE-cellulose) (Sober and Peterson, 1954; Peterson and Sober, 1956). Usdin and Porath (1957) also reported the separation of PteGlu, PteGlu$_2$, and PteGlu$_3$ by TEAE-cellulose chromatography and the identification of the PteGlu$_2$ by its growth-promoting activity for *S. faecium*. Using separation by ion-exchange chromatography and detection by microbiological assays, Usdin (1959) attempted the resolution of the folic acid-active substances present in human blood. His results were vitiated by the use of harsh extraction and concentration procedures which undoubtedly introduced substantial alterations in the structure of the folates naturally present in blood. Furthermore, Usdin did not assay his fractions before and after conjugase treatment and was therefore unable to detect long-chain polyglutamates. Silverman *et al.* (1961), in a study of the folates of leukemic mouse cells and of mouse liver, introduced a very valuable tool: the analytical DEAE-cellulose columns eluted with hyperbolic phosphate gradients prepared in 0.2% ascorbate. The fractions collected were analyzed with all three organisms and the elution position of standards PteGlu, H$_2$PteGlu, H$_4$PteGlu, 10-CHO—PteGlu, 10-CHO—H$_2$PteGlu, 10-CHO—H$_4$PteGlu, 5-CHO—H$_4$PteGlu, 5-CH$_3$—H$_4$PteGlu, and PteGlu$_3$ was determined and used as an additional criterion for the identification of the natural folates. The procedures of extraction involved heating the cell samples, or acetone powders of the cells or liver, in a potassium ascorbate pH 6.0 buffer to 75°C for 30 minutes. These conditions, selected to minimize the isomerization of 10-CHO—H$_4$PteGlu to 5-CHO—H$_4$PteGlu, were later shown by Bird *et al.* (1969) to result in pronounced conversion of H$_4$PteGlu to 10-CHO—H$_4$PteGlu and to promote the autolytic degradation of the polyglutamyl derivatives. This, plus the fact that the fractions were not treated with conjugase prior to the microbiological assays, led to the erroneous conclusion that polyglutamyl derivatives were not present in mouse leukemic cells, and also to an overestimation of the pool of 10-CHO—H$_4$PteGlu. 5-CH$_3$—H$_4$PteGlu was, however, recognized as the predominant one-carbon substituted folate in the liver samples.

A major methodological advance reported a year later by Noronha and Silverman (1962) was the addition of conjugase treatment to the use of analytical DEAE-cellulose chromatography and differential microbiological assays. In this report, they analyzed the folate forms of chicken liver before and after treating the effluent fractions with a chick pancreas conjugase preparation. Several major new peaks, not detectable before digestion, appeared in the elution pattern, indicating the presence of large amounts of polyglutamyl derivatives of varying complexity. An additional refinement in methodology was obtained by digesting the polyglutamate-containing peaks to their corresponding one-carbon substituted monoglutamates by the use of a conjugase preparation obtained from *Physalia physalis,* and rechromatographing the monoglutamates on the analytical DEAE-cellulose columns. Comparison of these elution positions with those of authentic one-carbon substituted monoglutamate standards facilitated the identification of the one-carbon substituents in the original polyglutamates. A second identification criterion was provided by the use of differential microbiological assays. This very important study provided the first evidence for the natural occurrence of at least four $5\text{-}CH_3\text{---}H_4PteGlu_n$ of increasing complexity. The major methodological limitations remaining were the inability to determine the length of the polyglutamyl moiety and the persistent occurrence of poorly understood interconversion reactions during the sample extraction procedures. The effects of the temperature of extraction upon tissue folate patterns was investigated by Wittenberg *et al.* (1962) who showed that at temperatures below 70°C, ascorbate extraction resulted in an increase in the proportion of $10\text{-}CHO\text{---}H_4PteGlu$ and a marked decrease in the content of polyglutamyl derivatives. Noronha and Aboobaker (1963), in a study of the folates of human blood, also noted the formation of *S. faecium* and *P. cerevisiae* active substances (either $H_4PteGlu$ or $10\text{-}CHO\text{---}H_4PteGlu$). These were evident even without exogenous conjugase digestion, when whole blood hemolyzed by freezing and thawing was allowed to stand at room temperature for 3 hours prior to chromatography. It was clear from these studies that besides having conjugase activity, cell extracts prepared at temperatures that did not produce rapid protein denaturation contained enzymes that altered the one-carbon moiety of the native polyglutamyl forms. Rapid heating to 95°C in 1% ascorbate, pH 6.0, eliminated these alterations and was therefore adopted as the most suitable extraction procedure. Bird *et al.* (1965) applied essentially the same extraction procedure (quick heating of a cold homogenate made in 1% ascorbate, pH 6.0, to 95°C for 10 minutes) to the study of the blood and liver folates of normal rats. These authors demonstrated that one of the most detrimental treatments was to store frozen a sample of tissue prior to analysis. Freezing ruptured the cells and, during thawing and homogenization, active conjugases and folate-interconverting enzymes rapidly modified the naturally occurring folates. Thus, chromatography of rapidly heated extracts of rat liver revealed at least seven folate derivatives, all but two of which were polyglutamates, while liver extracts obtained after freezing and thawing contained predominantly monoglutamates and showed a marked diminution in the content of $5\text{-}CH_3\text{--}H_4PteGlu_n$.

The determination of the number of glutamyl residues in the naturally occurring polyglutamates was made possible by the synthesis of polyglutamates of unequivocal structure that served as chromatographic standards. The separation of the homologous series of PteGlu to $PteGlu_7$ on DEAE-cellulose columns presented no difficulties and was reported by Krumdieck and Baugh in 1969. A second attractive approach was the use of gel-permeation chromatography through Sephadex or polyacrylamide columns of low exclusion limits. Indeed, Whitehead (1971) successfully used acrylamide gel columns (BioGel P-2) to demonstrate the existence of polyglutamates with more than three glutamyl residues in human liver, but did not attempt to determine their exact chain length. DEAE-cellulose and gel chromatography were utilized by Shin et al. (1972a) to identify for the first time the chain length of the polyglutamates of a biological sample. Rats were sacrificed 24 hours after administration of a dose of $[^3H]PteGlu$ to label the animal's folates. The liver folates were extracted by dropping slices of liver into 1.0% boiling ascorbate, as recommended by Bird et al. (1965), and the extracts were chromatographed on DEAE-cellulose by a modification of the procedure of Noronha and Silverman (1962). Ten radioactive peaks were resolved. Aliquots of the last four DEAE peaks, presumably the polyglutamates, were pooled and rechromatographed through a 0.75×200 cm column of Sephadex G-15, eluting as one single peak close to the void volume. Synthetic $PteGlu_7$, $PteGlu_6$, $PteGlu_5$, and $10\text{-}CHO\text{--}H_4PteGlu_5$ standards eluted from this column as an incompletely resolved peak in the same position as the DEAE pooled peaks. It was concluded, therefore, that the latter were polyglutamyl derivatives with chain lengths certainly longer than $PteGlu_3$. To better define their chain lengths the peaks were individually cochromatographed with synthetic standards of $PteGlu_7$, $PteGlu_6$, and $PteGlu_5$ through a 4-m-long Sephadex G-15 column. The natural polyglutamates eluted slightly ahead of the $PteGlu_5$ and behind the $PteGlu_6$ markers. Since the markers were fully oxidized folates and the naturally occurring compounds were, in all probability, reduced one-carbon substituted derivatives, no perfect cochromatographic behavior was expected. Next, aliquots of the DEAE peaks were compared to synthetic ^{14}C-labeled $10\text{-}CHO\text{--}H_4PteGlu_5$ by cochromatography through Sephadex G-15 and G-25 columns. Against this reduced and formylated pentaglutamate the agreement was perfect for one peak and quite close for the other three peaks. Based on this evidence, the authors concluded that all four peaks were pentaglutamyl derivatives. The nature of the one-carbon substituent in each peak was determined by differential microbiological assays. The major polyglutamate was identified as $5\text{-}CH_3\text{—}H_4PteGlu_5$. No longer polyglutamates were found in this study. In retrospect, the failure to recognize the existence of longer forms can be explained by the limited incorporation of [^{3}H]PteGlu into hexa- and longer polyglutamates that takes place when the animals are sacrificed only 24 hours after administration of the label.

Shin *et al.* (1972b) examined in greater detail the behavior of various mono- and polyglutamyl derivatives on Sephadex G-15 and G-25 columns. Pronounced adsorption artifacts retarded the elution of the monoglutamates $5\text{-}CHO\text{—}H_4PteGlu$, $5\text{-}CH_3\text{—}H_4PteGlu$, $H_4PteGlu$, and PteGlu. Adsorption to the gels increased as the concentrations of the eluting buffer (phosphate, pH 7.0) were increased. The behavior of the polyglutamates was not a mere function of their molecular weights. Adsorption artifacts were observed for the short-chain polyglutamates while longer chain derivatives appeared in the effluent sooner than expected based on their molecular weights. The presence of one-carbon substituents, and the reduction state of the pteridine moiety also markedly affected the position of elution. As in the case of the monoglutamates, increasing the concentration of the eluting phosphate buffer retarded the elution of the polyglutamates. These multiple interactions of the folates with the gels frustrated the hope of being able to separate the naturally occurring folates according to their polyglutamyl chain lengths. Had this been the case, the position of elution of polyglutamates of *equal chain length* should have overlapped, regardless of the presence or absence of one-carbon substituents, or of the oxidation state of the ring system.

In 1973, Osborne-White and Smith published a paper on the identification and measurement of the folates of sheep liver based on separation by anion-exchange chromatography and differential microbiological assays with *L. casei, S. faecium,* and *P. cerevisiae* before and after treatment of the fractions with hog kidney conjugase. These investigators were able to distinguish almost 30 forms of folates. Methyltetrahydrofolates, the unsubstituted tetrahydrofolates, and probably also the formyltetrahydrofolates eluted in seven successive peaks, that were separated from each other by constant increments in the logarithm of the phosphate concentration of the eluting buffer. This, plus the decreasing availability of the successive peaks to *L. casei* prior to conjugase treatment, led these authors to consider the series of seven peaks as consisting of mono- to heptaglutamates, each peak containing an unresolved mixture of 5-CH_3—H_4, unsubstituted tetrahydro-, and formyltetrahydrofolates of the same chain length. The quantitation of each of these within one peak was done by differential microbiological assays. This elegant work, which exploited to a maximum the possibilities of combined DEAE-cellulose chromatography and microbiological assays, did not, unfortunately, include the use of authentic synthetic markers and may have erred in the assignment of chain lengths of the isolated polyglutamyl peaks. For instance, of the seven 5-CH_3—$H_4PteGlu_n$ peaks, peak 3 is designated as 5-CH_3—$H_4PteGlu_3$ in spite of the fact that it had only a 39% growth-supporting activity for *L. casei* prior to conjugase treatment. Since the triglutamates are essentially fully utilized by *L. casei* (Tamura *et al.*, 1972a), it can be argued that this peak actually corresponds to a tetraglutamate pool. Whether or not the assignment of chain length was correct, these authors provided strong evidence for the existence of polyglutamyl pools with more than five glutamyl residues in the liver of mammals. Furthermore, it should be noted that their results did not depend on the assumption of equal incorporation of previously administered radioactive folic acid into the various polyglutamyl pools of the animals, but measured directly the steady-state distribution of endogenous folates. The observed relation between the logarithm of the phosphate concentration of the eluting buffer and the number of glutamyl residues in successive $PteGlu_n$ was confirmed by Rao and Noronha in 1978. These investigators described a procedure very similar to that of Osborne-White and Smith (1973) for the separation and characterization of the folylpolyglutamates occurring in nature. An important refinement was the use of marker polyglutamates of unequivocal structure to assist in establishing the chain length of the natural folates. These markers were obtained by bulk isolation from an acetone powder extract of Torula yeast (see Section VI). The straight-line proportionality observed when plotting log phosphate concentration against number of γ-glutamyl residues was verified using the purified 5-CH_3—H_4Pte-$Glu_{1,3, and 5}$ markers. Furthermore, it was shown that this relationship was also valid for homologous series of 5-CHO—$H_4PteGlu_n$ and 10-CHO—$H_4PteGlu_n$.

Undoubtedly the methods of Osborne-White and Smith (1973) and of Rao and Noronha (1978) are powerful analytical procedures that can provide information on the number of glutamyl residues, the state of reduction of the pteridine ring, and the nature of the attached one-carbon moiety of natural folates. They are, however, slow and extremely laborious since the differential microbiological assay of *each* fraction before and after conjugase treatment requires at least 18 bioassay tubes. The analysis of the 360 fractions collected by Osborne-White and Smith (1973) involved a staggering 6480 bioassays for the study of one tissue sample. Not surprisingly, the search for simpler methods continues.

A useful alternative to the DEAE-cellulose columns eluted with phosphate buffers was the introduction of QAE Sephadex A-25 as the exchanger and triethylammonium bicarbonate as the eluting buffer (Parker *et al.*, 1971). An important advantage of this system is the volatile nature of the buffer which can be completely eliminated by lyophilization.

The separation of substituted- and unsubstituted-pteroyl, mono- and polyglutamyl derivatives by high-pressure liquid chromatography (HPLC) was reported by Stout *et al.* in 1976. These authors used a siliceous anion exchanger, Partisil-10 SAX column, developed with a linear gradient of sodium chloride (0.02 to 2.0 M NaCl in 0.05 M $NaNH_4HPO_4$ buffer, pH 6.5) to resolve a mixture containing $PteGlu_{1,3,4, \text{ and } 7}$, $5\text{-}CH_3H_4$ $PteGlu_{1,3,5, \text{ and } 6}$ plus l $5\text{-}CHO\text{—}H_4PteGlu$, $10\text{-}CHO\text{—}PteGlu$, $H_2PteGlu$, and PteGlu. Only $5\text{-}CH_3\text{—}H_4PteGlu$ and $5\text{-}CHO\text{—}H_4PteGlu$ failed to be resolved. Detection was by UV absorption at 254 nm. The sensitivity of this detection system is too low to permit the direct analysis of tissue folates and no application of the method to biological samples was reported. A linear relationship between the retention time and the number of glutamyl residues in a homologous series of polyglutamates was found. Plots of adjusted retention times t'_R (defined as the retention time of a polyglutamate t_R, minus the retention time of mercaptoethanol, a nonsorbed solute) against $(n + 2)^{1/2}$, where n is the number of intercalary glutamyl residues in a homologous series, generate a straight line. It is suggested that this relationship may facilitate estimating the chain length of peaks belonging to a known series. With some modifications to extend the life of the column, Cashmore *et al.* (1980) applied the above procedure to biological samples in which the folates had been labeled with ^3H by prior administration of [^3H]folic acid. The elution was monitored at 254 nm to detect the reference standards added to the samples and 1-minute fractions were collected for estimating the natural folates by radioactivity counting. In the same article, Cashmore *et al.* (1980) described the separation of pteroyl and *p*-aminobenzoyl polyglutamates by reversed-phase chromatography. A Partisil-10 ODS2 column, eluted with a linear gradient of 0 to 7.5% acetonitrile in 0.1 M acetate buffer, pH 5.5, was used. The order of elution of the polyglutamates in the reversed-phase system is inverted, the longer forms eluting first. AL-Pellionex-WAX, a pellicular, weak anion-exchanger consisting of an aliphatic matrix with amino functional groups, was applied to the HPLC separation of monoglutamatyl derivatives by Reed and Archer (1976). The same column packing was used by Maruyama et al. (1978) to separate 10-CHO—PteGlu$_{1,3,6,}$ and $_7$. No attempt was made to apply this system to the analysis of polyglutamates in biological samples.

A very original approach to the determination of the chain length of the polyglutamyl derivatives of 5,10-CH$_2$—H$_4$PteGlu$_n$ has been introduced by Priest et al. (1980). Their method is based on the incorporation of 5,10-CH$_2$—H$_4$PteGlu$_n$ into a ternary complex with thymidylate synthetase and 5-fluoro-2-deoxy[^{3}H]uridylate ([^{3}H]FdUMP). These ternary complexes are covalently linked and stable enough to remain intact during polyacrylamide gel electrophoresis. The net negative charge of the complex formed with 5,10-CH$_2$—H$_4$PteGlu is −4 at a pH of 8.2. Two of the charges correspond to the carboxyl groups of the glutamyl moiety and the other two to the phosphate group of the [^{3}H]FdUMP. For each additional glutamyl residue added to the 5,10-CH$_2$—H$_4$PteGlu, the resulting ternary complex gains one additional negative charge. The complexes have different electrophoretic mobilities which are a linear function of the number of negative charges, that is to say, of the number of glutamyl residues in the 5,10-CH$_2$—H$_4$-PteGlu$_n$. After electrophoretic separation on polyacrylamide gel plates, the different complexes are detected with very high sensitivity by fluorography of the [^{3}H]FdUMP. This method possesses a number of advantages, among them, it is the only available method for the determination of 5,10-CH$_2$—H$_4$PteGlu$_n$; entrapment of tissue 5,10-CH$_2$—H$_4$PteGlu$_n$ into the ternary complexes stabilizes this labile coenzyme form and permits its accurate quantitation and characterization. Furthermore, the method permits the evaluation of H$_4$PteGlu$_n$ by its prior conversion to 5,10-CH$_2$—H$_4$PteGlu$_n$ by adding formaldehyde to the complex-forming mixture. The application of these procedures to the analysis of tissue samples has been described by Priest et al. (1981).

2. C-9–N-10 Cleavage Procedures

Kozloff et al. (1970) were the first to report and take advantage of the fact that p-aminobenzoic acid and p-aminobenzoylglutamate do not interact with polyacrylamide gels and elute from the columns according to their molecular weights. These authors succeeded in cleaving a dihydropteroylpolyglutamate present in Escherichia coli T-even bacteriophages to a p-aminobenzoylpoly-γ-glutamate (pABGlu$_n$) and in determining the molecular weight of the latter by gel-filtration chro-

matography. Detection of the $pABGlu_n$ was carried out by microbiological assay using a pABA-requiring $E.$ $coli$ strain. They concluded
that the viral dihydropteroylpolyglutamate had six glutamyl residues,
a fact later verified by the use of synthetic markers (Nakamura and
Kozloff, 1978). Since the work of Kozloff et $al.$ (1970), numerous studies
employing oxidative (Houlihan and Scott, 1972; Brown et $al.$, 1974a,b;
Hoffbrand et $al.$, 1976; Reed and Scott, 1980) and reductive (Baugh et
$al.$, 1974; Leslie and Baugh, 1974; Hintze and Farmer, 1975) treatments to cleave the C-9–N-10 bond of the folates, have been published.
In nearly all of these reports, detection of the $pABGlu_n$ resulting from
cleavage of the folates was carried out by prior in $vivo$ labeling of the
folates with [^{3}H]folic acid containing two tritium atoms in positions $3'$
and $5'$ of the p-aminobenzoyl moiety. The chain lengths of the resulting radioactive $pABGlu_n$ were determined by cochromatography with
synthetic markers. Recently both the oxidative and reductive cleavage
procedures have been critically examined and found wanting. Alkaline
permanganate oxidation, originally described by Houlihan and Scott
(1972), fails to cleave the C-9–N-10 of $5,10$-$CH{=}H_4PteGlu$, 10-
CHO—$H_4PteGlu$, and $5,10$-CH_2—$H_4PteGlu$ and, rather than produce
the expected pABGlu, results in the formation of 10-formylfolic acid
(10-CHO—$PteGlu$). Furthermore, 5-CH_3—$H_4PteGlu$ was oxidized to 5-
methyldihydrofolic acid (5-CH_3—$H_2PteGlu$), a form that cleaves to
$pABGlu_n$ only under acidic conditions (Maruyama et $al.$, 1978). Perhaps more disturbing, the alkaline permanganate treatment resulted
in considerable destruction of $pABGlu_n$ (Gapski et $al.$, 1971; Maruyama et $al.$, 1978). These results were confirmed and extended by
Lewis and Rowe (1979a,b) who demonstrated that only folic acid and
dihydrofolic acid were cleaved to pABGlu by the zinc-hydrochloric acid
reductive method described by Baugh et $al.$ (1974). Tetrahydrofolic
acid and 5-CH_3—$H_4PteGlu$ were stable to the reductive conditions and
$5,10$-$CH{=}H_4PteGlu$, 10-CHO—$H_4PteGlu$, and 5-CHO—$H_4PteGlu$
yielded N-methyl-pABGlu. The basic assumption that oxidative or reductive treatment of the various one-carbon substituted folates resulted in their conversion to a homologous series of $pABGlu_n$ differing
only in the length of the poly-γ-glutamyl chain was clearly not satis-
fied by either technique. Not surprisingly, the chromatographic resolution of the mixtures of $pABGlu_n$, uncleaved pteroylpolyglutamates,
and N-CH_3—$pABG_n$ was often poor, and strict cochromatography with
the synthetic $pABGlu_n$ markers was seldom observed. In most of these
experiments, the determination of the relative pool size of each chain
length $pABGlu_n$ was obtained by measuring the radioactivity of the
pool as a fraction of the total [^{3}H]$pABGlu_n$ eluted from the column.
Since the radioactive precursor commonly used to label the folates of

the experimental animals prior to their sacrifice is $[3',5',7,9$ (n)-^{3}H]folic acid, the presence of an uncleaved folate (still bearing the tritium atoms at positions 7 and 9) contaminating a fraction presumed to contain only a $3',5'$-^{3}H-labeled pABGlu$_n$ will result in a significant overestimation of the size of that pool. Data obtained with these early procedures of C-9–N-10 cleavage should therefore be interpreted with caution.

In 1977 Tyerman *et al.* published a modification of the Zn/HCl reductive cleavage procedure aimed at eliminating the need for prior radioactive labeling of the animal's folates, which would permit the determination of the chain lengths of the "endogenous" folates. To do this, the quantitation of the pABGlu$_n$ after separation by DEAE-cellulose chromatography was carried out by the colorimetric procedure of Bratton and Marshall (1939) for primary aromatic amines. Since this method is considerably less sensitive than the tritium-labeling approach, these authors introduced, after the Zn/HCl treatment, a charcoal adsorption step to desalt and concentrate the samples before column chromatography. This step permitted processing of much larger tissue samples, and, fortuitously, promoted the oxidation of 5-CH$_3$—H$_4$PteGlu$_n$ (otherwise stable to the reductive cleavage) to the acid labile 5-CH$_3$—H$_2$PteGlu$_n$ (Lewis and Rowe, 1979b). The latter cleaved during a subsequent acid wash of the charcoal. The main drawback of the reductive cleavage, namely, its failure to cleave the dominant mammalian tissue folate 5-CH$_3$—H$_4$PteGlu$_n$, was thus removed. It must be noted, however, that folates yielding N-CH_3—pABGlu$_n$ upon Zn/HCl treatment must have escaped detection by the Bratton–Marshall test. The endogenous rat liver and kidney patterns obtained by this procedure may have been distorted by loss of those chain lengths predominating in the formyl-substituted folates. Recently Eto and Krumdieck (1981) reported a predominance of hexaglutamates in the pool of folates bearing one-carbon substituents at the formyl oxidation level in rat liver. The loss of this pool in the procedure of Tyerman *et al.* (1977) may account for the much smaller proportion of hexaglutamates detected by these investigators.

A number of other modifications of the reductive procedure, aimed at ensuring the cleavage of the C-9–N-10 bond of all forms of folates have been published. Baugh *et al.* (1979a) described an alternative Zn/HCl cleavage method which consists of adding a treatment with a mixture of peracetic acid in trifluoroacetic acid. This mixture cleaves the C-9–N-10 bond of 5-CH$_3$—H$_4$PteGlu and will not attack the poly-γ-glutamyl chain, but still results in the formation of N-methyl-pABGlu$_n$ from 5-CHO—H$_4$PteGlu$_n$, 5,10-CH=H$_4$PteGlu$_n$, 5,10-CH$_2$—H$_4$PteGlu$_n$, and methotrexate (Baugh *et al.*, 1979b). The application of this procedure to biological samples has not been reported. Brody *et al.* (1979) introduced a method in which the formyl-substituted folates (10-CHO—H_4PteGlu$_n$ and 5-CHO—H_4PteGlu$_n$) are first converted to 5,10-CH=H_4PteGlu$_n$ by acid treatment and then reduced to 5-CH$_3$—H_4PteGlu$_n$ by NaBH$_4$. The mixture is then subjected to the standard Zn/HCl reductive cleavage followed by formation of the azo-dye derivatives of the pABGlu$_n$ (AzoGlu$_n$) by the Bratton–Marshall procedure. Since the Zn/HCl treatment does not cleave 5-CH$_3$—H_4PteGlu$_n$, it is hard to understand why the prior conversion of the formyl-substituted folates to 5-CH$_3$—H_4 derivatives should result in their cleavage to pABGlu$_n$. A possible explanation is that significant (but not quantitative) oxidation of 5-CH$_3$—H_4PteGlu$_n$ to 5-CH$_3$—H_2PteGlu$_n$ occurs in the strongly oxidizing environment of the Bratton–Marshall test. The 5-CH$_3$—H_2PteGlu$_n$ would then rapidly cleave in the strongly acidic reaction mixture (Eto and Krumdieck, 1980). An interesting chromatographic modification introduced by Brody *et al.* (1979) is the direct resolution of the AzoGlu$_n$ by BioGel P-4 polyacrylamide columns. A useful preliminary purification and desalting of the AzoGlu$_n$ derivatives is obtained by adsorbing them to a BioGel P-2 polyacrylamide column at an acid pH. Following an acidic wash and a neutralization wash, the adsorbed AzoGlu$_n$ are eluted from the column with water.

Foo *et al.* (1980) described a cleavage procedure which combined oxidative and reductive treatments to effect a quantitative conversion of all naturally occurring folates to pABGlu$_n$. Their method starts by treating the cell extracts, containing 100 mM mercaptoethanol, with HCl, adjusting the pH to 1.0. This converts 10-CHO—H_4PteGlu$_n$ and 5-CHO—H_4PteGlu$_n$ to 5,10-CH=H_4PteGlu$_n$. The latter is then reduced with NaBH$_4$ to 5-CH$_3$—H_4PteGlu$_n$ which adds to the 5-CH$_3$—H_4PteGlu$_n$ originally present in the extract. After removing the mercaptoethanol with HgCl$_2$, the solution is adjusted to pH 12 and allowed to oxidize under air to convert the 5-CH$_3$—H_4PteGlu$_n$ to 5-CH$_3$—H_2PteGlu$_n$. The base treatment also results in the deformylation of any 10-CHO—PteGlu$_n$ (if present) to PteGlu$_n$. A second acidification cleaves the 5-CH$_3$—H_2PteGlu$_n$ and, finally, Zn is added to reductively cleave the PteGlu$_n$. The pABGlu$_n$ are diazotized, converted to the azo dyes of naphthylethylenediamine (AzoGlu$_n$), and chromatographically resolved on BioGel P-4 columns as described by Brody *et al.* (1979). The "combined cleavage" procedure of Foo *et al.* (1980) is unquestionably superior to the original reductive cleavage. A comparison of both methods showed that the former increased the yield of pABGlu$_n$ derived from labeled bacterial intracellular folates from 60 to 90%. This method has been successfully applied to the study of the folates of *Corynebacterium* species (Shane, 1980).

A very interesting modification of the procedure of Foo *et al.* (1980) has been reported recently by Furness and Loewen (1981). These authors have followed the cleavage method of Foo *et al.* up to and including the Zn treatment. Their main contribution is the use of fluorescamine to detect and quantitate the $pABGlu_n$, following their separation by a DEAE-Sephadex A-25 anion-exchange column. The collected fractions treated with fluorescamine form an intensely fluorescent adduct. In preliminary experiments these authors showed that the fluorescamine adducts of pABA, pABGlu, and $pABGlu_7$ had the same relative fluorescence. It was more than 100 times greater than that of equimolar amounts of the fluorescamine–glutamate adduct.

Since the fluorescamine reaction requires a primary amine, Furness and Loewen (1981) either eliminated the $AzoGlu_n$ derivatization step of Foo *et al.* (1980) and applied the neutralized cleavage reaction mixture to the DEAE-Sephadex column, or, after forming the $AzoGlu_n$ derivatives, recovered the $pABGlu_n$ by reductively removing the naphthylethylenediamine moiety as outlined by Brody in 1976. This last approach permits a prepurification step obtained by adsorbing the $AzoGlu_n$ to a Dowex 50W-X8 column from which the $pABGlu_n$ are eluted with sodium hyposulfite which reductively cleaves the azo dyes.

The sensitivity of the fluorescamine reaction permits the detection of 25 pmol/ml of $pABGlu_n$. The analysis of "endogenous" patterns without the need for radioactive precursors is easily done. The method has been applied to the analysis of the folates of *S. faecium, L. casei, Staphylococcus aureus, Bacillus subtilis,* bakers' yeast, *E. coli,* the fungus *Achlya,* and rat liver.

Eto and Krumdieck (1980, 1981, 1982a) have taken advantage of the different susceptibility to oxidative cleavage of the various reduced, one-carbon substituted and unsubstituted folates to develop a "differential cleavage" approach by which the quantitation and/or determination of the poly-γ-glutamyl chain length of specific pools of folates can be carried out. The principle of this procedure is outlined in Fig. 8. The rectangle at the top includes all the one-carbon substituted and unsubstituted, reduced folates known to occur in biological samples grouped according to their behavior in acid. Pool 1 consists of folates which upon acidification and subsequent exposure to air cleave to $pABGlu_n$; pool 2 contains solely $5\text{-}CH_3\text{—}H_4PteGlu_n$ which is unaltered and stable to an acidic pH (prolonged, i.e., more than 2 hours, acid treatment under air converts $5\text{-}CH_3\text{—}H_4PteGlu$ to an unknown product); and pool 3 is composed of the folates that, in an acid medium,

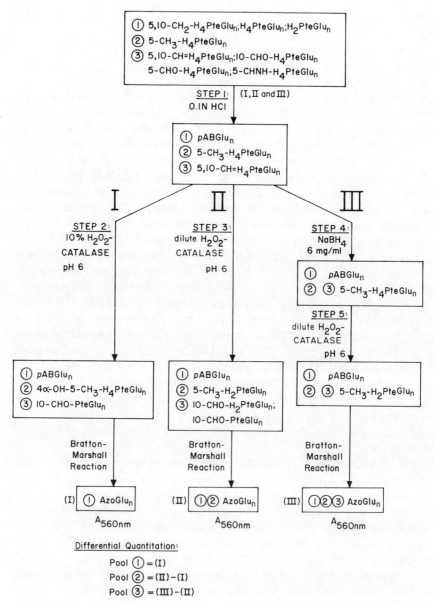

FIG. 8. Principle of the differential cleavage procedure. For explanation see text.

convert to the stable form $5,10\text{-}CH\!=\!H_4PteGlu_n$. The tissue sample is homogenized in acid, under argon, to convert the folates of pool 3 to $5,10\text{-}CH\!=\!H_4PteGlu_n$. This first step must be done anaerobically to prevent losses of $10\text{-}CHO\text{—}H_4PteGlu_n$ by air oxidation prior to its conversion to $5,10\text{-}CH\!=\!H_4PteGlu_n$. The sample is next divided into three aliquots which are then treated by procedures designed to cleave selectively the folates of pool 1 (route I in Fig. 8), of pools 1 + 2 (route II), and of all three pools 1 + 2 + 3 (route III). The cleaved folates are quantitated by diazotization of the resulting $pABGlu_n$ and formation of their corresponding azo dyes according to the Bratton–Marshall procedure. In routes I and II the uncleaved folates are excluded from the quantitation by conversion to Bratton–Marshall-negative products. To this end the $5\text{-}CH_3\text{—}H_4PteGlu_n$ are converted to $4\alpha OH\text{-}5\text{-}CH_3\text{—}H_4PteGlu_n$, and the $5,10\text{-}CH\!=\!H_4PteGlu_n$ to $10\text{-}CHO\text{—}PteGlu_n$. Cleavage of all forms (pools 1+2+3) in route III is achieved by air oxidation of pool I under acidic conditions followed by $NaBH_4$ reduction of the $5,10\text{-}CH\!=\!H_4PteGlu_n$ of pool 3 to $5\text{-}CH_3\text{—}H_4PteGlu_n$ and oxidation of the latter by mild H_2O_2 treatment to the acid labile $5\text{-}CH_3\text{—}H_2PteGlu_n$ which cleaves in the strongly acidic environment of the Bratton–Marshall test.

Chromatographic resolution of the $AzoGlu_n$ derivatives permits the determination of their corresponding chain lengths by comparison with synthetic $AzoGlu_n$ standards of known chain length. Initially, the separation was carried out as described by Brody et al. (1979) using BioGel P-4 polyacrylamide columns (Eto and Krumdieck, 1981). More recently a faster and much more sensitive high-performance liquid chromatographic procedure has been developed (Eto and Krumdieck, 1982a). The greater sensitivity of this procedure has permitted the direct colorimetric estimation and chain length determination of the three pools of endogenous folates from rat liver.

In a recent paper Shane (1982) reports the application of high-pressure liquid chromatography to the separation and quantitation of unlabeled $pABGlu_n$ cleaved from the folates of various biological extracts by the method of Foo et al. (1980). For the cleavage of bacterial cell extracts, the procedure of Foo et al. was followed strictly up to and including the BioGel P-2 purification of the $AzoGlu_n$. The purified azo dyes were then reductively cleaved with Zn/HCl to regenerate the $pABGlu_n$ which were then separated using a strong anion exchanger (Partisil-10 SAX) as done by Cashmore et al. (1980). The conditions for elution of the $pABGlu_n$ have been optimized so that excellent base-line separations of standard $pABGlu_{1-7}$ are obtained. Evidence indicating the resolution of $pABGlu_{8-11}$ from extracts of L. casei is also provided.

Detection and quantitation are done by monitoring UV absorption at 280 nm. Shane (1982) also describes the cleavage of the folates of rat liver accomplished by a simplified procedure which omits, from the method of Foo *et al.*, the mercaptoethanol in the initial trichloroacetic acid extract and the $NaBH_4$ and $HgCl_2$ steps. The rationale behind these modifications is that $HgCl_2$ becomes unnecessary in the absence of mercaptoethanol and that base treatment of the $5,10\text{-}CH\!=\!H_4Pte\text{-}Glu_n$ should rapidly convert them to $10\text{-}CHO\text{---}H_4PteGlu_n$ which would subsequently oxidize and deformylate to a mixture of $H_4PteGlu_n$, $H_2PteGlu_n$, and $PteGlu_n$. The two reduced folates are base labile and presumably cleave to $pABGlu_n$ in the alkaline solution. The $PteGlu_n$ are cleaved by the later Zn/HCl treatment of the procedure of Foo *et al.* (1980).

Whether using the complete or the simplified cleavage methods, the $AzoGlu_n$ derivation step is essential to prepurify and desalt the $pABGlu_n$ by P-2 gel chromatography. This step removes interfering UV-absorbing materials and permits concentrating the sample to a very small volume prior to injection into the HPLC column.

VIII. RESULTS

Table II summarizes the results of a number of studies on the distribution of chain lengths and one-carbon substituents among the folates of animal tissues and microorganisms. For a few tissues we have been able to include the percentage of a given polyglutamyl chain length that bears substituents at the oxidation levels of methyl, formyl, or methylene. The methylene pool includes, depending on the method, unsubstituted $H_2PteGlu_n$ and $H_4PteGlu_n$ [if the differential cleavage procedure of Eto and Krumdieck (1981, 1982a) was used] or just $H_4PteGlu_n$ [if the ternary complex method of Priest *et al.* (1981), was employed]. In some studies the proportion of unsubstituted folates is given separate from the $5,10\text{-}CH_2\text{---}H_4PteGlu_n$ pool. Some of the information included in the table may not be found in the original references cited. If that is the case, it is because the data have been recalculated by us, integrating peak areas under elution patterns published by the authors cited. No analysis of plant tissues or items of food has been included in the table.

Some generalizations can be made from the data in Table II.

1. The patterns of chain-length distribution of the polyglutamates vary considerably from species to species in microorganisms. Some bacteria exhibit a well-documented preponderance of short polygluta-

TABLE II

Distribution of Chain Lengths and One-carbon Substituents among the Folates in Animal Tissues and in Microorganisms

Source	Method — Intact	Method — C-9–N-10 cleavage[b]	Pattern — Endogenous[c]	Pattern — Exogenous[d]	1	2	3	4	5	6	7	8	≥9	Methyl	Formyl	Methylene	Unsubstituted	References
Human																		
Red cells	✓		A		⎡19⎤ (1–3)			19	39	23								Perry et al. (1976); Chanarin (1979)
Lymphocytes		B		72	22	2	13	21	20	16	6	1						Hoffbrand et al. (1976)
		B		72[e]	16	11	11	16	32	7	7							
Monkey																		
Liver	✓	B	A			2			24	46	15			60–80	20–40			Brown et al. (1974a); Scott and Weir (1976)
Liver		B		72	6	2	9	8	37	26	16							Tamura et al. (1981)
		C		72			5	7	64	15	3							Priest et al. (1981)
Liver	f	D							V=20	V=80								Priest et al. (1981)
Kidney		B		72				5	15	40	30	10						Brown et al. (1974a); Scott and Weir (1976)
Pig																		
Liver	f	D							V=15	V=85								Priest et al. (1981)
Rabbit																		
Liver	f	D							V=20	V=80								Priest et al. (1981)

(continued)

TABLE II (continued)

Source	Method — Intact	Method — C-9-N-10 cleav age[b]	Pattern — Endogenous[c]	Pattern — Exogenous[d]	1	2	3	4	5	6	7	8	≥9	Methyl	Formyl	Methylene	Unsubstituted	References
Sheep Liver	√		A		4	2	4	7	21	42	20			52		48		Osborne-White and Smith (1973)
					I=51	I=48	I=30	I=43	I=34	I=55	I=75							
Rat Liver	√				5				85–90									Shin et al. (1972a)
Liver		B	A	24	10				90					64	16			Houlihan et al. (1972); Houlihan et al. (1973)
Liver		C		1	68	9	11	10	2									Leslie and Baugh (1974)
				6	5	1	5	37	51	1	1							
				24			1	2	77	21								
				7 days				2	36	57	5							
				28 days					20	54	26							
Liver		B	B	24				9	66	25								Brown et al. (1974b); Scott and Weir (1976)
Liver		C	B					9	68	23								Shane et al. (1977)
Liver		C	B	24	3	2	10	21	52	8	4							Brody et al. (1979)
				48	1		3	6	64	21	5							
Liver	ƒ	C	D	2	45	5	14	23	12									Priest et al. (1981)
		C		48					100									
								V=40	V=60									

88

Tissue				h									Reference
Liver		A		72	4 (I=50, II=13, III=37)	56 (I=29, II=46, III=25)	40 (I=22, II=65, III=13)	1			27	50 ⌉ 23	Eto and Krumdieck (1981)
Liver		D	C		3	13	60	23					Furness and Loewen (1981)
Liver		A	B	72	3 (I=65, II=<10, III=30)	53 (I=42, II=36, III=24)	41 (I=30, II=60, III=10)	3 (I=25, II=75, III=0)			37	44 ⌉ 19	Eto and Krumdieck (1982a)
Liver		D	E		1	2	11	69	17	1			Shane (1982)
		D		4	10	38	16	13					
		D		24	1	3	3	23	66	4			
Liver (1) Folate sufficient (2) Folate deficient + sulfa		C		72	7	20	50	23	1				Cassady et al. (1980)
Liver regenerating (hours after partial hepatectomy)		D	B		1	9	21	40	28	2			Eto and Krumdieck (1982b)
0					3	53	42	2					
12					1	47	49	4					
72					2	23	57	19					
9 days					3	40	53	6					
21 days					3	55	39	2					
Kidney		C	B	24	16	2	8	22	53	42	2	37	45 ⌉ 19	Shane et al. (1977)
		C		48	6			24	47	49	4	41	43 ⌉ 12	
		C			8	2	5	18	57	13	7	I=30, IV=50		
Brain	√	A			I=100	42	14	7	4	IV=100, IV=100, IV=100, IV=100	18	16	66	Brody et al. (1976); Stokstad (1979)
					I=31, IV=69								
Red cells	√	A		24	50	50	35					>95	Shin et al. (1974)
					65								

(continued)

89

TABLE II (continued)

Source	Method		Pattern		Percentage distribution of chain length[a]									Percentage distribution of one-carbon substituents				References
	Intact	C-9–N-10 cleavage[b]	Endogenous[c]	Exogenous[d]	1	2	3	4	5	6	7	8	≥9	Methyl	Formyl	Methylene	Unsubstituted	
Mouse Liver	f		D						V=85	V=15								Priest et al. (1981)
Guinea pig Liver		B		24				5	85	10								Brown et al. (1974b); Scott and Weir (1976)
Hamster Liver		B		24				30	51	13	2	?						Brown et al. (1974b)
Chicken Liver	f		D					V=5	V=80	V=15								Priest et al. (1981)
Quail Liver		B		1/2	70		3	15	10									Thompson and Krundieck (1977)
				1	47		4	23	26									
				12	2			7	56	36								
				24				7	51	37	2							
				7 days				6	44	40	8							
Liver																		Thompson et al. (1977)
(1) Regular diet		B		72				12	56	26	6							
(2) High-protein diet		B		72				6	47	39	8							
(3) Low-methionine–choline diet		B		72				6	70	21	3							

90

	Fish	Liver				V=10	V=75	V=15						Reference
Microorganisms														
L. casei (low-folate medium)	√	D					8	14	42	19	26	10	39	Buehring *et al.* (1974)
L. casei (high-folate medium)		C	3	9	59	23	5							Baugh *et al.* (1974)
L. casei		C								100				Brody *et al.* (1979)
L. casei	f	D				V=55	V=45			⎦				Priest *et al.* (1981)
L. casei (low-folate medium)		C	4	2	1	V=45	4	20	61	15				Furness and Loewen (1981)
L. casei (low-folate medium)		D	4	1	2	1	4	5	37	46				Shane (1982)
S. faecium	√	D	17	4	61	24					0	45	25	Buehring *et al.* (1974)
S. faecium		C		20	55									Baugh *et al.* (1974)
S. faecium		D		6	90	4								Brody *et al.* (1979)
S. faecium		C		19	79	1								Furness and Loewen (1981)
S. faecium		D		5	77	19								Shane (1982)
S. faecium-MR (MTX resistant)		C	1	7	81	5	6							Baugh *et al.* (1974)
E. coli (1) Exponential phase		C	41	39	13	4	3	2						Furness and Loewen (1981)
(2) Stationary phase				15	18	11	19	20	14	3				
S. arizonae		D		21	32	23	19	5	1					Furness and Loewen (1981)

(continued)

TABLE II (continued)

Source	Method		Pattern		Percentage distribution of chain length[a]									Percentage distribution of one-carbon substituents				References
	C-9-N-10 cleav-age[b]	Intact	Endo-genous[c]	Exo-genous[d]	1	2	3	4	5	6	7	8	≥9	Methyl	Formyl	Methy-lene	Unsubsti-tuted	
S. aureus	D		C				20	80										Furness and Loewen (1981)
B. subtilis	D		C				93	7										Furness and Loewen (1981)
Clostridium thermoaceti-cum		√	D		12	35	47							95				Parker *et al.* (1971)
Corynebacte-rium sp.	D		B					100										Foo *et al.* (1980)
B. subtilis	C		D			3	88	6	1									Hintze and Farmer (1975)
Saccharomyces cerevisiae	B		D							16	71	13						Basset *et al.* (1976)
Neurospora crassa																		
(1) Regular medium	B		D						15	80			6					Chan and Cos-sins (1980)
(2) High gly-cine me-dium										56	24		20					
(3) High me-thionine medium										78			22					

92

Organism		I	II	III	IV	V=10	V=90	[b]	[c]	Reference
Yeast								f	D	Priest et al. (1981)
Bakers' yeast		1	3	3	15	64	14	D	C	Furness and Loewen (1981)
Achyla sp.	31	8	8	8	12	22	4	D	C	Furness and Loewen (1981)
Virus										
T2L phage					100			B	A	Kozloff et al. (1970)

[a]Number on top represents percentage of total polyglutamates with corresponding chain length. I, Percentage of given chain length with —CH$_3$ substituent; II, percentage of given chain length with —CHO (N-5 and/or N-10) substituent; III, percentage of given chain length with —CH$_2$— substituent and unsubstituted H$_2$ and H$_4$; IV, percentage of given chain length unsubstituted; V, percentage of given chain length with —CH$_2$— and unsubstituted H$_4$.

[b]A, Complete oxidative cleavage; B, incomplete oxidative cleavage; C, incomplete reductive cleavage; D, complete oxidative-reductive cleavage.

[c]A, Microbiological assay; B, Bratton–Marshall test; C, fluorometric; D, radioactive; E, UV absorption.

[d]Number indicates hours after administration (or duration of incubation) of/with labeled folic acid.

[e]Hours of incubation with ^{3}H-labeled 5-CHO—H$_4$PteGlu.

[f]Thymidylate synthetase, [^{3}H]FdUMP, 5,10-CH$_2$—H$_4$PteGlu$_n$ ternary complex.

mates (tetraglutamates in *S. faecium*) while others contain extremely long derivatives (octaglutamates and longer forms predominate in *L. casei*).

2. The interspecies variations in patterns of chain-length distribution among animals seem to be much less pronounced than among bacteria. Thus, the livers of primates, rodents, and birds all contain penta- and hexaglutamates as their predominant forms with much smaller quantities of tetra- and heptaglutamates.

3. Intraspecies variations in patterns of polyglutamate chain-length distribution are observed in animals from organ to organ. For example, in the rat, the kidney seems to contain a higher proportion of monoglutamate than the liver.

4. In both microorganisms and animals, the patterns have been shown to change significantly with circumstances likely to alter the steady-state of one-carbon metabolism. For example, the chain-length distribution in *L. casei* varies drastically with the concentration of folate in the medium (see Table II, *L. casei*). Shorter chains predominate when the folate content of the medium is high. The same phenomenon has been observed in rat liver (Table II). Other interesting examples are the changes observed in *E. coli* examined during the exponential and the stationary phases of growth, and the pattern changes in *Neurospora crassa*, which are grown in media of different compositions (Table II).

The most striking examples in animals were observed in the regenerating liver of rats (Table II, rat liver) and in the liver of quail fed high-protein and methionine-choline deficient diets (Table II, quail liver).

The significance of the above observations resides in the support they lend to the hypothesis that changes in the length of the polyglutamyl chain of the folates serve as an element of regulation of one-carbon metabolism. It is true that the demonstration of such changes does not in itself provide sufficient evidence to validate the hypothesis; on the other hand, if the changes had not been observed, the hypothesis of regulation would have been proven wrong.

ACKNOWLEDGMENTS

Partial support for the preparation of this manuscript was provided by NIH Grants NS 18350, GM 23453, and 5 PO1 CA 28103.

REFERENCES

Angier, R. B., Booth, J. H., Hutchings, B. L., Mowat, J. H., Semb, J., Stokstad, E. L. R., SubbaRow, Y., Waller, C. W., Cosulich, D. B., Fahrenbach, M. J., Hultquist, M. E., Kuh, E., Northey, E. H., Seeger, D. R., Sickels, J. P., and Smith, J. M., Jr. (1946). The structure and synthesis of the liver *L. casei* factor. *Science* **103**, 667–669.

Baggott, J. E., and Krumdieck, C. L. (1979). Folylpoly-γ-glutamates as cosubstrates of 10-formyltetrahydrofolate:5'-phosphoribosyl-5-amino-4-imidazolecarboxamide formyltransferase. *Biochemistry* **18**, 1036–1041.

Bakerman, H. A. (1961). A method for measuring the microbiological activity of tetrahydrofolic acid and other labile reduced folic acid derivatives. *Anal. Biochem.* **2**, 558–567.

Baril, L., and Carmel, R. (1978). Comparison of radioassay and microbiological assay for serum folate, with clinical assessment of discrepant results. *Clin. Chem.* **24**, 2192–2196.

Bassett, R., Weir, D. G., and Scott, J. M. (1976). The identification of hexa-, hepta- and octaglutamates as the polyglutamyl forms of folate found throughout the growth cycle of yeast. *J. Gen. Microbiol.* **93**, 169–172.

Baugh, C. M., and Krumdieck, C. L. (1971). Naturally occurring folates. *Ann. N. Y. Acad. Sci.* **186**, 7–28.

Baugh, C. M., Stevens, J. C., and Krumdieck, C. L. (1970). Studies on γ-glutamyl carboxypeptidase. I. The solid phase synthesis of analogs of polyglutamates of folic acid and their effects on human liver γ-glutamyl carboxypeptidase. *Biochim. Biophys. Acta* **212**, 116–125.

Baugh, C. M., Krumdieck, C. L., Baker, H. J., and Butterworth, C. E., Jr. (1971). Studies on the absorption and metabolism of folic acid. I. Folate absorption in the dog after exposure of isolated intestinal segments to synthetic pteroylpolyglutamates of various chain lengths. *J. Clin. Invest.* **50**, 2009–2021.

Baugh, C. M., Krumdieck, C. L., and Nair, M. G. (1973). Polygammaglutamyl metabolites of methotrexate. *Biochem. Biophys. Res. Commun.* **52**, 27–34.

Baugh, C. M., Braverman, E., and Nair, M. G. (1974). The identification of poly-γ-glutamyl chain lengths in bacterial folates. *Biochemistry* **13**, 4952–4957.

Baugh, C. M., Braverman, E. B., Nair, M. G., Horne, D. W., Briggs, W. T., and Wagner, C. (1979a). The peracid cleavage of 5-methyltetrahydrofolic acid at the C^9-N^{10} bridge. *Anal. Biochem.* **92**, 366–369.

Baugh, C. M., May, L., Braverman, E., and Nair, M. G. (1979b). Determination of the gammaglutamyl chain lengths in the folates by a combined zinc/acid-peracid procedure. *In* "Developments in Biochemistry Vol. 4: Chemistry and Biology of Pteridines" (R. L. Kisliuk and G. M. Brown, eds.), pp. 219–224. Elsevier, Amsterdam.

Binkley, S. B., Bird, O. D., Bloom, E. S., Brown, R. A., Calkins, D. G., Campbell, C. J., Emmett, A. D., and Pfiffner, J. J. (1944). On the vitamine B_c conjugate in yeast. *Science* **100**, 36–37.

Bird, O. D., and McGlohon, V. M. (1972). Differential assays of folic acid in animal tissues. *In* "Analytical Microbiology" (F. Kavanagh, ed.), Vol. 2, pp. 409–437. Academic Press, New York.

Bird, O. D., Binkley, S. B., Bloom, E. S., Emmett, A. D., and Pfiffner, J. J. (1945). On the enzymatic formation of vitamin B_c from its conjugate. *J. Biol. Chem.* **157**, 413–414.

Bird, O. D., McGlohon, V. M., and Vaitkus, J. W. (1965). Naturally occurring folates in the blood and liver of the rat. *Anal. Biochem.* **12**, 18–35.

Bird, O. D., McGlohon, V. M., and Vaitkus, J. W. (1969). A microbiological assay system for naturally occurring folates. *Can. J. Microbiol.* **15**, 465–472.

Boothe, J. H., Mowat, J. H., Hutchings, B. L., Angier, R. B., Waller, C. W., Stokstad, E. L. R., Semb, J., Gazzola, A. L., and SubbaRow, Y. (1948). Pteroic acid derivatives. II. Pteroyl-γ-glutamylglutamic acid and pteroyl-γ-glutamyl-γ-glutamylglutamic acid. *J. Am. Chem. Soc.* **70**, 1099–1102.

Boothe, J. H., Semb, J., Waller, C. W., Angier, R. B., Mowat, J. H., Hutchings, B. L.,

Stokstad, E. L. R., and SubbaRow, Y. (1949). Pteroic acid derivatives. III. Pteroyl-γ-glutamylglutamic acid and pteroyl-γ-glutamyl-γ-glutamylglutamic acid. *J. Am. Chem. Soc.* **71**, 2304–2308.

Bratton, A. C., and Marshall, E. K., Jr. (1939). A new coupling component for sulfanilamide determination. *J. Biol. Chem.* **128**, 537–550.

Brody, T. (1976). New assay method for folate polyglutamate synthesizing enzymes. *Fed. Proc. Fed. Am. Soc. Biol. Chem.* **35**, 1544.

Brody, T., Shin, Y. S., and Stokstad, E. L. R. (1976). Rat brain folate identification. *J. Neurochem.* **27**, 409–413.

Brody, T., Shane, B., and Stokstad, E. L. R. (1979). Separation and identification of pteroylpolyglutamates by polyacrylamide gel chromatography. *Anal. Biochem.* **92**, 501–509.

Brown, J. P., Davidson, G. E., and Scott, J. M. (1974a). The identification of the forms of folate found in the liver, kidney and intestine of the monkey and their biosynthesis from exogenous pteroylglutamate (folic acid). *Biochim. Biophys. Acta* **343**, 78–88.

Brown, J. P., Davidson, G. E., and Scott, J. M. (1974b). Comparative biosyntheses of folate polyglutamates in hamster, guinea-pig and rat. *Int. J. Biochem.* **5**, 735–739.

Buehring, K. U., Tamura, T., and Stokstad, E. L. R. (1974). Folate coenzymes of *Lactobacillus casei* and *Streptococcus faecalis*. *J. Biol. Chem.* **249**, 1081–1089.

Butterworth, C. E., Jr., Baugh, C. M., and Krumdieck, C. (1969). A study of folate absorption and metabolism in man utilizing carbon-14-labeled polyglutamates synthesized by the solid phase method. *J. Clin. Invest.* **48**, 1131–1142.

Cashmore, A. R., Dreyer, R. N., Horvath, C., Knipe, J. O., Coward, J. K., and Bertino, J. R. (1980). Separation of pteroyl-oligo-γ-L-glutamates by high-performance liquid chromatography. *In* "Methods in Enzymology" (D. B. McCormick and L. D. Wright, eds.), Vol. 66, pp. 459–468. Academic Press, New York.

Cassady, I. A., Budge, M. M., Healy, M. J., and Nixon, P. F. (1980). An inverse relationship of rat liver folate polyglutamate chain length to nutritional folate sufficiency. *Biochim. Biophys. Acta* **633**, 258–268.

Chan P. -Y., and Cossins, E. A. (1980). Polyglutamylfolate synthesis in *Neurospora crassa:* Changes in pool size following growth in glycine- and methionine-supplemented media. *Arch. Biochem. Biophys.* **200**, 346–356.

Chanarin, I. (1979). "The Megaloblastic Anaemias." Blackwell, Oxford.

Chanarin, I., and Perry, J. (1967). A simple method for the preparation of 5-methyltetrahydropteroylglutamic acid. *Biochem. J.* **105**, 633–634.

Cichowicz, D. J., Foo, S. K., and Shane, B. (1981). Folylpoly-γ-glutamate synthesis by bacteria and mammalian cells. *Mol. Cell. Biochem.* **39**, 209–228.

Colman, N., and Herbert, V. (1979). Kinetic and chromatographic evidence for heterogeneity of the high affinity folate binding proteins in serum. *In* "Developments in Biochemistry Vol. 4: Chemistry and Biology of Pteridines" (R. L. Kisliuk and G. M. Brown, eds.), pp. 525–530. Elsevier, Amsterdam.

Covey, J. M. (1980). Polyglutamate derivatives of folic acid coenzymes and methotrexate. *Life Sci.* **26**, 665–678.

Coward, J. K., Chello, P. L., Cashmore, A. R., Parameswaran, K. N., DeAngelis, L. M., and Bertino, J. R. (1975). 5-Methyl-5,6,7,8-tetrahydropteroyl oligo-γ-L-glutamates: Synthesis and kinetic studies with methionine synthetase from bovine brain. *Biochemistry* **14**, 1548–1552.

Curthoys, N. P., Scott, J. M., and Rabinowitz, J. C. (1972). Folate coenzymes of *Clostridium acidi-urici*. *J. Biol. Chem.* **247**, 1959–1964.

Day, P. L. (1944). The nutritional requirements of primates other than man. *Vitam. Horm.* **2**, 71–105.

Donaldson, K. O., and Keresztesy, J. C. (1962). Naturally occurring forms of folic acid. III. Characterization and properties of 5-methyldihydrofolate, an oxidation product of 5-methyltetrahydrofolate. *J. Biol. Chem.* **237**, 3815–3819.

Drey, C. N. C., and Priestley, G. P. (1978). A model folate synthesis incorporating the basic picolyl ester group. *J. Chem. Soc. Perkin Trans.* **I**, 800–804.

Drey, C. N. C., and Priestley, G. P. (1979). Improved synthesis of folate conjugates. Part 2. *J. Chem. Res.* June 6, 3055–3071.

Eto, I., and Krumdieck, C. L. (1980). Determination of three different pools of reduced one-carbon-substituted folates. I. A study of the fundamental chemical reactions. *Anal. Biochem.* **109**, 167–184.

Eto, I., and Krumdieck, C. L. (1981). Determination of three different pools of reduced one-carbon-substituted folates. II. Quantitation and chain-length determination of the pteroylpolyglutamates of rat liver. *Anal. Biochem.* **115**, 138–146.

Eto, I., and Krumdieck, C. L. (1982a). Determination of three different pools of reduced one-carbon-substituted folates. III. Reversed-phase high-performance liquid chromatography of the azo dye derivatives of p-aminobenzoylpoly-γ-glutamates and its application to the study of unlabeled endogenous pteroylpolyglutamates of rat liver. *Anal. Biochem.* **120** 323–329.

Eto, I., and Krumdieck, C. L. (1982b). Changes in the chain length of folylpolyglutamates during liver regeneration. *Life Sci.* **30**, 183–189.

Farina, P. R., Farina, L. J., and Benkovic, S. J. (1973). Stereoselective chemical reduction of 5,10-methyltetrahydrofolate. *J. Am. Chem. Soc.* **95**, 5409–5411.

Foo, S. K., Cichowicz, D. J., and Shane, B. (1980). Cleavage of naturally occurring folates to unsubstituted p-aminobenzoylpoly-γ-glutamates. *Anal. Biochem.* **107**, 109–115.

Francis, K. T., Thompson, R. W., and Krumdieck, C. L. (1977). Reaction of tetrahydrofolic acid with cyanate from urea solutions: Formation of an inactive folate derivative. *Am. J. Clin. Nutr.* **30**, 2028–2032.

Furness, R. A. H., and Loewen, P. C. (1981). Detection of p-aminobenzoylpoly(γ-glutamates) using fluorescamine. *Anal. Biochem.* **117**, 126–135.

Futterman, S. (1957). Enzymatic reduction of folic acid and dihydrofolic acid to tetrahydrofolic acid. *J. Biol. Chem.* **228**, 1031–1038.

Gapski, G. R., Whiteley, J. M., and Huennekens, F. M. (1971). Hydroxylated derivatives of 5-methyl-5,6,7,8-tetrahydrofolate. *Biochemistry* **10**, 2930–2934.

Gawthorne, J. M., and Smith, R. M. (1973). The synthesis of pteroylpolyglutamates by sheep liver enzymes *in vitro. Biochem. J.* **136**, 295–301.

Ghitis, J. (1967). The folate binding in milk. *Am. J. Clin. Nutr.* **20**, 1–4.

Givas, J. K., and Gutcho, S. (1975). pH Dependence of the binding of folates to milk binder in radioassay of folates. *Clin. Chem.* **21**, 427–428.

Godwin, H. A., Rosenberg, I. H., and Ferenz, C. R., Jacobs, P. M., and Meienhofer, J. (1972). The synthesis of biologically active pteroyloligo-γ-L-glutamates (folic acid conjugates). Evaluation of [³H] pteroylheptaglutamate for metabolic studies. *J. Biol. Chem.* **247**, 2266–2271.

Goldman, I. D., Chabner, B. A., and Bertino, J. R. (eds.). (1983). "Proceedings of the Workshop on Folyl- and Antifolyl-Polyglutamates, Airlie, Virginia, 1981. Plenum, New York.

Halsted, C. H., Gandhi, G., and Tamura, T. (1981). Sulfasalazine inhibits the absorption of folates in ulcerative colitis. *N. Engl. J. Med.* **305**, 1513–1517.

Hakala, M. T., and Welch, A. D. (1957). A polyglutamate form of citrovorum factor synthesized by *Bacillus subtilis. J. Bacteriol.* **73**, 35–41.

Hatefi, Y., Talbert, P. T., Osborn, M. J., and Huennekens, F. M. (1960). Tetrahydrofolic acid (5,6,7,8-tetrahydropteroylglutamic acid). *Biochem. Prep.* **7**, 89–92.

Herbert, V. (1959). Studies on the role of intrinsic factor in vitamin B_{12} absorption, transport, and storage. *Am. J. Clin. Nutr.* **7**, 433–443.

Hillcoat, B. L., and Blakley, R. L. (1964). The reduction of folate by borohydride and by dithionite. *Biochem. Biophys. Res. Commun.* **15**, 303–307.

Hintze, D. N., and Farmer, J. L. (1975). Identification of poly-γ-glutamyl chain lengths in folates of *Bacillus subtilis*. *J. Bacteriol.* **124**, 1236–1239.

Hoffbrand, A. V., Tripp, E., and Lavoie, A. (1976). Synthesis of folate polyglutamates in human cells. *Clin. Sci. Mol. Med.* **50**, 61–68.

Hogan, A. G., and Parrott, E. M. (1940). Anemia in chicks caused by a vitamin deficiency. *J. Biol. Chem.* **132**, 507–517.

Hogan, A. G., Boucher, R. V., and Kempster, H. L. (1935). Adequacy of simplified rations for the complete life cycle of the chick. *J. Nutr.* **10**, 535–547.

Houlihan, C. M., and Scott, J. M. (1972). The identification of pteroylpentaglutamate as the major folate derivative in rat liver and the demonstration of its biosynthesis from exogenous [^{3}H] pteroylglutamate. *Biochem. Biophys. Res. Commun.* **48**, 1675–1681.

Houlihan, C. M., Boyle, P. H., and Scott, J. M. (1972). Preparation and purification of pteroic acid from folic acid. *Anal. Biochem.* **46**, 1–6.

Houlihan, C. M., Davidson, G. E., Scott, J. M., and Brown, J. P. (1973). Distribution of pteroylpoly-γ-L-glutamates in rat liver. *Biochem. Soc. Trans.* **1**, 297–299.

Huennekens, F. M., Mathews, C. K., and Scrimgeour, K. G. (1963). Preparation and properties of tetrahydrofolic acid. *In* "Methods in Enzymology" (S. P. Colowick and N. O. Kaplan, eds.), Vol. 6, pp. 802–806. Academic Press, New York.

Hutchings, B. L., Bohonos, N., and Peterson, W. H. (1941a). Growth factors for bacteria. XIII. Purification and properties of an eluate factor required by certain lactic acid bacteria. *J. Biol. Chem.* **141**, 521–528.

Hutchings, B. L., Bohonos, N., Hegsted, D. M. Elvehjem, C. A., and Peterson, W. H. (1941b). Relation of a growth factor required by Lactobacillus casei to the nutrition of the chick. *J. Biol. Chem.* **140**, 681–682.

Hutchings, B. L., Stokstad, E. L. R., Bohonos, N., and Slobodkin, N. H. (1944). Isolation of a new Lactobacillus casei factor. *Science* **99**, 371.

Hutchings, B. L., Stokstad, E. L. R., Bohonos, N., Sloane, N. H., and SubbaRow, Y. (1948a). The isolation of the fermentation *Lactobacillus casei* factor. *J. Am. Chem. Soc.* **70**, 1–3.

Hutchings, B. L., Stokstad, E. L. R., Mowat, J. H., Boothe, J. H., Waller, C. W., Angier, R. B., Semb, J., and SubbaRow, Y. (1948b). Degradation of the fermentation *L. casei* factor. II. *J. Am. Chem. Soc.* **70**, 10–13.

Johnson, I., Guilford, H., and Rose, M. (1977). Measurement of serum folate: Experience with ^{75}Se-selenofolate radioassay. *J. Clin. Pathol.* **30**, 645–648.

Jones, P., Grace, C. S., and Rozenberg, M. C. (1979). Interpretation of serum and red cell folate results. A comparison of microbiological and radioisotopic methods. *Pathology* **11**, 45–52.

Jongejan, J. A., Mager, H. I. X., and Berends, W. (1979). Autoxidation of 5-alkyltetrahydropteridines. The oxidation product of 5-methyl-THF. *In* "Developments in Biochemistry Vol. 4: Chemistry and Biology of Pteridines" (R. L. Kisliuk and G. M. Brown, eds.), pp. 241–246. Elsevier, Amsterdam.

Kaufman, B. T., Donaldson, K. O., and Keresztesy, J. C. (1963). Chromatographic separation of the diastereoisomers of *dl,* L-5, 10-methylenetetrahydrofolate. *J. Biol. Chem.* **238,** 1498–1500.

Kay, L. D., Osborn, M. J., Hatefi, Y., and Huennekens, F. M. (1960). The enzymatic conversion of N^5-formyl tetrahydrofolic acid (folinic acid) to N^{10}-formyl tetrahydrofolic acid. *J. Biol. Chem.* **235,** 195–201.

Keresztesy, J. C., and Donaldson, K. O. (1961). Synthetic prefolic A. *Biochem. Biophys. Res. Commun.* **5,** 286–288.

Kisliuk, R. L. (1981). Pteroylpolyglutamates. *Mol. Cell. Biochem.* **39,** 331–345.

Kisliuk, R. L., Gaumont, Y., and Baugh, C. M. (1974). Polyglutamyl derivatives of folate as substrates and inhibitors of thymidylate synthetase. *J. Biol. Chem.* **249,** 4100–4103.

Kozloff, L. M., Lute, M., Crosby, L. K., Rao, N., Chapman, V. A., and DeLong, S. S. (1970). Bacteriophage tail components. I. Pteroyl polyglutamates in T-even bacteriophages. *J. Virol.* **5,** 726–739.

Krumdieck, C. L., and Baugh, C. M. (1969). The solid-phase synthesis of polyglutamates of folic acid. *Biochemistry* **8,** 1568–1572.

Krumdieck, C. L., and Baugh, C. M. (1970). Radioactive assay of folic acid polyglutamate conjugase(s). *Anal. Biochem.* **35,** 123–129.

Krumdieck, C. L., and Baugh, C. M. (1980). Solid-phase synthesis of pteroylpolyglutamates. *In* "Methods in Enzymology" (D. B. McCormick, and L. D. Wright, eds.), Vol. 66, pp. 523–529. Academic Press, New York.

Krumdieck, C. L., Boots, L. R., Cornwell, P. E., and Butterworth, C. E., Jr. (1976). Cyclic variations in folate composition and pteroylpolyglutamyl hydrolase (conjugase) activity of the rat uterus. *Am. J. Clin. Nutr.* **29,** 288–294.

Lankelma, J. , van der Kleijn, E., and Jamsen, M. J. Th. (1980). Determination of 5-methyltetrahydrofolic acid in plasma and spinal fluid by high-performance liquid chromatography, using on-column concentration and electrochemical detection. *J. Chromatogr.* **182,** 35–45.

Larrabee, A. R., and Buchanan, J. M. (1961). A new intermediate of methionine biosynthesis. *Fed. Proc. Fed. Am. Soc. Biol. Chem.* **20,** 9.

Laskowski, M., Mims, V., and Day, P. L. (1945). Studies on the enzyme which produces the Streptococcus lactis R-stimulating factor from inactive precursor substance in yeast. *J. Biol. Chem.* **157,** 731–739.

Leslie, G. I., and Baugh, C. M. (1974). The uptake of pteroyl[^{14}C]-glutamic acid into rat liver and its incorporation into the natural pteroyl poly-γ-glutamates of that organ. *Biochemistry* **13,** 4957–4961.

Levy, C. C., and Goldman, P. (1967). The enzyme hydrolysis of methotrexate and folic acid. *J. Biol. Chem.* **242,** 2933–2938.

Lewis, G. P., and Rowe, P. B. (1979a). Oxidative and reductive cleavage of folates—a critical appraisal. *In* "Developments in Biochemistry Vol. 4: Chemistry and Biology of Pteridines" (R. L. Kisliuk and G. M. Brown, eds.), pp. 253–254. Elvesier, Amsterdam.

Lewis, G. P., and Rowe, P. B. (1979b). Oxidative and reductive cleavage of folates—a critical appraisal. *Anal. Biochem.* **93,** 91–97.

Liu, J.-K., and Dunlap, R. B. (1974). Implication of a tryptophyl residue in the active site of dihydrofolate reductase. *Biochemistry* **13,** 1807–1814.

Longo, D. L., and Herbert, V. (1976). Radioassay for serum and red cell folate. *J. Lab. Clin. Med.* **87,** 138–151.

McBurney, M. W., and Whitmore, G. F. (1974a). Isolation and biochemical characterization of folate deficient mutants of Chinese hamster cells. *Cell* **2,** 173–182.

McBurney, M. W., and Whitmore, G. F. (1974b). Characterization of a Chinese hamster cell with a temperature-sensitive mutation in folate metabolism. *Cell* **2**, 183–188.

McGown, E. L., Lewis, C. M., Dong, M. H., and Sauberlich, H. E. (1978). Results with commerical radioassay kits compared with microbiological assay of folate in serum and whole-blood. *Clin. Chem.* **24**, 2186–2191.

McGuire, J. J., and Bertino, J. R. (1981). Enzymatic synthesis and function of folylpolyglutamates. *Mol. Cell. Biochem.* **38**, 19–48.

MacKenzie, R. E., and Baugh, C. M. (1980). Tetrahydropteroylpolyglutamate derivatives as substrates of two multifunctional proteins with folate-dependent enzyme activities. *Biochim. Biophys. Acta* **611**, 187–195.

Marshall, G. R., and Merrifield, R. B. (1965). Synthesis of angiotensins by the solid-phase method. *Biochemistry* **4**, 2394–2401.

Maruyama, T., Shiota, T., and Krumdieck, C. L. (1978). The oxidative cleavage of folates. A critical study. *Anal. Biochem.* **84**, 227–295.

Mathews, C. K., and Huennekens, F. M. (1960). Enzymic preparation of the *l*, L-diastereoisomer of tetrahydrofolic acid. *J. Biol. Chem.* **235**, 3304–3308.

Matthews, R. G., and Baugh, C. M. (1980). Interactions of pig liver methylenetetrahydrofolate reductase with methylenetetrahydropteroylpolyglutamate substrates and with dihydropteroylpolyglutamate inhibitors. *Biochemistry* **19**, 2040–2045.

May, M., Bardos, T. J., Barger, F. L., Lansford, M., Ravel, J. M., Sutherland, G. L., and Shive, W. (1951). Synthetic and degradative investigations of the structure of folinic acid-SF. *J. Am. Chem. Soc.* **73**, 3067–3075.

Meienhofer, J., Jacobs, P. M., Godwin, H. A., and Rosenberg, I. H. (1970). Synthesis of hepta-γ-L-glutamic acid by conventional and solid-phase techniques. *J. Org. Chem.* **35**, 4137–4140.

Mills, R. C., Briggs, G. M., Jr., Elvehjem, C. A., and Hart, E. B. (1942). *Lactobacillus casei* $_E$ factor in the nutrition of the chick. *Proc. Soc. Exp. Biol. Med.* **49**, 186–189.

Mims, V., and Laskowski, M. (1945). Studies on vitamin B_c conjugase from chicken pancreas. *J. Biol. Chem.* **160**, 493–503.

Mims, V., Totter, J. R., and Day, P. L. (1944). A method for the determination of substances enzymatically convertible to the factor stimulating Streptococcus lactis R. *J. Biol. Chem.* **155**, 401–405.

Mitchell, G. A., Pochron, S. P., Smutny, P. V., and Guity, R. (1976). Decreased radioassay values for folate after serum extraction when pteroylglutamic acid standards are used. *Clin. Chem.* **22**, 647–649.

Mitchell, H. K., Snell, E. E., and Williams, R. J. (1941). The concentration of "folic acid." *J. Am. Chem. Soc.* **63**, 2284.

Moran, R. G., Werkheiser, W. C., and Zakrzewski, S. F. (1976). Folate metabolism in mammalian cells in culture. I. Partial characterization of the folate derivatives present in L1210 mouse leukemia cells. *J. Biol. Chem.* **251**, 3569–3575.

Mowat, J. H., Hutchings, B. L., Angier, R. B., Stokstad, E. L. R., Boothe, J. H., Waller, C. W., Semb, J., and SubbaRow, Y. (1948). Pteroic acid derivatives. I. Pteroyl-α-glutamylglutamic acid and pteroyl-α,γ-glutamyldiglutamic acid. *J. Am. Chem. Soc.* **70**, 1096–1098.

Mowat, J. H., Gazzola, A. L., Hutchings, B. L., Boothe, J. H., Waller, C. W., Angier, R. B., Semb, J., and SubbaRow, Y. (1949). Pteroic acid derivatives. IV. Pteroyl-α,γ-glutamyldiglutamic acid. *J. Am. Chem. Soc.* **71**, 2308–2310.

Nair, M. G., and Baugh, C. M. (1973). Synthesis and biological evaluation of poly-γ-glutamyl derivatives of methotrexate. *Biochemistry* **12**, 3923–3927.

Nakamura, K., and Kozloff, L. M. (1978). Folate polyglutamates in T4D bacteriophage and T4D-infected *Escherichia coli. Biochim. Biophys. Acta* **540**, 313–319.

Noronha, J. M., and Aboobaker, V. S. (1963). Studies on the folate compounds of human blood. *Arch. Biochem. Biophys.* **101**, 445–447.

Noronha, J. M., and Silverman, M. (1962). Distribution of folic acid derivatives in natural material. I. Chicken liver folates. *J. Biol. Chem.* **237**, 3299–3302.

O'Dell, B. L., and Hogan, A. G. (1943). Additional observations on the chick antianemia vitamin. *J. Biol. Chem.* **149**, 323–337.

Osborn, M. J., Talbert, P. T., and Huennekens, F. M. (1960). The structure of "active formaldehyde" (N^5,N^{10}-methylene tetrahydrofolic acid). *J. Am. Chem. Soc.* **82**, 4921–4927.

Osborne-White, W. S., and Smith, R. M. (1973). Identification and measurement of the folates in sheep liver. *Biochem. J.* **136**, 265–278.

Parker, D. J., Wu, T.-F., and Wood, H. G. (1971). Total synthesis of acetate from CO_2: Methyltetrahydrofolate, an intermediate, and a procedure for separation of the folates. *J. Bacteriol.* **108**, 770–776.

Perry, J., Lumb, M., Laundy, M., Reynolds, E. H., and Chanarin, I. (1976). Role of vitamin B_{12} in folate coenzyme synthesis. *Br. J. Haematol.* **32**, 243–248.

Peterson, E. A., and Sober, H. A. (1956). Chromatography of proteins. I. Cellulose ion-exchange adsorbents. *J. Am. Chem. Soc.* **78**, 751–755.

Pfiffner, J. J., Binkley, S. B., Bloom, E. S., Brown, R. A., Bird, O. D., Emmitt, A. D., Hogan, A. G., and O'Dell, B. L. (1943). Isolation of the antianemia factor (vitamin B_c) in crystalline form from liver. *Science* **97**, 404–405.

Pfiffner, J. J., Calkins, D. G., O'Dell, B. L., Bloom, E. S., Brown, R. A., Campbell, C. J., and Bird, O. D. (1945). Isolation of an antianemia factor (vitamin B_c conjugate) in crystalline form from yeast. *Science* **102**, 228–230.

Pfiffner, J. J., Calkins, D. G., Bloom, E. S., and O'Dell, B. L. (1946). On the peptide nature of vitamin B_c conjugate from yeast. *J. Am. Chem. Soc.* **68**, 1392.

Phillips, D. R., and Wright, A. J. A. (1982). Studies on the response of *Lactobacillus casei* to different folate monoglutamates. *Br. J. Nutr.* **47**, 183–189.

Piper, J. R., and Montgomery, J. A. (1977). Preparation of 6-(bromomethyl)-2,4-pteridinediamine hydrobromide and its use in improved synthesis of methotrexate and related compounds. *J. Org. Chem.* **42**, 208–211.

Piper, J. R., and Montgomery, J. A. (1983). A synthetic approach to poly-γ-glutamyl analogs of methotrexate. "Proceedings of the Workshop on Folyl- and Antifolyl-Polyglutamates," Airlie, VA (I. D. Goldman, B. A. Chabner, and J. R. Bertino, eds.). Plenum, New York (in press).

Piper, J. R., Montgomery, J. A., Sirotnak, F. M., and Chello, P. L. (1982) Syntheses of α- and γ-substituted amides, peptides, and esters of methotrexate and their evaluation as inhibtors of folate metabolism. *J. Med. Chem.* **25**, 182–187.

Poe, M., Greenfield, N. J., Hirshfield, J. M., Williams, M. N., and Hoogsteen, K. (1972). Dihydrofolate reductase. Purification and characterization of the enzyme from an amethopterin-resistant mutant of *Escherichia coli. Biochemistry* **11**, 1023–1030.

Priest, D. G., Happel, K. K., and Doig, M. T. (1980). Electrophoretic identification of poly-γ-glutamate chain-lengths of 5,10-methylenetetrahydrofolate using thymidylate synthetase complexes. *J. Biochem. Biophys. Methods* **3**, 201–206.

Priest, D. G., Happel, K. K., Mangum, M., Bednarek, J. M., Doig, M. T., and Baugh, C. M. (1981). Tissue folylpolyglutamate chain-length characterization by electrophoresis as thymidylate synthetase-fluorodeoxyuridylate ternary complexes. *Anal. Biochem.* **115**, 163–169.

Rao, K. N., and Noronha, J. M. (1978). A general method for characterizing naturally occurring folate compounds, illustrated by characterizing Torula yeast (*Candida utilis*) folates. *Anal. Biochem.* **88**, 128–137.

Reed, L. S., and Archer, M. C. (1976). Separation of folic acid derivatives by high-performance liquid chromatography. *J. Chromatogr.* **121**, 100–103.

Reed, B., and Scott, J. M. (1980). Identification of the intracellular folate coenzymes of different cell types. *In* "Methods in Enzymology," (D. B. McCormick and L. D. Wright, Eds.), Vol. 66, pp. 501–507. Academic Press, New York.

Robinson, D. R., and Jencks, W. P. (1967). Mechanism and catalysis of the hydrolysis of methenyltetrahydrofolic acid. *J. Am. Chem. Soc.* **89**, 7098–7103.

Rosenberg, I. H. (1976). Absorption and malabsorption of folates. *Clin. Haematol.* **5**, 589–618.

Rothenberg, S. P., da Costa, M., Lawson, J., and Rosenberg, Z. (1974). The determination of erythrocyte folate concentration using a two-phase ligand-binding radioassay. *Blood* **43**, 437–443.

Rowe, P. B. (1968). A simple method for the synthesis of N^5, N^{10}-methenyltetrahydrofolic acid. *Anal. Biochem.* **22**, 166–168.

Ruddick, J. E., Vanderstoep, J., and Richards, J. F. (1978). Folate levels in food—a comparison of microbiological assay and radioassay methods for measuring folate. *J. Food Sci.* **43**, 1238–1241.

Salem, M. E., Lewis, G. P., and Rowe, P. B. (1979). The preparative electrochemical reduction of pteroylpentaglutamate. *Anal. Biochem.* **97**, 48–50.

Sauberlich, H. E., and Baumann, C. A. (1948). A factor required for the growth of Leuconostoc citrovorum. *J. Biol. Chem.* **176**, 165–173.

Schumacher, A. E., Heuser, G. F., and Norris, L. C. (1940). The complex nature of the alcohol precipitate factor required by the chick. *J. Biol. Chem.* **135**, 313–320.

Scott, J. M. (1980). Preparation and purification of pteroic acid from pteroylglutamic acid (folic acid). *In* "Methods in Enzymology" (D. B. McCormick and L. D. Wright, eds.), Vol. 66, pp. 657–660. Academic Press, New York.

Scott, J. M., and Weir, D. G. (1976). Folate composition, synthesis and function in natural materials. *Clin. Haematol.* **5**, 547–568.

Semb, J., Boothe, J. H., Angier, R. B., Waller, C. W., Mowat, J. H., Hutchings, B. L., and SubbaRow, Y. (1949). Pteroic acid derivatives. V. Pteroyl-α-glutamyl-α-glutamylglutamic acid, pteroyl-γ-glutamyl-α-glutamylglutamic acid, pteroyl-α-glutamyl-γ-glutamylglutamic acid. *J. Am. Chem. Soc.* **71**, 2310–2315.

Shane, B. (1980). Pteroylpoly(γ-glutamate) synthesis by *Corynebacterium* species. *In vitro* synthesis of folates. *J. Biol. Chem.* **255**, 5649–5654.

Shane, B. (1982). High performance liquid chromatography of folates: Identification of poly-γ-glutamate chain lengths of labeled and unlabeled folates. *Am. J. Clin. Nutr.* **35**, 599–608.

Shane, B., Watson, J. E., and Stokstad, E. L. R. (1977). Uptake and metabolism of [³H] folate by normal and by vitamin B-12- and methionine-deficient rats. *Biochim. Biophys. Acta* **497**, 241–252.

Shane, B., Tamura, T., and Stokstad, E. L. R. (1980). Folate assay: A comparison of radioassay and microbiological methods. *Clin. Chim. Acta* **100**, 13–19.

Shin, Y. S., Williams, M. A., and Stokstad, E. L. R. (1972a). Identification of folic acid compounds in rat liver. *Biochem. Biophys. Res. Commun.* **47**, 35–43.

Shin, Y. S., Buehring, K. U., and Stokstad, E. L. R. (1972b). Separation of folic acid compounds by gel chromatography on Sephadex G-15 and G-25. *J. Biol. Chem.* **247**, 7266–7269.

Shin, Y. S., Buehring, K. U., and Stokstad, E. L. R. (1974). Studies of folate compounds in nature. Folate compounds in rat kidney and red blood cells. *Arch. Biochem. Biophys.* **163,** 211–224.

Shioiri, T., Ninomiya, K., and Yamada, S. (1972). Diphenylphosphoryl azide. A new convenient reagent for a modified Curtius reaction and for peptide synthesis. *J. Am. Chem. Soc.* **94,** 6203–6205.

Silverman, M., and Wright, B. E. (1956). Microbiological aspects of the diglutamyl derivatives of citrovorum factor and N^{10} formylfolic acid. *J. Bacteriol.* **72,** 373–377.

Silverman, M., Law, L. W., and Kaufman, B. (1961). The distribution of folic acid activities in lines of leukemic cells of the mouse. *J. Biol. Chem.* **236,** 2530–2533.

Snell, E. E., and Peterson, W. H. (1940). Growth factors for bacteria. X. Additional factors required by certain lactic acid bacteria. *J. Bacteriol.* **39,** 273–285.

Sober, H. A., and Peterson, E. A. (1954). Chromatography of proteins on cellulose ion-exchangers. *J. Am. Chem. Soc.* **76,** 1711–1712.

Stokstad, E. L. R. (1979). Overview of folic acid derivatives in animal tissues. *In* "Folic Acid in Neurology, Psychiatry, and Internal Medicine" (M. I. Botez and E. H. Reynolds, eds.), pp. 35–45. Raven, New York.

Stokstad, E. L. R., and Manning, P. D. V. (1938). Evidence of a new growth factor required by chicks. *J. Biol. Chem.* **125,** 687–696.

Stokstad, E. L. R., and Koch, J. (1967). Folic acid metabolism. *Physiol. Rev.* **47,** 83–116.

Stokstad, E. L. R., Hutchings, B. L., and SubbaRow, Y. (1948). The isolation of the *Lactobacillus casei* factor from liver. *J. Am. Chem. Soc.* **70,** 3–5.

Stout, R. W., Cashmore, A. R., Coward, J. K., Horvath, C. G., and Bertino, J. R. (1976). Separation of substituted pteroyl monoglutamates and pteroyl oligo-γ-L-glutamates by high pressure liquid chromatography. *Anal. Biochem.* **71,** 119–124.

Tamura, T., Shin, Y. S., Williams, M. A., and Stokstad, E. L. R. (1972a). *Lactobacillus casei* response to pteroylpolyglutamates. *Anal. Biochem.* **49,** 517–521.

Tamura, T., Buehring, K. U., and Stokstad, E. L. R. (1972b). Enzymatic hydrolysis of pteroylpolyglutamates in cabbage. *Proc. Soc. Exp. Biol. Med.* **141,** 1022–1025.

Tamura, T., Romero, J. J., Watson, J. E., Gong, E. J., and Halsted, C. H. (1981). Hepatic folate metabolism in the chronic alcoholic monkey. *J. Lab. Clin. Med.* **97,** 654–661.

Tatum, C. M., Jr., Benkovic, P. A., Benkovic, S. J., Potts, R., Schleicher, E., and Floss, H. G. (1977). Stereochemistry of methylene transfer involving 5,10-methylenetetrahydrofolate. *Biochemistry* **16,** 1093–1102.

Tatum, C. M., Fernald, M. G., and Schimel, J. P. (1980). Facile new synthesis and purification of 5,10-methenyltetrahydrofolate from folic acid. *Anal. Biochem.* **103,** 255–257.

Temple, C., Jr., Rose, J. D., and Montgomery, J. A. (1981). Chemical conversion of folic acid to pteroic acid. *J. Org. Chem.* **46,** 3666–3667.

Thompson, R. W., and Krumdieck, C. L. (1977). Time course study of the in vivo synthesis of avian liver pteroylpoly-γ-glutamates. *Am. J. Clin. Nutr.* **30,** 1576–1582.

Thompson, R. W., Leichter, J., Cornwell, P. E., and Krumdieck, C. L. (1977). Alterations in the chain length of pteroylpoly-γ-glutamates and in the activity of pteroylpoly-γ-glutamate hydrolase in response to changes in the steady state of one carbon metabolism. *Am. J. Clin. Nutr.* **30,** 1583–1590.

Tigner, J., and Roe, D. A. (1979). Tissue folacin stores in rats measured by radioassay. *Proc. Soc. Exp. Biol. Med.* **160,** 445–448.

Totter, J. R., Mims, V., and Day, P. L. (1944). Further studies on the relationship between xanthopterin, folic acid and vitamin M. *Science* **100,** 223–225.

Tyerman, M. J., Watson, J. E., Shane, B., Schultz, D. E., and Stokstad, E. L. R. (1977).

Identification of glutamate chain lengths of endogenous folylpoly-γ-glutamates in rat tissues. *Biochim. Biophys. Acta* **497**, 234–240.

Usdin, E. (1959). Blood folic acid studies. VI. Chromatographic resolution of folic acid-active substances obtained from blood. *J. Biol. Chem.* **234**, 2373–2376.

Usdin, E., and Porath, J. (1957). Separation of folic acid and derivatives by electrophoresis and anion exchange chromatography. *Ark. Kemi* **11**, 41–46.

Uyeda, K., and Rabinowitz, J. C. (1965). Metabolism of formiminoglycine. Gylcine formiminotransferase *J. Biol. Chem.* **240**, 1701–1710.

Waller, C. W., Hutchings, B. L., Mowat, J. H., Stokstad, E. L. R., Boothe, J. H., Angier, R. B., Semb, J., SubbaRow, Y., Cosulich, D. B., Fahrenbach, M. J., Hultquist, M. E., Kuh, E., Northey, E. H., Seeger, D. R., Sickels, J. P., and Smith, J. M., Jr. (1948). Synthesis of pteroylglutamic acid (liver *L. casei* factor) and pteroic acid. I. *J. Am. Chem. Soc.* **70**, 19–22.

Waxman, S., and Schreiber, C. (1973). Measurement of serum folate levels and serum folic acid-binding protein by ^{3}H-PGA radioassay. *Blood* **42**, 281–290.

Waxman, S., and Schreiber, C. (1980). Determination of folate by use of radioactive folate and binding proteins. *In* "Methods in Enzymology" (D. B. McCormick and L. D. Wright, eds.), Vol. 66, pp. 468–483. Academic Press, New York.

Whitehead, V. M. (1971). Study of the folate polyglutamates in liver from animals and man. *Blood* **38**, 809.

Wieland, O. P., Hutchings, B. L., and Williams, J. H. (1952). Studies on the natural occurrence of folic acid and the citrovorum factor. *Arch. Biochem. Biophys.* **40**, 205–217.

Wills, L. (1931). Treatment of "pernicious anaemia of pregnancy" and "tropical anaemia." With special reference to yeast extract as a curative agent. *Br. Med. J.* **1**, 1059–1064.

Wills, L., and Bilimoria, H. S. (1932). Studies in pernicious anaemia of pregnancy. Part V. Production of a macrocytic anaemia in monkeys by deficient feeding. *Indian J. Med. Res.* **20**, 391–404.

Winsten, W. A., and Eigen, E. (1950). Bioautographic studies with use of Leuconostoc citrovorum 8081. *J. Biol. Chem.* **184**, 155–161.

Wittenberg, J. B., Noronha, J. M., and Silverman, M. (1962). Folic acid derivatives in the gas gland of *Physalia physalis* L. *Biochem. J.* **85**, 9–15.

Wright, L. D., and Welch, A. D. (1943). The production of folic acid by rat liver in vitro. *Science* **98**, 179–182.

Vitamin A and Cancer

DAVID E. ONG AND FRANK CHYTIL

Department of Biochemistry, Vanderbilt University School of Medicine,
Nashville, Tennessee

I. INTRODUCTION

Recently investigators have sought to elucidate possible relationships between the incidence of cancer and the intake of vitamin A and vitamin A analogs, now commonly called retinoids. Indeed, a body of evidence has accumulated over the years that the vitamin A status of human beings as well as experimental animals appears to be one of the many factors that can influence the development of malignant growths of diversified site, morphology, and consequence to the host. This diversity, which extends to the known or presumed inducing agent, argues vigorously against the possibility of a simple explanation of the processes involved. In spite of considerable progress toward describing molecular events associated with malignant transformation and growth there is still too little understanding to allow treatment or prevention. It is not surprising therefore that serious consideration has been given to the possible effect of dietary factors on cancer incidence or development.

Over 20 reviews covering diverse aspects of the relationship between vitamin A and cancer have appeared in the recent scientific literature.

The mechanism of vitamin A action at the cellular level is currently under intensive study and our article will attempt to apply our particular biases to the problem with the hope of stimulating new experimental approaches. We believe that successful application of retinoids to prevention and therapy of some cancer will require an understanding of the physiological function of the vitamin. We are not dealing with a drug that interferes with the metabolism of both normal and neoplastic tissue but a nutrient necessary for the proper function of diverse tissues of the body, ranging from the mucous-secreting epithelium of the trachea to the sperm-producing epithelium of the testes. Since the tissues requiring vitamin A are diverse, the effects of vitamin A on these tissues are diverse and effects of vitamin A on the neoplasms of these tissues are not uniform. Only increased understanding of the role(s) of vitamin A in normal tissue would seem to offer hope of improving our understanding of effects of vitamin A on cancer.

II. HISTORY

Soon after this micronutrient was discovered in 1919, Wyard (1922) tried a vitamin A-deficient diet for the treatment of patients suffering from cancer but without success. This early interest may have been prompted by the similarities of lesions in vitamin A-deficient animals to morphological changes observed in tumors. Histopathological studies on the vitamin A-deficient rat revealed in many tissues the replacement of the columnar and transitional epithelium by squamous, frequently keratinizing epithelial cells that multiplied rapidly (Wolbach and Howe, 1925). In their classical paper Wolbach and Howe (1925) made the following observation.

> In the epithelium of the bladder, ureters, and pelvis of the kidney the original epithelium becomes replaced by keratinizing epithelium which develops as in other locations from underlying nests of cells. In the kidneys, the apices of the pyramids become covered by a thick layer of keratinizing epithelium, while the epithelium of the pelvis, ureters, and bladder show the most remarkable pictures encountered in this study. In these latter locations there is evidence of very rapid growth of the epithelium: in some instances keratinization ceased. Mitotic figures are to be found in every field of a 3 mm immersion objective and frequently there are two to four mitoses per field. In the bladder invaginations and dermoid cyst-like formations occur. In ureter, pelvis, and bladder epithelial downgrowth resulting in the incorporation of blood vessels is frequent. The behaviours indicate growth power suggestive of neoplastic potentiality.

The dramatic changes described above are fully reversed by restoring a normal diet containing vitamin A (Wolbach and Howe, 1933).

These early studies may also have suggested that lower intake of vitamin A might lead to an elevated susceptibility of the animal to cancerogenic insult. Fujimaki (1926) reported that rats receiving a vitamin A-deficient diet had a higher frequency of spontaneous gastric carcinomas. The failure of Sugiura and Benedict (1930a,b) to reproduce Fujimaki's observation indicated the difficulty of research on spontaneous tumors occurring at very low frequency. Consequently, the later introduction of the use of chemical carcinogens to produce experimental tumors with high frequency in laboratory animals has shown more successfully the existence of a relationship between vitamin A and cancer.

Several earlier reviewers have discussed the evidence that an inadequate supply of retinol (vitamin A alcohol) or its esters brings about a higher frequency of tumors (e.g., Caspari and Ottensooser, 1929; Gordonoff and Ludwig, 1935; Vollmar, 1939; Harding and Leech, 1940). After a survey of the experimental data, Burk and Winzler (1944) concluded: "sufficient evidence has accumulated which makes it desirable to seek further a peculiar and perhaps specific relationship between vitamin A and malignant growth. This evidence consists of the demonstration of hyperplastic lesions of epithelial linings in vitamin A deficiency, possible alteration of viamin A metabolism in tumor bearing patients, the effect of carcinogens on vitamin A metabolism, and occasional experiments that the dietary vitamin A level may influence the growth and incidence of experimental cancer."

These conclusions were based in part on the finding that vitamin A deficiency was an essential condition for production of epithelial metaplasia by mechanical irritation in rats (McCullough and Dalldorf, 1937). It became apparent that metabolism of vitamin A may be altered in tumors when it was found that little or no vitamin A was detectable in many tumors (for review, see Burk and Winzler, 1944) and that malignant tissue contained less retinol than the tissue of origin. It also became clear that the extent of "depletion" of vitamin A depended on the tumor and which carcinogen was used for its induction.

Early workers also attempted to influence the incidence of various types of experimental tumors by altering vitamin A content of the diet. Not surprisingly, as in many other fields of biological endeavor, contradictory results have been obtained in attempting to relate low vitamin A content in the diet to higher occurrences of some tumors or the effects of an excess of dietary vitamin A on the growth of transplantable tumors (for review, see Burk and Winzler, 1944).

Recently a considerable body of evidence has been published that retinoids can influence the development of some epithelial tumors

(Bollag, 1970a,b, 1972, 1979, 1981; Bollag and Hanck, 1977; Clamon, 1980; Elias and Williams, 1981; Hill and Grubbs, 1982; Israel and Aquilera, 1980; Mayer et al., 1978; Meyskens, 1981; Nettesheim, 1980; Peck, 1981; Schroder and Black, 1980; Sporn, 1976, 1977, 1978a,b, 1980; Sporn and Newton, 1979; Sporn et al., 1976a; Visek et al., 1978; Young and Newberne, 1981). This evidence has been generated from epidemiological studies in man and from effects of retinoids on experimental tumors in animals. Related to this question but not discussed in this article has been the evidence that retinoids can influence organs and transformed cells in culture.

III. Vitamin A Deficiency and Human Cancer

Several epidemiological studies have produced evidence that a lower intake of total vitamin A, the preformed vitamin and/or the provitamin, is associated with a higher risk for development of cancer (Table I). In most studies, however, the dietary data collected focused primarily on foods containing the provitamin carotenes (vegetables, fruits), rather than preformed vitamin A (retinyl esters) as found in liver or vitamin pills. As observed by Peto et al. (1981) much of the available data may indicate a protective effect due to high levels of carotene and this protection seems to be unrelated to the carotenes as a potential source of vitamin A. It is still possible, however, that a low intake of vitamin A, with subsequent low levels of retinol in the body, also alters the risk of developing cancer. For example, a high intake of provitamin A should provide high circulating levels of carotenes that may have a protective effect compared to the same blood level of retinol but lower carotene. A low intake of carotene will very likely be associated with low concentrations of retinol as well as carotene in blood. So, two factors may be operating: some protection provided by high levels of carotenes, some increased risk from low levels of retinol.

A potential bias in this area is the expectation that a low intake of vitamin A will be associated with a higher incidence of cancer. Of particular interest is the Bjelke (1975) study on lung cancer, smoking, and intake of vitamin A. When the lung cancers were grouped according to histology, all six confirmed adenocarcinomas occurred in the higher vitamin A group. Of the other 19 carcinomas (primarily squamous cell, 11, or small cell, 7), only 5 were in the high group. The overall conclusion was increased risk with low intake but certainly when adenocarcinomas alone are considered the reverse appears to be true.

One may bypass the problem of assessing diet by examining the

TABLE I

Epidemiological Studies on the Relationship between Dietary Intake of
Vitamin A and Cancer

Cancer site	Dietary intake-substance determined	Relationship observed	Reference
Bladder	Primarily carotenes	Higher risk with lower intake	Mettlin and Graham (1979)
Cervical displasia	Total vitamin A β-carotene	Higher risk with lower intake (both)	Romney et al. (1981)
Gastrointestinal	Total vitamin A	None	Modan et al. (1981)
Larynx	Primarily carotenes	Higher risk with lower intake (males only)	Graham et al. (1981)
Pulmonary	Primarily carotenes	Higher risk with lower intake	Bjelke (1975); Mettlin, et al. (1979)
Pulmonary	Retinol and carotenes	Higher risk with low carotene intake only	Shekelle et al. (1981)
Various (other than pulmonary)	Retinol and carotenes	None	Shekelle et al. (1981)
Various	Regular use of vitamin A preparations	None	Smith and Jick (1978)

retinol content of blood directly. This has been done in a number of studies (Table II), wherein serum concentration of vitamin A from subjects with cancer were compared to an appropriate control population. There is the problem that differences observed may be due in part to the presence of the cancer rather than reflecting a condition that existed prior to the development of cancer. Cancers might cause lower blood levels of retinol by changing intake, absorption, release from liver stores, or rate of utilization. Even with that caveat, it is of interest that most of the studies indicate that in cancer patients circulating levels of retinol are lower than in control subjects.

Of even more interest are several studies with data on vitamin A levels prior to development or diagnosis of cancer. Again in these studies (Kark et al. 1981, 1982; Wald et al., 1980; Stähelin et al., 1982), low concentrations of serum retinol correlate with a higher risk of developing cancer. In each study the average content did not classify groups as truly vitamin A deficient, as the average was within the normal range. However this lower average value reflects the fact that a significant

TABLE II

VITAMIN A IN THE SERUM OF PATIENTS WITH CANCER

Site of cancer	Serum vitamin A compared to control subjects	References
Bladder	Lower	Basu et al. (1982); Mahmoud and Robinson (1982)
Breast	Lower	Basu et al. (1982)
Female reproductive system	Lower	Kark et al. (1982); Basu et al. (1982)
Gastrointestinal	Lower	Abels et al. (1941); Kark et al. (1981); Staehelin et al. (1982)
Leukemia and Hodgkins disease	Normal	Kark et al. (1982)
Lung bronchial	Lower	Basu et al. (1976); Atukorala et al. (1979); Wald et al. (1980); Kark et al. (1982); Basu et al. (1982)
Lung bronchial	Normal	Cohen et al. (1977); Staehelin et al. (1982)
Myeloma	Lower	Basu et al. (1982)
Oral	Lower	Wahi et al. (1965)
Oral and oro-pharynx	Lower	Ibrahim et al. (1977)
Prostate	Lower	Kark et al. (1982)
Skin and lip	Lower	Kark et al. (1982)

proportion of the group that developed cancer was indeed truly deficient (Ibrahim et al., 1977).

This apparent increase in susceptibility could be due to several reasons, including altered metabolism of carcinogens or altered immunocompetency when vitamin A is low. A state of vitamin A deficiency might simulate that produced by comitogens such as phorbol esters, which increase the efficacy of carcinogens possibly through enhanced DNA synthesis. Many tissues in vitamin A-deficient animals develop not only altered states of differentiation but also increased rates of proliferation (particularly lung, kidney, and bladder in rat, for example), which may make any carcinogen more potent. This effect then would not be specifically related to the function of vitamin A, but simply due to the increased DNA synthesis that occurs in some tissues in its absence. For example, more benzopyrene binds to the DNA of trachea, explanted to organ culture, from vitamin A-deficient hamsters than to trachea from controls (Genta et al., 1974), and this increased binding appeared to be in the areas of rapid proliferation.

IV. VITAMIN A DEFICIENCY AND EXPERIMENTAL CANCER IN ANIMALS

The effect of vitamin A deficiency on susceptibility to carcinogens in experimental animals is perhaps even less clear than the effects on human beings discussed previously. The poor health and rapid decline of animals truly deficient in the vitamin make such studies quite difficult, as the time required for induction of tumors by carcinogens is long compared to the time of decline in general health of the truly deficient animal. However, several studies have suggested that rat bladder (Capurro et al., 1960; Cohen et al., 1976), hamster cheek pouch (Rowe and Gorlin, 1959), and rat salivary gland (Rowe et al., 1970) may be more susceptible to carcinogens in the deficient animal. The remainder of the studies with deficient animals concern the colon, in which the results are quite mixed. Newberne and Rogers (1973) observed that a significant number of rats on a low intake of vitamin A unexpectedly developed colon tumors when given the known liver carcinogen aflatoxin B_1. This was not observed in rats with adequate vitamin A intake. However when the experiments were extended to DMH,[1] a known colon carcinogen, no significant enhancement due to low vitamin A intake was found (Newberne and Suphakarn, 1977). In fact, in the study by Narisawa et al. (1976), there was clear evidence that rats truly deficient in vitamin A developed significantly fewer colon tumors than normally nourished rats when challenged with the colon carcinogen MNNG, introduced intrarectally. The effect of vitamin A status on colon carcinogenesis may be quite different depending on the carcinogen employed. The study by Narisawa et al. (1976) suggests that some tumors may well be vitamin A dependent, in the same way that some tumors are steroid hormone dependent.

[1]Abbreviations: BCPN, (N-butyl-N-(3-carboxypropyl)nitrosamine; BOP, N-nitrosobis(2-oxopropyl)amine; BP, benzo[a]pyrene; DBN, dibutylnitrosamine; DMBA, 7,12-dimethylbenz[a]anthracene; DMH, dimethylhydrazine; ER, ethylretinamide; FANFT, N-[4-(5-nitro-2-furyl)-2-thiazolyl]formamide; 2-HER, 2-hydroxyethylretinamide; 4-HPR, N-(4-hydroxyphenyl)retinamide; MCA, 3-methylcholanthrene; 3-MDAB, 3-methyl-4-dimethylaminoazobenzene; MNNG, N-methyl-N'-nitro-N-nitrosoguanadine; MNU, N-methyl-N-nitrosourea; OH-BBN, N-butyl-N-(4-hydroxybutyl)nitrosamine; 4-PPR, N-4-propionyloxyphenylretinamide; R, all-trans-retinol; RA, all-trans-retinoic acid; 13-RA, 13-cis-retinoic acid; RD, retinylidene dimedone; RME, retinyl methyl ether; RO13-6298, arotinoid; ROAc, retinyl acetate; RPalm, retinyl palmitate; TMMP, all-trans-9-(4-methoxy-2,3,6-trimethylphenyl)-3,7-dimethyl-2,4,6,8-nonatetranoate-RO-10-1670; TMMP-EA, RO-11-1430 ethylamide of TMMP; TMMP-EE, RO-10-9359 ethyl ester of TMMP.

V. Effects of Administration of Retinoids and Carcinogens to Experimental Animals

There are many studies on providing natural or synthetic retinoid in pharmacological amounts to animals exposed to known carcinogens. In a number of these studies treatment with retinoids has reduced the number of tumors induced by these carcinogens. We have summarized these studies in a series of tables.

An early experimental system was the induction of skin papillomas by chemical carcinogens, ultraviolet light, or virus (Table III). This system has shown a remarkable sensitivity to retinoids and several retinoid compounds are effective in inhibiting the appearance or hastening the disappearance of these skin tumors. The retinoids have been effective when provided orally, parenterally, or topically.

Considerable interest in the therapeutic potential of retinoids developed after it was shown that administration of large amounts of retinyl palmitate could markedly reduce lung neoplasia induced by benzopyrene (Saffiotti et al., 1967). Other retinoids have also been effective against experimentally induced lung tumors (Table IV).

Successful reduction of DMBA-induced mammary gland tumors by

TABLE III

PREVENTION OR REGRESSION OF SKIN PAPILLOMAS[a] BY RETINOIDS

Retinoid used	Administration	Species	References
RPalm	ip	Rabbit[b]	McMichael (1965)
R	Oral	Mouse	Davies (1967)
RA	Topical	Rabbit	Prutkin (1968, 1971, 1975)
RPalm, RA	Oral or ip	Mouse	Bollag (1970a)
ROAc,R	Topical	Mouse	Shamberger (1971)
RA	Topical, oral	Mouse	Bollag (1972); Bollag and Ott (1975)
RA, TMMP-EE	Oral, ip	Mouse	Bollag (1974, 1975)
RA, TMMP	Topical	Mouse	Pawson et al. (1977)
TMMP-EE	im	Rabbit[b]	Ito (1981)
RO13-6298[c]	Oral, ip	Mouse	Bollag (1981)
RA	Topical	Mouse[d]	Epstein and Grenkin (1981); Kligman and Kligman (1981)

[a]Induced by DMBA unless otherwise noted.
[b]Shoppe virus induced.
[c]Carotinoid.
[d]UV light induced.

TABLE IV
PREVENTION OF TUMORS OF THE RESPIRATORY TRACT BY RETINOIDS

Carcinogenic agent	Retinoid used	Administration	Reference
BP-Fe$_2$O$_3$	RPalm	Intragastric	Saffiotti et al. (1967)
MCA	ROAc	Oral	Cone and Nettesheim (1973)
MCA	ROAc	Diet	Nettesheim et al. (1976)
MCA	ROAc	Diet	Nettesheim and Williams (1976)
MCA	ROAc	Diet	Nettesheim et al. (1979)

retinyl acetate (Moon et al., 1976) has led to a number of further studies. In some, the retinoids have been specifically "targeted" to the tissue by modifications that make them more lipid soluble (Table V). These new compounds include retinyl methyl ether and 4-hydroxyphenylretinamide.

Bladder tumors, induced by a variety of carcinogens, have proven quite susceptible to prevention by retinoids (Table VI). Analogs of retinoic acid have been studied extensively in these systems.

Tumor induction at other sites, including liver, tongue, forestomach, cervix, pancreas, and salivary gland has proven to be sensitive to inhibition by retinoids (Table VII).

In contrast to the above examples, induction of carcinomas at some sites appears to be unaffected by retinoids or in some cases even en-

TABLE V
PREVENTION OF MAMMARY GLAND TUMORS IN RATS BY RETINOIDS IN THE DIET

Carcinogenic agent	Retinoid used	Reference
DMBA	ROAc	Moon et al. (1976); McCormick et al. (1980); Thompson et al. (1982)
DMBA	RME, ROAc	Grubbs et al. (1977)
MNU	ROAc	Moon et al. (1977); Thompson et al. (1979); Welsch et al. (1980)
MNU	ROAc, 4-HPR	Moon et al. (1979)
BP	ROAc	McCormick et al. (1981)
MNU	ROAc, or ROAc + selenium	Thompson et al. (1981b)
DMBA, MNU	4-HPR + ovarectomy	McCormick et al. (1982)

TABLE VI
PREVENTION OF BLADDER TUMORS BY RETINOIDS IN THE DIET

Carcinogenic agent	Retinoid	Reference
FANFT[a]	RPalm	Cohen *et al.* (1976)
OH-BBN	13-RA	Grubbs *et al.* (1977)
MNU	13-RA	Sporn *et al.* (1977)
MNU	13-RA	Squire *et al.* (1977)
OH-BBN	ROAc	Miyata *et al.* (1978)
OH-BBN	13-RA	Becci *et al.* (1978, 1979, 1981)
FANFT	ROAc	Dawson *et al.* (1979)
BCPN	TMMP	Miyata *et al.* (1980)
OH-BBN	TMMP	Murasaki *et al.* (1980)
FANFT	ER, 2-HER	Croft *et al.* (1981a)
FANFT	13-RA	Croft *et al.* (1981b)
OH-BBN	13-RA, ER, 2-HER	Thompson *et al.* (1981a)

[a]Promoted by vitamin A deficiency.

hanced. A particular site of interest is the colon, because of the high incidence of colon cancer in humans. High levels of retinyl palmitate appear to have no effect on colon carcinomas induced by DMH (Rogers *et al.*, 1973; Rogers and Newberne 1975). Similarly, derivatives of retinoic acid have not been effective against colon cancer induced by several carcinogens (Ward *et al.*, 1978; Wenk *et al.*, 1981; Nigro *et al.*, 1982).

TABLE VII
PREVENTION OF MALIGNANT GROWTH BY RETINOIDS

Site	Inducing agent	Retinoid	Administration	Reference
Forestomach and cervix (hamster)	DMBA or BP	RPalm	Diet	Chu and Malmgren (1965)
Liver	3-MDAB	13-RA	Diet	Daoud and Griffin (1980)
Pancreas	BOP	ER, 13-RA, 2-HER, 4-HPR	Diet	Birt *et al.* (1981)
Pancreas	Azaserine	2-HER, 4-PPR, RD	Diet	Longnecker *et al.* (1982)
Tongue (hamster)	DMBA	13-RA	Oral	Shklar *et al.* (1980)
Skin (rat)	DMBA	RPalm	im	Brown *et al.* (1977)

TABLE VIII

EFFECT OF RETINOIDS ON CHEMICALLY INDUCED MALIGNANT GROWTH

Location of tumor	Carcinogenic agent	Species	Retinoid used	Effect[a]	Mode of administration	Reference
Cheek pouch	DMBA	Hamster	RPalm	E	Topical	Levij and Polliack (1968); Levij et al. (1969); Polliack and Levij (1969); Polliack et al. (1971)
Cheek pouch	DMBA	Hamster	ROAc	E	Topical	McGaughey et al. (1977); McGaughey and Jensen (1980)
Bladder	BBN	Rat	TMMP	No effect	Oral	Schmaehl and Habs (1978)
Colon	DMH	Rat	TMMP	No effect	Oral	Schmaehl and Habs (1978)
Colon	MNU, DMH	Rat	ER, ROAc 2-HER, 4-HPR	No effect	Diet	Silverman et al. (1981)
Colon	MNU	Rat	ER, 2-HER, RD	No effect	Diet	Wenk et al. (1981)
Colon	MNU	Rat	13-RA, TMMP, EA	No effect	Diet	Ward et al. (1978)
Colon, liver, kidney	DMH	Rat	RA	No effect	Oral	Schmaehl et al. (1976)
Respiratory	BP+Fe₂O₃	Hamster	ROAc	E	Intragastric	Smith et al. (1975a)
Skin	BP	Rat	RA, RPalm	No effect	Oral	Schmaehl et al. (1972)
Bladder, liver	DBN	Rat	RPalm	No effect	Oral	Schmaehl et al. (1972)
Mammary gland	DMBA	Rat	RPalm	No effect	Oral	Schmaehl et al. (1972)
Trachea	MNU	Hamster	13-RA, ER	E	Diet	Stinson et al. (1981)
Wing	RSVI[b]	Chicken	RPalm	E	Topical	Polliack and Sasson (1972)
Mammary gland	Spontaneous	Mouse	ROAc	No effect	Diet	Maiorana and Gullino (1980)
Mammary gland	Estrogen, progesterone	Mouse	ROAc	E	Diet	Welsch et al. (1981)

[a] E, Enhancement.
[b] RSV, Rous sarcoma virus.

The variety of approaches employed, coupled with the notable lack of success, suggests that there may be something different about induced tumors in the colon compared to those in the sites already discussed. The observation of Narisawa *et al.* (1976) that animals with adequate intake of vitamin A develop significantly more tumors than animals deprived of vitamin A opened the possibility that the tumors in that study may even require vitamin A. Other examples of retinoids either having no effect or enhancing the efficacy of carcinogens are given in Table VIII.

The effects of retinoids on several transplantable tumors are shown in Table IX. It is of interest that a number of well-established tumor lines are unaffected by retinoids that are effective in other systems.

In summary, it is clear that tumor induction at some organ sites can be affected by administration of pharmacological amounts of retinoids,

TABLE IX

EFFECT OF RETINOIDS ON TRANSPLANTABLE TUMORS

Tumor type	Species	Retinoid used	Effect	Mode	Reference
Adenocarcinoma	Mice	R	Inhibitory	ip	Brandes *et al.* (1966)
Chondrosarcoma	Rat	TMMP-A TMMP-EA TMMP-EE	Inhibitory	Oral, ip	Trown *et al.* (1976)
Crocker sarcoma					
Ehrlich carcinoma (solid)	Mice	TMMP-EE	NE	ip	Bollag (1974)
Ehrlich carcinoma (ascites)					
Leukemia (L1210)	Mice	R	Inhibitory[a]	ip	Cohen (1972); Cohen and Carbone (1972)
Leukemia (L1210)	Mice	TMMP-EE	NE	ip	Bollag (1974)
Leukemia (L1210)	Mice	RA or RPalm	NE	sc	Stewart *et al.* (1979)
Melanoma S91	Mice	RA	Inhibitory	ip	Patek *et al.* (1979)
Lung	Mice	RP	NE	Diet	Smith *et al.* (1972)
Lung (Lewis)	Mice	RPalm	Inhibitory	ip	Pavelic *et al.* (1980)
Morris hepatoma	Rat	RPalm	NE	ip	Cameron *et al.* (1979)

[a]Enhanced antitumor effect of 1,3-bis(2-chloroethyl)-1-nitrosourea.

but this effect is not always to reduce tumor incidence. Also, tumor induction at some sites has so far been resistant to modification by retinoids. There may be no one experimental tumor system which can be used to predict the efficacy of the various retinoids in other tumor systems.

VI. Effects of Administration of Retinoids to Human Cancer Patients

The successes achieved with laboratory animals have provided the impetus to bring retinoids to bear on established human carcinomas. The published results are shown in Table X. There has been only limited success so far. Whether increased success can be obtained by the use of new analogs or by an earlier or even prophylactic treatment is of considerable interest of course. No studies of prophylactic treatment have been reported.

VII. Vitamin A and Differentiation of Normal Tissue

A summary of our current understanding of vitamin A metabolism in the normal animal will be presented in an attempt to assimilate the wealth of evidence on the influences of vitamin A on cancer. Little is known, except in the visual process, about the mechanisms of vitamin A action at the molecular level, but one may say with certainty that the "action" of vitamin A is shown most dramatically in its ability to control and direct differentiation of epithelial tissues. This phenomenon was revealed most clearly from the striking histological studies by Wolbach and Howe (1925) of morphological changes in the rat occurring during vitamin A deficiency and during refeeding with the vitamin (Wolbach and Howe, 1933). Although some species differences in susceptibility to vitamin A deficiency do exist, it is fair to conclude that in all species studied thus far, including humans, vitamin A exerts a profound effect on differentiation. And although the process of induction of malignant growth is still not understood, particularly in humans, it is clear that malignant tumors have altered cellular differentiation when compared with normal tissues. The complexity of the malignant process is emphasized by the variety of tumor types, even within the same tissue of orgin. Thus it is not surprising that vitamin A-like compounds influence these malignant growths not only to a different extent but more importantly in diverse ways.

TABLE X

RESULTS OF TREATMENT WITH RETINOIDS IN MAN

Malignancy	Retinoid used	Administration	Effect	References
Basal cell carcinoma	RA	Topical	Some regression	Bollag and Ott (1971a,b, 1975)
Bladder papillomas (recurrent)	RA	Oral	Some regression	Evard and Bollag (1972)
Bronchial metaplasia	TMMP	Oral	Some regression	Gouveia et al. (1982)
Bronchogenic carcinoma	RPalm	Oral	Some regression	Miksche et al. (1974); Kokron et al. (1982)
	RPalm, 13-RA[a]	Oral	Increased immune response	Miksche et al. (1977)
	13-RA	Oral	Degenerative alterations in abnormal cells in the sputum	Saccomanno et al. (1982)
Cervix (inoperable)	RPalm[a]	Oral	Relapse rates lower but nonsignificantly reduced	Kucera (1980)
Cervix	RA	Topical	Complete regression (33%)	Surwit et al. (1982)
Leukoplakia (oral cavity)	RA	Oral	Regression	Ryssel et al. (1971)
	RA, 13-RA,[b] TMMP, RA	Oral	Some regression	Koch (1978)
		Topical	Some regression	Kurka et al. (1978)
Melanoma	RA	Topical	Some regression	Levine and Meyskens (1980)
Squamous cell carcinomas (head and neck)	RPalm[c]	Oral	Some regression	Thatcher et al. (1980)
Various	13-RA	Oral	Some regression	Meyskens et al. (1982)

[a] In combination with irradiation therapy.
[b] In combination with fluorouracil.
[c] In combination with bleomycin, 5FU, Me.

Even normal tissue "reacts" to vitamin A deficiency in a diversified manner. For example, the tracheal epithelium undergoes a squamous metaplasia resulting in a keratinized epidermoid-like epithelium in deficient animals. In testes no keratinization of epithelia occurs, but the germinal epithelium simply disappears (Wolbach and Howe, 1925). Consequently, although vitamin A is necessary for the proper cellular differentiation of most, if not all, epithelial tissues, the effects of vitamin A are specific in that each tissue reacts to the deficiency in its own way. Such tissue specificity to vitamin A action may be important when effects of vitamin A on various tumors are considered.

The improper differentration and overproliferation of cells observed in vitamin A deficiency begin at foci rather than throughout the tissue. This suggests that some condition or stimulus in addition to lack of vitamin A is involved in this process. However, the stem cells are not irreversibly altered in this process, as all affected tissues retain the ability to regenerate their normal epithelium (Wolbach and Howe, 1933; Wong and Buck, 1971).

We must assume that the cell nucleus is influenced by vitamin A as it is the cell particle whose products are ultimately responsible for the state of differentiation. We should expect that the metabolism of the nucleus as reflected by these products, that is, the expression of the genome, should then be affected by the vitamin A status of the cell. Here again we can draw a parallel with cancer as the nucleus and its genomic expression is clearly altered in all cancers (Koller, 1963).

VIII. FATE OF VITAMIN A-ACTIVE COMPOUNDS *in Vivo*

In the vitamin A or retinoid family, the natural compounds of particular interest are retinol and retinoic acid. Retinol in the diet allows the animal to maintain all physiological functions requiring vitamin A, such as vision, reproduction, growth, and differentiation. Retinoic acid (vitamin A acid), a natural metabolite of retinol (Ito *et al.*, 1974), when provided to a retinol-deprived animal, maintains the growth and proper differentiation of most tissues, but not vision (Dowling and Wald, 1960) or reproductive capacity in either the male or female (Thompson *et al.*, 1964). Evidence for a physiological role for retinoic acid has only been circumstantial (Appling and Chytil, 1981).

Several hundred synthetic retinoids have been prepared with the goal of obtaining more efficient and/or less toxic compounds to be used pharmacologically. To our knowledge none of these synthetic retinoids displays antivitamin activity. The various modifications of the molecule produce different pharmacokinetics as well as different toxicities, activities, and tissue distribution when compared to the natural compounds (Moon et al., 1979: Wang et al., 1980; Sporn et al., 1976b). It should be stressed that although modification of the polar end group (e.g., by esterification or amidation) results in different pharmacokinetic and higher activity in some testing systems, there is no evidence that these derivatives work as such. It appears that the action of retinoids on the cellular and molecular level involves compounds with the free alcoholic or carboxylic group.

The form of the vitamin that with appropriate metabolic transformation, satisfies all needs of the animal is all-trans-retinol. The vitamin is obtained in the diet primarily as either a pro-vitamin, a carotene such as β-carotene, or as long-chain fatty acyl esters of retinol. Carotene is absorbed directly into the intestinal mucosal cell where a specific enzyme oxidatively cleaves it into two molecules of retinal (Thompson et al., 1950; Olson, 1961; Goodman and Huang, 1965; Olson and Hayaishi, 1965). The retinal is then reduced to retinol (Fidge and Goodman, 1967).

Esters of retinol are not absorbed well and first must be cleaved to free retinol either by pancreatic esterases or a brush border esterase (Mahadevan et al., 1961, 1963) for absorption. Once within the intestinal cell the retinol, whether from hydrolyzed retinyl esters or from carotene cleavage and reduction, is esterified with long-chain fatty acids, primarily palmitate (Huang and Goodman, 1965), and is then incorporated into chylomicrons, which are released to the lymph.

These chylomicrons or their remnants containing the retinol esters are taken up by the liver, the storage organ for vitamin A. It appears there may be an obligatory hydrolysis to retinol involved (Goodman et al., 1965). Retinol is stored in the ester form, however, and is esterified primarily with saturated long-chain fatty acids (Futterman and Andrews, 1964).

The release of retinol from the liver and its transport to target tissues have been worked out in the last 15 years, primarily by work from D. S. Goodman's and P. A. Peterson's laboratories (for recent reviews, see Smith and Goodman, 1979; Rask et al., 1980.) Briefly, retinyl esters are hydrolyzed and the retinol combines with a specific protein, called retinol-binding protein or RBP. This protein (MW about 20,000) is synthesized in the liver and is not released to the blood until it combines with retinol. Consequently, it will accumulate in the liver if the animal is vitamin A deficient as retinol status does not appear to regulate the synthesis of the protein (Soprano *et al.*, 1982). Once in the blood the retinol–RBP complex binds with prealbumin to form a circulating ternary complex. Normally nourished animals appear to maintain a relatively constant level of retinol, equivalent to about 30–60 µg/dl. The mechanism by which this level is maintained is not known.

Target cells appear to have specific plasma membrane receptors for this circulating complex (Heller, 1975; Bok and Heller, 1976; Rask and Peterson, 1976; McGuire *et al.*, 1981). Only the retinol, not RBP, enters the cell. The RBP does not appear to be recycled after delivering the retinol, but is degraded in the kidney (Glover, 1973). RBP is not only necessary for efficient uptake of retinol (e.g., Maraini and Gozzoli, 1975), but may also prevent deleterious effects that can arise from the detergent-like properties of the ligand (e.g., Dingle *et al.*, 1972). This elaborate transport system apparently delivers only all-*trans*-retinol to the plasma membrane. Although RBP is able to bind retinal or retinoic acid *in vitro* (Glover *et al.*, 1974), only retinol is bound to serum RBP *in vivo*. In contrast, administered [^{14}C]retinoic acid is found bound to serum albumin (Smith *et al.*, 1973) and appears to have no specific transport system. There is also no storage capability for the compound. Administered retinoic acid is metabolized rapidly and excreted (Dunagin *et al.*, 1964; Roberts and DeLuca, 1967). In normal animal tissue the concentration of retinoic acid is very low, and it is doubtful that it is obtained in the diet in significant quantities. These observations suggest to us that cells which utilize retinoic acid most likely obtain it by synthesis from the retinol delivered to the cells. However, there is no direct evidence to support this hypothesis.

The growth-promoting activity of retinoic acid has been studied over the years. Due to the rapid metabolism and excretion of retinoic acid it has sometimes appeared to have a considerably lower biological activity than retinol. Zile and DeLuca (1968) found however, that when retinoic acid was given orally in small multiple doses (0.5 µg at 6-hour intervals) to deficient rats, a growth effect was seen that was equivalent to that obtained with a single dose of 2 µg of retinol. Consequently, when a retinoid related to retinoic acid is administered it may be more effective if it is given repeatedly in small doses. These and other observations have shown very clearly that the disposition of administered retinoic acid in the whole animal is quite different from that of administered retinol. This fact has perhaps received too little attention when retinoic acid derivatives have been used as cancer preventing agents.

IX. Cellular Retinoid Binding Proteins

In recent years considerable effort has been directed to the detection, isolation, and characterization of intracellular proteins that specifically bind compounds with vitamin A activity. This area of research was initiated by the discovery of a widely distributed, cellular, and specific retinol-binding protein, detected in the soluble extracts of all vitamin A-sensitive organs examined (Bashor *et al.*, 1973). Subsequently, a different protein, that specifically binds retinoic acid, was also discovered in extracts of diverse animal tissues (Ong and Chytil, 1975a; Sani and Hill, 1976). The two proteins are quite distinct. The cellular retinol-binding protein, CRBP, binds retinol with high specificity and affinity, but does not bind retinal or retinoic acid. The cellular retinoic acid-binding protein, CRABP, has high affinity for retinoic acid but does not bind retinol or retinal. These proteins also differ from RBP by a number of criteria including amino acid sequence. CRBP and CRABP are present in most fetal tissues, but tissue levels vary during perinatal development, indicating that they are not regulated in a synchronous manner and suggesting that they are not interchangeable in function (Ong and Chytil, 1976a).

There is a body of evidence from our work, as well as that of many others, that these proteins play an important role in vitamin A action. For example, CRBP carries all-*trans*-retinol, the natural form of the vitamin, *in vivo* (Ong and Chytil, 1974, 1975a; Ross *et al.*, 1978; Saari *et al.*, 1982) and is depleted of this natural form during vitamin A deficiency (Ong *et al.*, 1976). In the normal animal the protein is 40–100% saturated with retinol. The binding specificity of CRBP for isomers of retinol reflects the activity of these isomers either when tested for growth promotion in the whole animal or in tissue culture (Ong and Chytil, 1975b). This would suggest that CRBP has an important role in the action of retinol *in vivo*. It was also clearly shown that C-15 of the retinol must be present as the free alcohol; retinyl acetate or retinyl palmitate do not bind. The implication is that if CRBP is responsible for retinol action, then the esters, which are dietary and storage forms of retinol, must be hydrolyzed in order to exert their action.

Finally, with retinol bound to CRBP, specific binding of retinol to nuclei can be observed and the amount of the binding is greater in nuclei from vitamin A-deficient animals than from chow-fed (control) animals. Two hours after refeeding vitamin A to deficient animals nuclei from the refed animals show a decrease in binding sites to levels observed with control animals (Takase *et al.,* 1979). Interestingly, CRBP does not remain with the nucleus but is the vehicle necessary for the delivery of retinol to these specific binding sites. These binding sites are present on the chromatin and, we suggest, may be important in regulation of genomic expression (Liau *et al.,* 1981).

Similar observations have also been made for CRABP. For example, the endogenous ligand of CRABP appears to be retinoic acid (Saari *et al.,* 1982). The binding specificity of CRABP for a number of analogs of retinoic acid correlates well with the activity of the analogs as evaluated by others in either of two systems: ability to maintain mouse-skin epidermal cell cultures or ability to reverse the metaplasia of tracheas explanted to organ culture from vitamin A-deficient hamsters (Chytil and Ong, 1976). The availability of the free carboxyl group in the C-15 position appears to be a necessary condition for CRABP to bind a retinoic acid derivative (Sani and Hill, 1976; Lotan *et al.,* 1980; Trown *et al.,* 1980). The very existence of a specific binding protein carrying endogenous retinoic acid implies that retinoic acid, in addition to retinol, has a physiological function.

Interaction of CRABP with retinoic acid has been suggested as a preliminary screening step to identify derivatives with potential activity (Chytil and Ong, 1976). Subsequent similar correlations of binding with activity have been described for other experimental systems (Jetten and Jetten, 1979; Trown *et al.,* 1980; Bollag and Matter, 1981).

Several studies have been directed to the potential nuclear interaction of CRABP. Wiggert *et al.* (1976) have reported that cultured retinoblastoma cells contain CRBP and CRABP in the cytosol, but that extracts of their nuclei did not. Preincubation of cells with [^{3}H]retinoic acid provided evidence for translocation of CRABP to the nucleus. The appearance of CRABP in the nucleus has also been observed for an embryonal carcinoma cell line (Jetten and Jetten, 1979) and chick embryo skin (Sani and Donovan, 1979). The fact that CRABP apparently remains in the nucleus with its ligand, while CRBP transfers retinol and then leaves, suggests a fundamental difference in mechanisms by which the proteins exert their effects.

The indication of a nuclear function for retinoids (Fuchs and Green, 1981; Omori and Chytil, 1982), perhaps mediated by these specific binding proteins, suggests a means by which vitamin A can direct differentiation of tissues. The potential exists to activate or supress expression of any gene, making these proteins of interest in the interactions of vitamin A with neoplastic tissue, and with the cell nucleus in particular.

X. Effects of Retinoids on Differentiation and Proliferation of Tumor Tissue

A particularly intriguing possibility is that part of the inhibition of tumor growth by retinoids may be mediated through restoration of control over the rate of proliferation or direction of differentiation, a control that is altered or lost in the carcinogenic process. This might be a physiological effect, even though pharmacological amounts of the retinoid may be needed to bring about that effect.

This process might be similar to the repair of lesions caused by vitamin A deficiency in normal tissue. Morphological studies on the process of tumor regression have been few, but there are several studies on retinoid-induced (DMBA) regression of mouse papillomas. There is some suggestion that this regression is similar to the repair process in the deficient animal as described by Wolbach and Howe (1933). In both cases the "improper" cells showed vacuolization and loss of cytoplasm (Matter and Bollag, 1977). The papillomas developed necrotic cells (Frigg and Torhorst, 1977; Matter and Bollag, 1977), while in repair of normal epithelium the abnormal cells disappear rapidly by a lytic process. In both cases, the repair proceeds with little change in DNA synthesis as determined by a labeling index for the papillomas (Frigg and Torhorst, 1977).

Increased proliferation of cells is accompanied by increases in ornithine decarboxylase activity. Also, the topical administration of phorbol ester (12-O-tetradecanoylphorbol 13-acetate or TPA) induces the activity of ornithine decarboxylase (ODC). This action of TPA is believed to be essential for tumor promotion. It is of interest that a number of natural retinoids topically applied were found to inhibit this increase in activity of ODC (Verma and Boutwell, 1977). The degree of inhibition depends on the dose and time of application of the retinoids. The inhibition appears to be specific to ODC as retinoids did not affect the induction of S-adenonsylmethionine decarboxylase, the other enzyme in polyamine synthesis induced by phorbol esters. There is a difference in potency of natural retinoids which follows the order: retinoic acid > retinal > retinol > retinyl acetate > retinyl palmitate (Verma and Boutwell, 1977). It is of interest that the relative potency is related to the probable sequence in which retinoids are metabolized to retinoic acid. Synthetic retinoids tested in this system show striking differences in potency (Verma et al., 1978, 1980; Weeks et al., 1979; Astrup and Paulsen, 1982), indicating that the system responsible for inhibiting ODC in epidermis by retinoids is dependent on other structural features of the retinoids. Since the role of this enzyme in cellular proliferation is not known, the significance of these findings is not clear.

XI. ROLE OF THE INTRACELLULAR BINDING PROTEINS IN RETINOID ACTION IN TUMOR TISSUE

The possibility that retinoid effects on tumors are similar to vitamin A action in normal tissue has directed our attention to the intracellular binding proteins for retinoids previously discussed. There is some indication that the binding protein for retinoic acid, CRABP, may be important in the action of retinoic acid analogs on tumor tissue. In particular, there is evidence that the binding specificity of this protein for analogs agrees strikingly well with the potency of these analogs in several tumor test systems. To our knowledge all retinoids effective in these studies either as administered or as an easily postulated metabolite bind well to CRABP.

CRABP derived from mouse papilloma showed affinities for retinoid analogs that fit the potency of those analogs in causing regression of the papillomas (Chytil and Ong, 1976). Similar results have been obtained with a more extensive group of analogs using both the mouse papilloma test system and a transplantable chondrosarcoma to assess activity (Trown et al., 1980). Several tissue culture systems that can be induced to differentiate by retinoids also show a remarkable similarity between retinoid activity and the affinity of CRABP from the same cells for retinoid (Jetten and Jetten, 1979; Lotan, 1980).

A number of studies have analyzed for intracellular binding proteins for retinoids in tumor tissue. The presence of CRABP in tumors was first reported for carcinomas from human lung and breast (Ong et al., 1975). A particularly interesting point was that this binding protein was not detectable in the histologically normal tissue adjacent to the tumor, suggesting either a dramatic increase in the numbers of a cell type which normally contains this protein or an altered expression of the genome. This early communication did not comment on the presence/absence of CRBP in these tumors. This may have caused more attention to be directed to CRABP than CRBP, but subsequently, we have found that both proteins can show dramatic changes in concentration in malignant tumors of animals (Ong and Chytil, 1976b) or man (Ong et al., 1982; Chytil and Ong, 1979, 1982). A better understanding of the role of binding proteins in the effect of retinoids on tumor tissue will require that both proteins be analyzed. Efforts in several laboratories have been directed to the detection and quantitation of CRABP, and occasionally CRBP, in human carcinomas (Table XI). Higher concentrations than normal may be found for one or both binding proteins in tumor tissue. However, the effect of malignancy on the existence or quantity of these binding proteins is quite variable even with tumors arising from similar organs. At this point it seems safe to say that each tumor should be evaluated individually for binding protein content. Also we should not assume that high concentrations of either binding protein necessarily indicate that the tumor tissue requires or is utilizing more retinol or retinoic acid than normal tissue. Proteins may be expressed in higher amounts in tumors without necessarily influencing metabolism of the tumor (Abelev, 1971; Schapira, 1973).

These binding proteins have also been determined in animal tumors, both transplantable and carcinogen induced (Table XII). CRBP was frequently not determined. In several examples of carcinogen-induced tumor, it was observed, as for some "spontaneous" human tumors, that amounts of binding protein in the tumor were considerably higher than in adjacent grossly normal tissue. These examples include CRABP in mouse papilloma (Chytil and Ong, 1976) and CRBP in colon adenocarcinoma (Ong et al., 1978). CRABP from tumors including mouse papillomas, human breast carcinomas (Chytil and Ong, 1976), and rat mammary tumors (Trown et al., 1980) has been evaluated for binding specificity and found to be quite similar, if not identical, to CRABP from normal tissue and there is little species difference in binding specifity.

If indeed these proteins are involved in mediating the effects of these compounds on tumors, the evaluation of analogs by interaction with CRBP or CRABP may be a useful preliminary step to identify those with potential growth or antitumor activity. Further, knowledge of structural requirements for binding would then provide help in the design of new compounds of interest.

We have proposed that the presence of the binding proteins may be necessary, although not sufficient for tumor sensitivity to retinoid therapy (Ong and Chytil, 1976b). If this proves to be true, then screening tumors for the presence of the binding protein will be a useful step to select those that would be candidates for retinoid therapy.

The occasional potentiation of carcinogen action by pharmacological amounts of retinoids led us to determine whether the binding proteins might be important in this effect. The several studies on colorectal carcinomas induced in rats by carcinogens suggested that these tumors might be of interest. As mentioned before, not only has there been little or no success in preventing this induction, it appears that a

TABLE XI

Cellular Retinol-(CRBP) and Retinoic Acid-Binding (CRABP) Proteins in Human Carcinomas

Tumor site	CRBP	Reference	CRABP	Reference
Breast	+	Chytil and Ong (1982)	+	Ong et al. (1975); Huber et al. (1978); Chytil and Ong (1978); Palan and Romney (1979, 1980); Kueng et al. (1980); Mehta et al. (1982a)
Colon	+	Palan et al. (1980)	+	Sani et al. (1980a,b); Palan et al. (1980)
Endometrium	+	Palan and Romney (1980)	+	Palan and Romney (1980)
Kidney	+	Chytil and Ong (1978)	+	Chytil and Ong (1978)
Liver	+	Muto et al. (1979)	+	Muto et al. (1979)
Lung	NT[a]		+	Ong et al. (1975); Clamon et al. (1981); Palan and Romney (1980)
Oral cavity	+	Ong et al. (1982)	+	Ong et al. (1982); Bichler and Daxenbichler (1982)
Ovary	+	Palan and Romney (1980)	+	Palan and Romney (1980)
Uterus (cervix)	+	Palan and Romney (1980)	+	Palan and Romney (1980)

[a]NT, not tested.

TABLE XII

Cellular Retinol-Binding (CRBP) and Retinoic Acid-Binding Protein (CRABP) in Experimental Tumors

Tumor	Host	Type	CRBP	Reference	CRABP	Reference
Carcinosarcoma	Rat	Walker 256	+	Ong and Chytil (1976b)	+[a]	Ong and Chytil (1976b)
Chondrosarcoma	Rat		ND[b]	Ong and Chytil (1976b)	+	Ong and Chytil (1976b)
Colon	Mice	26 and 57 metastatic	NT[c]		+	Sani and Corbett (1977); Sani and Titus (1977)
	Mice	36 and 58 (nonmetastatic)	NT		ND	Sani and Corbett (1977); Sani and Titus (1977)
	Rat	DMH induced	+	Ong et al. (1978)	+	Ong et al. (1978)
Ehrlich carcinoma	Mice	Ascites	ND	Bashor and Chytil (1975)	ND	Ong (unpublished)
		Solid carcinoma	ND	Ong and Chytil (1976b)	ND	Ong and Chytil (1976b)
Hepatoma	Rat	AS-300 ascites	ND	Bashor and Chytil (1975)	NT	
		Novikoff	ND	Bashor and Chytil (1975)	NT	
Leukemia	Mice	L1210	ND	Ong and Chytil (1976b)	ND	Ong and Chytil (1976b)
	Rat	Dunning	+	Ong and Chytil (1976b)	+	Ong and Chytil (1976b)
Lung	Mice	Lewis	NT		+	Sani and Corbett (1977); Sani and Titus (1977)
Melanoma	Mice	B16	NT		+	Sani and Corbett (1977); Sani and Titus (1977)

Tumor	Species	Cell line				Reference
Mammary metastatic	Mice	C3H 13/C/24, C3H 04/A/64, C3H 16/C/13	NT		+	Sani and Corbett (1977); Sani and Titus (1977)
Mammary	Rat		+	Ong and Chytil (1976b)	+	Ong and Chytil (1976b)
		MAC-1 adenocarcinoma CMBA induced	NT		+	Mehta et al. (1980, 1982b); Moon and Mehta (1981)
Prostatic carcinoma	Mice	Transplantable R-3327H	NT		+	
		R-3327HI	NT		+	
		R-3327-AT	NT		+	Gesell et al. (1982)
		R-3327-Lylw	NT		+	
		MNU induced	NT		+	Mehta et al. (1980)
Sarcoma	Mice	180	ND	Ong and Chytil (1976b)	ND	Ong and Chytil (1976b)
Skin papilloma	Rat	Ridgeway osteogenic	NT		+	Sani and Titus (1977)
	Mice	DMBA induced	+	Ong and Chytil (1976b)	+	Sani and Corbett (1977)
	Rabbit	Shope	NT		+	Ong and Chytil (1976b)
Urinary bladder	Mice	AC1/N	+	Kawamura and Hashimoto (1980)	NT	Rattanapanone et al. (1981)

[a]Not detectable in another sample.
[b]ND, not detectable.
[c]NT, not tested.

normally nourished animal develops significantly more tumors than a deficient animal, suggesting these tumors may require vitamin A. Examination of the colorectal adenocarcinomas induced by DMH showed that they contained significantly higher amounts of CRBP than the adjacent, grossly normal tissue (Ong *et al.*, 1978). This increase in CRBP occurred only upon tumor appearance and not with the general hyperplasia of the intestinal crypts associated with carcinogen administration. In normal tissue CRBP carries endogenous retinol and the protein becomes depleted of retinol with institution of vitamin A deficiency (Ong *et al.*, 1976). This implies that the active form is the retinol–CRBP complex and not CRBP alone. In colon tumors CRBP was found to be virtually saturated with retinol and presumably capable of function. This was consistent with the idea that these tumors may require retinol for growth. Recently we examined a transplantable colon adenocarcinoma which contained CRBP and found the protein to be charged with retinol. In preliminary experiments this tumor did not grow in rats deficient in vitamin A but instead became necrotic. This suggests that this transplantable tumor also requires vitamin A. This possibility of vitamin A-requiring tumors is obviously of importance should retinoids be considered for therapy (Schroder and Black, 1980).

In summary, it is clear that the mere presence or amount of these binding proteins may not explain the effects of retinoids on cancers. We must consider all aspects of vitamin A metabolism.

XII. Possible Alterations of Vitamin A Metabolism Related to Malignancy

We would suggest that a number of alterations might occur in vitamin A metabolism due to malignancy or might occur and contribute to the development of malignancy.

Among these alterations are

1. Deficiency of the vitamin, due either to diet or inadequacy in absorption, may cause an altered susceptibility to carcinogenic agents or an altered proliferation rate for established neoplasms. This might be due to altered metabolism of carcinogens or an altered immune response, neither of which has been discussed here.

2. Cancer itself may affect the overall vitamin A status, by reducing intake (diet), absorption, storage, or transport, with a potential effect on the further development of that cancer.

3. The amount of vitamin A or the form or effectiveness of vitamin A may be altered in neoplastic tissue, irrespective of concentrations in blood of retinol, due to (A) the plasma membrane or, more specifically, the plasma membrane receptor responsible for the transit of retinol being altered, leading to a low or nonexistent content of retinol in neoplastic tissue; or (B) an alteration in the postulated oxidation of retinol to retinoic acid in cancer tissue.

4. The content of either of the two retinoid-binding proteins might be altered in cancer tissue, leading to a changed ability to respond to vitamin A.

5. The properties of these proteins in cancer tissue may be altered (e.g., reduced binding affinity, reduced ability to interact with the nucleus), leading to a changed ability to respond to vitamin A.

6. The properties of the nucleus of a cancer cell may be altered, so that its interaction with the retinoids and their binding proteins is changed.

The possible changes within neoplastic tissue detailed here have the potential to affect genes, leading to an expression different from that in normal tissue. In addition, one may envision that the administration of pharmacological amounts of retinoids could reverse the effect of the lesion. For example, administration of pharmacological amounts of retinol would lead to high blood concentrations of retinol not bound to RBP. This retinol could then penetrate cells nonspecifically. If neoplastic tissue were defective in the physiological uptake mechanism for retinol, nonspecific entry could restore cellular concentrations with consequent effects on cellular metabolism. Another possibility is that if the postulated oxidation of retinol to retinoic acid were blocked it might be overcome by administering large amounts of retinoic acid. Other possibilities can be imagined.

It is entirely conceivable that more than one of the above phenomena could occur at the same time. Consequently, we would suggest that a universal mechanism for the effect of vitamin A on cancer tissue may not exist and, even more discouraging, each example of neoplastic tissue may have to be evaluated individually. Considerably more work on the mechanism of vitamin A action will be necessary before the picture can be clarified.

ACKNOWLEDGMENTS

Supported by grants from the U.S. Public Health Service HD 09195, HL 1531, and CA 20850. The authors thank D. Wadkins for her help with the manuscript.

REFERENCES

Abelev, G. I. (1971). Alpha-fetoprotein in ontogenesis and its association with malignant tumors. *Adv. Cancer Res.* **14,** 295–358.

Abels, J. C., Gorham, A. T., Pack, G. T., and Rhoads, C. P. (1941). Metabolic studies in patients with cancer of the gastrointestinal tract. I. Plasma vitamin A levels in patients with malignant neoplastic disease, particularly of the gastro-intestinal tract. *J. Clin. Invest.* **20,** 749–764.

Appling, D. R., and Chytil, F. (1981). Evidence of a role for retinoic acid (vitamin-A acid) in the maintenance of testosterone production in male rats. *Endocrinology* **108,** 2120–2123.

Astrup, E. G., and Paulsen, J. E. (1982). Effect of retinoic acid pretreatment on 12-O-tetradecanoylphorbol-13-acetate-induced cell population kinetics and polyamine biosynthesis in hairless mouse epidermis. *Carcinogenesis* **3,** 313–320.

Atukorala, S., Basu, T. K., Dickerson, J. W. T., Donaldson, D., and Sakula, A. (1979). Vitamin A, zinc and lung cancer. *Br. J. Cancer* **40,** 927–931.

Bashor, M. M., and Chytil, F. (1975). Cellular retinol-binding protein. *Biochim. Biophys. Acta* **411,** 87–96.

Bashor, M. M., Toft, D. E., and Chytil, F. (1973). In vitro binding of retinol to rat-tissue components. *Proc. Natl. Acad. Sci. U.S.A.* **70,** 3483–3487.

Basu, T. K., Donaldson, D., Jenner, M., Williams, D. C., and Sakula, A. (1976). Plasma vitamin A in patients with bronchial carcinoma. *Br. J. Cancer* **33,** 119–121.

Basu, T. K., Rowlands, L., Jones, L., and Kohn, J. (1982). Vitamin A and retinol-binding protein in patients with myelomatosis and cancer of epithelial origin. *Eur. J. Cancer Clin. Oncol.* **18,** 339–342.

Becci, P. J., Thompson, H. J., Grubbs, C. J., Squire, R. A., Brown, C. C., Sporn, M. B., and Moon, R. C. (1978). Inhibitory effect of 13-cis-retinoic acid on urinary bladder carcinogenesis induced in C57BL/6 mice by N-butyl-N-(4-hydroxybutyl)-nitrosamine. *Cancer Res.* **38,** 4463–4466.

Becci, P. J., Thompson, H. J., Grubbs, C. J., Brown, C. C., and Moon, R. C. (1979). Effect of delay in administration of 13-cis-retinoic acid on the inhibition of urinary bladder carcinogenesis in the rat. *Cancer Res.* **39,** 3141–3144.

Becci, P. J., Thompson, H. J., Strum, J. M., Brown, C. C., Sporn, M. B., and Moon, R. C. (1981). N-Butyl-N-(4-hydroxybutyl)nitrosamine-induced urinary bladder cancer in C57BL/6X DBA/2 F_1 mice a useful model for study of chemoprevention of cancer with retinoids. *Cancer Res.* **41,** 927–932.

Bichler, E., and Daxenbichler, G. (1982). Retinoic acid binding protein in human squamous cell carcinomas of the ORL region. *Cancer* **49,** 619–622.

Birt, D. F., Sayed, S., Davies, M. H., and Pour, P. (1981). Sex differences in the effects of retinoids on carcinogenesis by N-nitrosobis (2-oxopropyl)amine in Syrian hamster. *Cancer Lett.* **14,** 13–21.

Bjelke, E. (1975). Dietary vitamin A and human lung cancer. *Int. J. Cancer* **15,** 561–565.

Bok, D., and Heller, J. (1976). Transport of retinol from blood to the retina: An autoradiographic study of the pigment epithelial cell surface for plasma retinol-binding protein. *Exp. Eye Res.* **22,** 395–402.

Bollag, W. (1970a). Therapy of chemically induced skin tumors of mice with vitamin A palmitate and vitamin A acid. *Experientia* **27,** 90–92.

Bollag, W. (1970b). Vitamin A and vitamin A acid in the prophylaxis and therapy of epithelial tumors. *Int. J. Vitam. Nutr. Res.* **40,** 299–314.

Bollag, W. (1972). Prophylaxis of chemically induced benign and malignant epithelial tumors by vitamin A acid (retinoic acid). *Eur. J. Cancer* **8,** 689–693.

Bollag, W. (1974). Therapeutic effects of an aromatic retinoic acid analog on chemically induced skin papillomas and carcinomas of mice. *Eur. J. Cancer* **10**, 731–737.

Bollag, W. (1975). Prophylaxis of chemically induced epithelial tumors with an aromatic retinoid acid analog (Ro 10-9359). *Eur. J. Cancer* **11**, 721–724.

Bollag, W. (1979). Retinoids and cancer. *Cancer Chemother. Pharmacol.* **3**, 207–215.

Bollag, W. (1981). Arotinoids. A new class of retinoids with activities in oncology and dermatology. *Cancer Chemother. Pharmacol.* **7**, 27–29.

Bollag, W., and Hanck, A. (1977). From vitamin A to retinoids. Modern trends in the field of oncology and dermatology. *Acta Vitaminol. Enzymol.* **31**, 113–123.

Bollag, W., and Matter, A. (1981). From vitamin A to retinoids in experimental and clinical oncology: Achievements, failures, and outlook. *Ann. N.Y. Acad. Sci.* **359**, 9–23.

Bollag, W., and Ott, F. (1971a) Therapy of actinic keratoses and basal cell carcinomas with local application of vitamin A acid (NSC-122758). *Cancer Chemother. Rep.* **55**, 59–60.

Bollag, W., and Ott, F. (1971b). Vitamin A Saure in der Tumortherapie. *Schweiz. Med. Wochenschr.* **101**, 17–18.

Bollag, W., and Ott, F. (1975). Vitamin A acid in benign and malignant epithelial tumors of the skin. *Acta Derm. Venereol. Suppl.* **74**, 163–166.

Brandes, D., Anton, E. Schofield, B., and Barnard, S. (1966). Role of lysosomal labilizers in treatment of mammary gland carcinomas with cyclophosphamide (NSC-26271): Preliminary report. *Cancer Chemother. Rep.* **50**, 47–53.

Brown, I. V., Lane, B. P., and Pearson, J. (1977). Effects of depot injections of retinyl palmitate on 7,12-dimethylbenz(a)anthracene-induced preneoplastic changes in rat skin. *J. Natl. Cancer Inst.* **58**, 1347–1355.

Burk, D., and Winzler, R. J. (1944). Vitamins and cancer. *Vitam. Horm.* **2**, 305–352.

Cameron, I., Grubbs, B., and Rogers, W. (1979). High-dose methylprednisolone, vitamin A, and vitamin C in rats bearing the rapidly growing Morris 7777 hepatoma. *Cancer Treat. Rep.* **63**, 477–483.

Capurro, P., Angrist, A., Black, J., and Moumgis, B. (1960). Studies in squamous metaplasia in rat bladder. I. Effect of hypovitaminosis A, foreign bodies, and methylcholanthrene. *Cancer Res.* **20**, 563–567.

Caspari, W., and Ottensooser, F. (1929). Ueber den Einfluss der Kost auf das Wachstum von Impfgeschwuelsten. Bedeutung der Vitamin A and B. *Z. Krebsforsch.* **30**, 1–23.

Chu, E. W., and Malmgren, R. A. (1965). An inhibitory effect of vitamin A on the induction of tumors of forestomach and cervix in the Syrian hamster by carcinogenic polycyclic hydrocarbons. *Cancer Res.* **25**, 884–895.

Chytil, F., and Ong, D. E. (1976). Mediation of retinoic acid induced growth and antitumor activity. *Nature (London)* **260**, 49–51.

Chytil, F., and Ong, D. E. (1978). Cellular vitamin A binding proteins. *Vitam. Horm.* **36**, 1–32.

Chytil, F., and Ong, D. E. (1979). Cellular retinol and retinoic acid-binding proteins in vitamin A action. *Fed. Proc. Fed. Am. Soc. Exp. Biol.* **38**, 2510–2513.

Chytil, F., and Ong, D. E. (1982). Retinoid binding proteins and human cancer. *In* "Molecular Interrelations of Nutrition and Cancer" (M. S. Arnott, J. van Eys, and Y. M. Wang, eds.), pp. 409–417. Raven, New York.

Clamon, G. H. (1980). Retinoids for the prevention of epithelial cancers: Current status and future potential. *Med. Pediatr. Oncol.* **8**, 177–185.

Clamon, G. H., Nugent, K. M., and Rossi, N. P. (1981). Cellular retinoic acid-binding protein in human lung carcinomas. *J. Natl. Cancer Inst.* **67**, 61–63.

Cohen, M. H. (1972). Enhancement of the antitumor effects of 1,3-bis (2-chloroethyl)-1-nitrosourea by vitamin A and caffeine. *J. Natl. Cancer Inst.* **48**, 927–932.

Cohen, M. H., and Carbone, P. P. (1972). Enhancement of the antitumor effects of 1,3-bis(2-chloroethyl)-1-nitrosourea and cyclophosphamide by vitamin A. *J. Natl. Cancer Inst.* **48**, 921–926.

Cohen, M. H., Primack, A., Broder, L. E., and Williams, L. R. (1977). Vitamin A serum levels and dietary vitamin A intake in lung cancer patients. *Cancer Lett.* **4**, 51–54.

Cohen, S. M., Wittenberg, J. F., and Bryan, G. T. (1976). Effect of avitaminosis A and hypervitaminosis A on urinary bladder carcinogenicity of N-[4-(5-nitro-2-furyl)-2-thiazolyl] formamide. *Cancer Res.* **36**, 2334–2339.

Cone, M. V., and Nettesheim, P. (1973). Effects of vitamin A on 3-methyl-cholanthrene-induced squamous metaplasias and early tumors in the respiratory tract of rats. *J. Natl. Cancer Inst.* **50**, 1599–1606.

Croft, W. A., Croft, M. A., Paulus, K. P., Williams, J. H., Wang, C. Y., and Lower, G. M., Jr. (1981a). Synthetic retinamides: Effect on urinary bladder carcinogenesis by FANFT in Fisher rats. *Carcinogenesis* **2**, 515–517.

Croft, W. A., Croft, M. A., Paulus, K. P., Williams, J. H., Wang, C. Y., and Lower, G. M., Jr. (1981b). 13-cis-Retinoic acid: Effect on urinary bladder carcinogenesis by N-[4-(5-nitro-2-furyl)-2-thiazolyl]-formamide in Fisher rats. *Cancer Lett.* **12**, 355–360.

Daoud, A. H., and Griffin, A. C. (1980). Effect of retinoic acid, butylated hydroxytoluene, selenium and sorbic acid on axo-dye hepatocarcinogenesis. *Cancer Lett.* **9**, 299–304.

Davies, D. E. (1967). Effect of vitamin A on 7,12-dimethylbenz(a)anthracene-induced papillomas in rhino mouse skin. *Cancer Res.* **27**, 237–241.

Dawson, W. D., Miller, W. W., and Liles, W. B. (1979). Retinyl acetate prophylaxis in cancer of the urinary bladder. *Invest. Urol.* **16**, 376–377.

Dingle, J. T., Fell, H. B., and Goodman, D. S. (1972). The effect of retinol and retinol-binding protein on embryonic skeletal tissue in organ culture. *J. Cell Sci.* **11**, 393–402.

Dowling, J. E., and Wald, G. (1960). The role of vitamin A acid. *Vitam. Horm.* **18**, 515–541.

Dunagin, P. E., Jr., Zachman, R. D., and Olson, J. A. (1964). Identification of free and conjugated retinoic acid as product of retinal (vitamin A aldehyde) metabolism in the rat in vivo. *Biochim. Biophys. Acta* **90**, 432–434.

Elias, P. M., and Williams, M. L. (1981). Retinoids, cancer, and the skin. *Arch. Dermatol.* **117**, 160–180.

Epstein, J. H., and Grenkin, D. A. (1981). Inhibition of ultraviolet-induced carcinogenesis by all-trans retinoic acid. *J. Invest. Dermatol.* **76**, 178–180.

Evard, J. P., and Bollag, W. (1972). Konservative Behandlung der rezidivierenden Harnblasenpapillomatose mit Vitamin-A-Saure. *Schweiz. Med. Wochenschr.* **102**, 1880–1883.

Fidge, N. H., and Goodman, D. S. (1967). Enzymatic reduction of retinal to retinol in rat intestinal mucosa. *Fed. Proc. Fed. Am. Soc. Exp. Biol.* **26**, 849.

Frigg, M., and Torhorst, J. (1977). Autoradiographic and histopathologic studies on the mode of action of an aromatic retinoid (RO 10-9359) on chemically induced epithelial tumors in Swiss mice. *J. Natl. Cancer Inst.* **58**, 1365–1371.

Fuchs, E., and Green, H. (1981). Regulation of terminal differentiation of cultured human keratinocytes by vitamin A. *Cell* **25**, 617–625.

Fujimaki, Y. (1926). Formation of gastric carcinoma in albino rats fed on deficient diets. *J. Cancer Res.* **10**, 469–477.

Futterman, S., and Andrews, J. S. (1964). The composition of liver vitamin A ester and the synthesis of vitamin A ester by liver microsomes. *J. Biol. Chem.* **239**, 4077–4080.

Genta, V. M., Kaufman, D. G., Harris, C. C., Smith, J. M., Sporn, M. B., and Saffiotti, U. (1974). Vitamin A enhances binding of benzo(a)pyrene to tracheal epithelial DNA. *Nature (London)* **247**, 48–49.

Gessel, M. S., Brandes, M. J., Arnold, E. A., Isaacs, J. T., Ueda, H., Millan, J. C., and Brandes, D. (1982). Retinoic acid binding protein in normal and neoplastic rat prostate. *Prostate* **3**, 131–138.

Glover, J. (1973). Retinol binding proteins. *Vitam. Horm.* **31**, 1–42.

Glover, J., Jay, C., and White, G. H. (1974). Distribution of retinol-binding protein in tissues. *Vitam. Horm.* **32**, 215–235.

Goodman, D. S., and Huang, H. S. (1965). Biosynthesis of vitamin A with rat intestinal enzymes. *Science* **149**, 879–880.

Goodman, D. S., Huang, H. S., and Shiratori, T. (1965). Tissue distribution and metabolism of newly absorbed vitamin A in the rat. *J. Lipid. Res.* **6**, 390–396.

Gordonoff, Y., and Ludwig, F. (1935). Ueber den Einfluss der Vitamine auf das Wachstum von Gewebe und von Impfgeschwuelsten. *Z. Vitaminforsch.* **4**, 213–223.

Gouveia, J., Hercend, P., Lemaigre, G., Mathê, G., Gros, F. Santelli, G., Homasson, J. P., Angebault, M., Lededente, A., Parrot, R., Gaillard, J. P., Bonniot, J. P., Marsac, J., and Pretet, S. (1982). Degree of bronchial metaplasia in heavy smokers and its regression after treatment with a retinoid. *Lancet* **1**, 710–712.

Graham, S., Mettlin, C., Marshall, J., Priore, R., Rzepka, T., and Sheed, D. (1981). Dietary factors in the epidemiology of cancer of the larynx. *Am. J. Epidemiol.* **113**, 675–680.

Grubbs, C. J., Moon, R. C., Sporn, M. B., and Newton, D. L. (1977). Inhibition of mammary cancer by retinyl methyl ether. *Cancer Res.* **37**, 599–602.

Harding, W. G., and Leech, W. D. (1940). The influence of vitamins on neoplasma. *Z. Vitaminforsch.* **10**, 295–311.

Heller, J. (1975). Interaction of plasma retinol-binding protein with its receptor. *J. Biol. Chem.* **250**, 3613–3619.

Hill, D. L., and Grubbs, C. J. (1982). Retinoids as chemopreventive and anticancer agents in intact animals. (Review). *Anticancer Res.* **2**, 111–124.

Huang, H. S., and Goodman, D. S. (1965). Vitamin A and carotenoids. I. Intestinal absorption and metabolism of ^{14}C labelled vitamin A alcohol and β-carotene in the rat. *J. Biol. Chem.* **240**, 2839–2844.

Huber, P. R., Geyer, E., Kung, W., Matter, A., Torhorst, J., and Eppenberger, U. (1978). Retinoic acid binding protein in human breast cancer and dysplasia. *J. Natl. Cancer Inst.* **61**, 1375–1378.

Ibrahim, K., Jafarey, N. A., and Zuberi, D. J. (1977). Plasma vitamin "A" and carotene levels in squamous cell carcinoma of oral cavity and oro-pharynx. *Clin. Oncol.* **2**, 203–207.

Israel, L., and Aguilera, J. (1980). Vitamine A et cancer. *Pathol. Biol.* **28**, 253–259.

Ito, Y. (1981). Effect of an aromatic retinoic acid analog (Ro 10-9359) on growth of virus-induced papilloma (Shope) and related neoplasia of rabbits. *Eur. J. Cancer* **17**, 35–42.

Ito, Y., Zile, M., DeLuca, H. F., and Ahrens, H. M. (1974). Metabolism of retinoic acid in vitamin A-deficient rats. *Biochim. Biophys. Acta* **369**, 338–350.

Jetten, A. M., and Jetten, M. E. R. (1979). Possible role of retinoic acid binding protein in retinoid stimulation of embryonal carcinoma cell differentiation. *Nature London* **278**, 180–182.

Kark, J. D., Smith, A. H., Switzer, B. R., and Hames, C. G. (1981). Serum vitamin A (retinol) and cancer incidence in Evans County, Georgia. *J. Natl. Cancer Inst.* **66**, 7–16.

Kark, J. D., Smith, A. H., and Hames, C. G. (1982). Serum retinol and the inverse relationship between serum cholesterol and cancer. *Br. Med. J.* **284**, 152–154.

Kawamura, H., and Hashimoto, Y. (1980). Vitamin A receptor in cancers and in vitro-transformed epithelial cells of the rat urinary bladder: Its implication in the preventive effect of vitamin A on in vitro keratinization. *Gann* **71**, 507–513.

Kligman, L. H., and Kligman, A. M. (1981). Lack of enhancement of experimental photocarcinogenesis by topical retinoic acid. *Arch. Dermatol. Res.* **270**, 453–462.

Koch, H. F. (1978). Biochemical treatment of precancerous oral lesions: The effectiveness of various analogues of retinoic acid. *J. Max. Fac. Surg.* **6**, 59–63.

Kokron, O., Alth, G., Cerni, C., Denck, H., Fischer, M., Karrer, K., Micksche, M., Orgis, E., Titscher, R., and Wrba, H. (1982). Ergebnisse einer vergleichenden Therapiestudie bein inoperable Bronchuskarzinom. *Onkologie* **5**, 20–22.

Koller, P. C. (1963). The nucleus of the cancer cell. A historical review. *Exp. Cell Res. Suppl.* **9**, 3–14.

Kucera, H. (1980). Adjuvancity of vitamin A in an advanced irradiated cervical cancer. *Wien. Klin. Wochenschr. Suppl. 118,* **92**, 1–20.

Kueng, W. M., Geyer, E., Eppenberger, U., and Huber, P. R. (1980). Quantitative estimation of cellular retinoic acid binding protein activity in normal, dysplastic and neoplastic human breast tissue. *Cancer Res.* **40**, 4265–4269.

Kurka, M., Orfanos, C. E., and Pullman, H. (1978). Vitamin A Saure zur Lokalbehandlung epithelialer Neoplasien. *Hautarzt* **29**, 313–318.

Levij, I. S., and Polliack, A. (1968). Potentiating effect of vitamin A on 9-10 dimethyl 1-2 benzanthracene carcinogenesis in the hamster cheek pouch. *Cancer* **22**, 300–306.

Levij, I. S., Rwomushana, J. W., and Polliack, A. (1969). Enhancement of chemical carcinogenesis in the hamster cheek pouch by prior topical application of vitamin A palmitate. *J. Invest. Dermatol.* **53**, 228–231.

Levine, N., and Meyskens, F. L. (1980). Topical vitamin-A-acid therapy for cutaneous metastatic melanoma. *Lancet* **2**, 224–226.

Liau, G., Ong, D. E., and Chytil, F. (1981). Interaction of the retinol/cellular retinol-binding protein complex with isolated nuclei and nuclear components. *J. Cell. Biol.* **91**, 63–68.

Longnecker, D. S., Curphey, T. J., Kuhlmann, E. T., and Roebuck, B. D. (1982). Inhibition of pancreatic carcinogenesis by retinoids in azaserine-treated rats. *Cancer Res.* **42**, 19–24.

Lotan, R. (1980). Effects of vitamin A and its analogs (retinoids) on normal and neoplastic cells. *Biochim. Biophys. Acta* **605**, 33–91.

Lotan, R., Neumann, G., and Lotan, D. (1980). Relationship among retinoid structure, inhibition of growth and cellular retinoic acid-binding protein in cultured S91 melanoma cells. *Cancer Res.* **40**, 1097–1102.

McCormick, D. L., Burns, F. J., and Albert, R. E. (1980). Inhibition of rat mammary carcinogenesis by short dietary exposure to retinyl acetate. *Cancer Res.* **40**, 1140–1143.

McCormick, D. L., Burns, F. J., and Albert, R. E. (1981). Inhibition of benzo(a)pyrene-induced mammary carcinogenesis by retinyl acetate. *J. Natl. Cancer Inst.* **66**, 559–564.

McCormick, D. L., Mehta, R. G., Thompson, C. A., Dinger, N., Caldwell, J. A., and Moon, R. C. (1982). Enhanced inhibition of mammary carcinogenesis by combined treatment with N-(4-hydroxyphenyl)retinamide and ovariectomy. *Cancer Res.* **42**, 508–512.

McCullough, K., and Dalldorf, G. (1937). Epithelial metaplasia. *Arch. Pathol.* **24**, 486–496.

McGaughey, C., and Jensen, J. L. (1980). Effects of the differentiating agents (inducers) dimethylacetamide, di-and tetramethylurea on epidermal tumor promotion by retinyl (vitamin A) acetate and croton oil in hamster cheek pouch. *Oncology* **37**, 65–70.

McGaughey, C., Jensen, J. L., and Stowell, E. C. (1977). Effects of adenosine and guanosine cyclic phosphates and their corresponding nucleotides and nucleosides on vitamin A-induced epidermal tumor promotion and growth in hamster cheek pouch. *J. Med.* **8**, 443–456.

McGuire, B. W., Orgebin-Crist, M. C., and Chytil, F. (1981). Autoradiographic localization of serum retinol-binding protein in rat testis. *Endocrinology* **108**, 658–667.

McMichael, H. (1965). Inhibition of growth of Shope rabbit papilloma by hyper-vitaminosis A. *Cancer Res.* **25**, 947–955.

Mahadevan, S., Murthy, S. K., Krishnamurthy, S., and Ganguly, J. (1961). Studies on vitamin A esterase. 4. Hydrolysis and synthesis of vitamin A esters by rat intestinal mucosa. *Biochem. J.* **79**, 416–424.

Mahadevan, S., Sastry, P. S., and Ganguly, J. (1963). Studies on metabolism of vitamin A. 4. Studies on the mode of absorption of vitamin A by rat intestine in vitro. *Biochem. J.* **88**, 534–539.

Mahmoud, L. A. N., and Robinson, W. A. (1982). Vitamin A levels in human bladder cancer. *Int. J. Cancer* **30**, 143–145.

Maiorana, A., and Gullino, P. M. (1980). Effect of retinyl acetate on the incidence of mammary carcinomas and hepatomas in mice. *J. Natl. Cancer Inst.* **64**, 655–663.

Maraini, G., and Gozzoli, F. (1975). Binding of retinol to isolated retinal pigment epithelium in the presence and absence of retinol-binding protein. *Invest. Ophthalmol.* **14**, 785–787.

Matter, A., and Bollag, W. (1977). A fine structural study on the therapeutic effects on an aromatic retinoid on chemically-induced skin papillomas of the mouse. *Eur. J. Cancer* **13**, 831–838.

Mayer, H., Bollag, W., Hänni, R., and Rüegg, R. (1978). Retinoids, a new class of compounds with prophylactic and therapeutic activities in oncology and dermatology. *Experientia* **34**, 1105–1246.

Mehta, R. G., Cerny, W. L., and Moon, R. C. (1980). Distribution of retinoic acid binding protein in normal and neoplastic mammary tissues. *Cancer Res.* **40**, 47–49.

Mehta, R. G., Kute, T. E., Kopkins, M., and Moon, R. C. (1982a). Retinoic acid binding proteins and steroid receptor levels in human breast cancer. *Eur. J. Cancer Clin. Oncol.* **18**, 221–226.

Mehta, R. G., McCormick, D. L., Cerny, W. L., and Moon, R. C. (1982b). Correlation between retinoid inhibition of N-methyl-N-nitrosourea-induced mammary carcinogenesis and levels of retinoic acid binding proteins. *Carcinogenesis* **3**, 89–91.

Mettlin, C., and Graham, S. (1979). Dietary risk factors in human bladder cancer. *Am. J. Epidemiol.* **110**, 255–263.

Mettlin, C., Graham, S., and Swanson, M. (1979). Vitamin A and lung cancer. *J. Natl. Cancer Inst.* **62**, 1435–1438.

Meyskens, F. L. (1981). Modulation of abnormal growth by retinoids: A clinical perspective of the biological phenomena. *Life Sci.* **28**, 2323–2327.

Meyskens, F. L., Gilmartin, E., Alberts, D. S., Levine, N. S., Brooks, R., Salmon, S. E., and Surwit, E. A. (1982). Activity of isotretinoin against squamous cell cancers and preneoplastic lesions. *Cancer Treat. Rep.* **66**, 1315–1319.

Micksche, M., Kokron, O., Cerni, C., Titscher, R., and Wrba, H. (1974). Klinische und immunologische Verlaubsbeobachtung der hochdosierten Vitamin-A-Therapie bei Bronchuskarzinomen. *Osterreich. Z. Onkol.* **3–4**, 70–76.

Micksche, M., Cerni, C., Kokron, O., Titscher, R., and Wrba, H. (1977). Stimulation of immune response in lung cancer patients by vitamin A therapy. *Oncology* **34**, 234–238.

Miyata, Y., Tsuda, H., Matayoshi-Miyasato, K., Fukushima, S., Murasaki, G., Ogiso, T., and Ito, N. (1978). Effect of vitamin A acetate on urinary bladder carcinogenesis induced by N-butyl-N-(4-hydroxybutyl)nitrosamine in rats. *Gann* **69**, 845–848.

Miyata, Y., Nakatsuka, T., Arai, M., Murasaki, G., Nakanishi, K., and Ito, N. (1980). Inhibition by an aromatic retinoid of DNA damage induced by the bladder carcinogen N-butyl-N(3-carboxypropyl)nitrosamine. *Gann* **71**, 341–348.

Modan, B., Cuckle, H., and Lubin, F. (1981). A note on the role of dietary retinol and carotene in human gastro-intestinal cancer. *Int. J. Cancer,* **28**, 421–424.

Moon, R. C., and Mehta, R. G. (1981) Retinoid binding in normal and neoplastic mammary tissue. *Adv. Exp. Med. Biol.* **183**, 231–249.

Moon, R. C., Grubbs, C. J., and Sporn, M. B. (1976). Inhibition of 7,12-dimethyl-benz(a)anthracene-induced mammary carcinogenesis by retinyl acetate. *Cancer Res.* **36**, 2626–2630.

Moon, R. C., Grubbs, C. J., Sporn, M. B., and Goodman, D. G. (1977). Retinyl acetate inhibits mammary carcinogenesis induced by N-methyl-N-nitroso-urea. *Nature London* **267**, 620–621.

Moon, R. C., Thompson, H. J., Becci, P. J., Grubbs, C. J., Gander, R. J., Newton, D. L., Smith, J. M., Phillips, S. L., Henderson, W. R., Mullen, L. T., Brown, C. C., and Sporn, M. B. (1979). N-(4-Hydroxyphenyl)retinamide, a new retinoid for prevention of breast cancer in the rat. *Cancer Res.* **39**, 1339–1346.

Murasaki, G., Miyata, Y., Babaya, K., Arai, M., Fukushima, S., and Ito, N. (1980). Inhibition effect of an aromatic retinoic acid analog on urinary bladder carcinogenesis in rat treated with N-butyl-N-(4-hydroxybutyl)nitrosamine. *Gann* **71**, 333–340.

Muto, Y., Omori, M., and Sugawara, K. (1979). Demonstration of a novel cellular retinol-binding protein F-type, in hepatocellular carcinoma. *Gann* **70**, 215–222.

Narisawa, T., Reddy, B. S., Wong, C. O., and Weisburger, J. H. (1976). Effect of vitamin deficiency on rat colon carcinogenesis by N'methyl-N'-nitro-N-nitroso-guanidine. *Cancer Res.* **36**, 1379–1383.

Nettesheim, P. (1980). Inhibition of carcinogenesis by retinoids. *Can. Med. Assoc. J.* **122**, 757–765.

Nettesheim, P., and Williams, M. L. (1976). The influence of vitamin A on the susceptibility of the rat lung to 3-methylcholanthrene. *Int. J. Cancer* **17**, 351–357.

Nettesheim, P., Cone, M. V., and Snyder, C. (1976). The influence of retinyl acetate on the postinitiation phase of preneoplastic lung nodules in rats. *Cancer Res.* **36**, 996–1002.

Nettesheim, P., Snyder, C., and Kim, J. C. S. (1979). Vitamin A and the susceptibility of respiratory tract tissues to carcinogenic insult. *Environ. Health Perspect.* **29**, 89–93.

Newberne, P. M., and Rogers, A. E. (1973). Rat colon carcinomas, associated with aflatoxin and marginal vitamin A. *J. Natl. Cancer Inst.* **50**, 439–448.

Newberne, P. M., and Suphakarn, V. (1977). Preventive role of vitamin A in colon carcinogenesis in rats. *Cancer* **40**, 2553–2556.

Nigro, N. D., Bull, A. W., Wilson, P. S., Soullier, B. K., and Alousi, M. A. (1982). Combined inhibitors of carcinogenesis: Effect of azoxymethane-induced intestinal cancer in rats. *J. Natl. Cancer Inst.* **69**, 103–107.

Olson, J. A. (1961). The conversion of radioactive β-carotene into vitamin A by the rat intestine in vivo. *J. Biol. Chem.* **236**, 349–356.

Olson, J. A., and Hayaishi, O. (1965). The enzymatic cleavage of β-carotene into vitamin A by soluble enzymes of rat liver and intestine. *Biochemistry* **54**, 1364–1370.

Omori, M., and Chytil, F. (1982). Mechanism of vitamin A action: Gene expression in retinol deficient rats. *J. Biol. Chem.* **257**, 14370–14374.

Ong, D. E., and Chytil, F. (1974). Multiple retinol binding proteins in rabbit lung, *Biochem. Biphys. Res. Commun.* **59**, 221–229.

Ong, D. E., and Chytil, F. (1975a). Retinoic acid binding protein in rat tissue. *J. Biol. Chem.* **250**, 6113–6116.

Ong, D. E., and Chytil, F. (1975b). Specificity of cellular retinol-binding protein for compounds with vitamin A activity. *Nature (London)* **255**, 74–75.

Ong, D. E., and Chytil, F. (1976a). Changes in levels of cellular retinol and retinoic-acid-binding proteins of liver and lung during perinatal development of rat. *Proc. Natl. Acad. Sci. U.S.A.* **73**, 3976–3978.

Ong, D. E., and Chytil, F. (1976b). Presence of cellular retinol and retinoic acid binding proteins in experimental tumors. *Cancer Lett.* **2**, 25–30.

Ong, D. E., Page, D. L., and Chytil, F. (1975). Retinoic acid binding protein: Occurrence in human tumors. *Science* **190**, 60–61.

Ong, D. E., Tsai, C. H., and Chytil, F. (1976). Cellular retinol-binding protein and retinoic acid-binding protein in rat testes: Effect of retinol depletion. *J. Nutr.* **106**, 204–211.

Ong, D. E., Markert, C., and Chiu, J. F. (1978). Cellular binding proteins for vitamin A in colorectal adenocarcinoma of rat. *Cancer Res.* **38**, 4422–4426.

Ong, D. E., Goodwin, W. J., Jesse, R. H., and Griffin, A. C. (1982). Presence of cellular retinol and retinoic acid-binding proteins in epidermoid carcinoma of the oral cavity and oropharynx. *Cancer* **49**, 1409–1412.

Palan, P. R., and Romney, S. L. (1979). Cellular binding proteins for vitamin A in normal human uterine cervix and in dysplasia. *Cancer Res.* **39**, 3114–3118.

Palan, P. R., and Romney, S. L. (1980). Cellular binding proteins for vitamin A in human carcinomas and in normal tissues. *Cancer Res.,* **40**, 4221–4224.

Palan, P. R., Duttagupta, C., and Romney, S. L. (1980). Sex difference in cellular retinol- and retinoic acid-binding proteins in human colon adenocarcinomas. *Cancer Lett.* **11**, 97–101.

Patek, P. Q., Collins, J. L., Yogeeswaran, G., and Dennert, G. (1979). Antitumor potential of retinoic acid: Stimulation of immune mediated effectors. *Int. J. Cancer* **24**, 624–628.

Pavelic, Z. P., Dave, S., Bialkowski, S., Priore, R. L., and Greco, W. P. (1980). Antitumor activity of Corynebacterium parvum and retinyl palmitate used in combination on the Lewis lung carcinoma. *Cancer Res.* **40**, 4617–4621.

Pawson, B. A., Cheung, H. C., Han., R. L., Trown, P. W., Buck, M., Hansen, R., Bollag, W., Ineichen, U., Pleil, H., Ruegg, R., Dunlop, N. M., Newton, D. L., and Sporn, M. B. (1977). Dihydroretinoic acids and their derivatives. Synthesis and biological activity. *J. Med. Chem.* **20**, 918–925.

Peck, G. L. (1981). Chemoprevention of cancer with retinoids. *Gynecol. Oncol.* **12,** S331–S340.

Peto, R., Doll, R., Buckley, J. D., and Sporn, M. B. (1981). Can dietary beta-carotene materially reduce human cancer rates? *Nature (London)* **290,** 201–208.

Polliack, A., and Levij, I. S. (1969). The effect of topical vitamin A on papillomas and intraepithelial carcinomas induced in hamster cheek pouches with 9,10-dimethyl-1,2-benzanthracene. *Cancer Res.* **29,** 327–332.

Polliack, A., and Sasson, Z. B. (1972). Enhancing effect of excess topical vitamin A on Rous sarcomas in chickens. *J. Natl. Cancer Inst.* **48,** 407–416.

Polliack, A., Rwomushana, J. W., and Levij, I. S. (1971). Treatment of experimental benign hyperkeratotic lesions of the hamster cheek pouch with topical vitamin A palmitate. *Pharmacol. Ther. Dent.* **1,** 63–70.

Prutkin, L. (1968). The effect of vitamin A acid on tumorigenesis and protein production. *Cancer Res.* **28,** 1021–1030.

Prutkin, L. (1971). Modification of the effect of vitamin A acid on the skin tumor keratoacanthoma by applications of actinomycin D. *Cancer Res.* **31,** 1080–1083.

Prutkin, L. (1975). Inhibition of tumorigenesis by topical application of low doses of vitamin A acid and fluorouracil. *Experientia* **31,** 494.

Rask, L., and Peterson, P. A. (1976). In vitro uptake of vitamin A from the retinol-binding plasma protein to mucosal epithelial cells from the monkey's small intestine. *J. Biol. Chem.* **251,** 6360–6366.

Rask, L., Anundi, H., Boehme, J., Erikson, J., Fredriksson, A., Nilsson, S. F., Ronne, H., Vahlquist, A., and Peterson, P. A. (1980). The retinol binding protein. *Scand. J. Clin. Lab. Invest. Suppl. 154,* **40,** 45–61.

Rattanapanone, V., Tashiro, S., Tokuda, H., Rattanapanone, N., and Ito, Y. (1981). Cellular retinoic acid-binding protein in virus-induced papillomas (Shope) of rabbit skin. *Cancer Res.* **41,** 1483–1487.

Roberts, A., and DeLuca, H. F. (1967). Pathways of retinol and retinoic acid metabolism in the rat. *Biochem. J.* **102,** 600–605.

Rogers, A. E., and Newberne, P. M. (1975). Dietary effects on chemical carcinogenesis in animal models for colon and liver tumors. *Cancer Res.* **35,** 3427–3432.

Rogers, A. E., Herndon, B. J., and Newberne, P. M. (1973). Induction by dimethylhydrazine of intestinal carcinoma in normal rats and rats fed high or low levels of vitamin A. *Cancer Res.* **33,** 1003–1009.

Romney, S. L., Palan, P. R., Duttagupta, C., Wassertheil-Smoller, S., Wylie, J., Miller, G., Slagle, N. S., and Lucido, D. (1981). Retinoids and the prevention of cervical dysplasia. *Am. J. Obstet. Gynecol.* **141,** 890–894.

Ross, A. C., Takahashi, Y. I., and Goodman, D. S. (1978). The binding protein for retinol from rat testis cytosol. Isolation and partial characterization. *J. Biol. Chem.* **253,** 6591–6598.

Rowe, N. H., and Gorlin, R. J. (1959). The effect of a deficiency upon experimental oral carcinogenesis. *J. Dent. Res.* **38,** 72–83.

Rowe, N. H., Grammer, F. C., Watson, F. R., and Nickerson, N. H. (1970). A study of environmental influence upon salivary gland neoplasia in rats. *Cancer* **26,** 436–444.

Ryssel, M. J., Brunner, K. W., and Bollag, W. (1971). Die perorale Anwendung von Vitamin A-Saure bei Leukoplakien, Hyperkeratosen und Plastenepithelkarzinomen: Ergebnisse und Wertraglichkeit. *Schweiz. Med. Wochenschr.* **101,** 1027–1030.

Saari, J. C., Bredberg, L., and Garwin, G. (1982). Identification of the endogenous retinoids associated with three cellular retinoid binding proteins from bovine retina and retinal pigment epithelium. *J. Biol. Chem.* **257,** 13329–13333.

Saccomanno, G., Moran, P. G., Schmidt, R., Hartshorn, D. F., Brian, D. A., Dreher, W. H., and Sowada, B. J. (1982). Effects of 13-cis retinoids on premalignant and malignant cells of lung origin. *Acta Cytol.* **26**, 78–85.

Saffiotti, U., Montesano, R., Sellakumar, A. R., and Borg, S. A. (1967). Experimental cancer of the lung. Inhibition by vitamin A of induction of tracheobronchial squamous metaplasia and squamous cell tumors. *Cancer* **20**, 857–864.

Sani, B. P., and Corbett, T. H. (1977). Retinoic acid-binding protein in normal and experimental tumors. *Cancer Res.* **37**, 209–213.

Sani, B. P., and Donovan, M. K. (1979). Localization of retinoic acid-binding protein in nuclei and the nuclear uptake of retinoic acid. *Cancer Res.* **39**, 2492–2496.

Sani, B. P., and Hill, D. L. (1976). A retinoic acid-binding protein from chick embryo skin. *Cancer Res.* **36**, 409–413.

Sani, B. P., and Titus, B. C. (1977). Retinoic acid-binding protein in experimental tumors and in tissues with metastatic tumor foci. *Cancer Res.* **37**, 4031–4034.

Sani, B. P., Banerjee, C. K., and Peckham, J. C. (1980a). The presence of binding proteins for retinoic acid and dihydrotestosterone in murine and human colon tumors. *Cancer* **46**, 2421–2429.

Sani, B. P., Condon, S. M., Brockman, R. W., Weiland, L. H., and Schutt, A. J. (1980b). Retinoic acid binding protein in experimental and human tumors. *Cancer* **45**, 1199–1206.

Schapira, F. (1973). Isozymes and cancer. *Adv. Cancer Res.* **18**, 77–153.

Schmaehl, D., and Habs, M. (1978). Experiments on the influence of an aromatic retinoid on the chemical carcinogenesis in rats by butyl-butanol-nitrosamine and 1,2-dimethylhydrazine. *Arzneim. Forsch.* **28**, 49–51.

Schmaehl, D., Kruger, C., and Preissler, P. (1972). Versuche zur Krebsprophylaxe mit Vitamin A. *Arzneim. Forsch.* **22**, 946–949.

Schmaehl, D., Danisman, A., Habs, M., and Diehl, B. (1976). Experimental investigations on the influence upon the chemical carcinogenesis. *Z. Krebsforsch.* **86**, 89–94.

Schroder, E. W., and Black, P. H. (1980). Retinoids: Tumor preventors or tumor enhancers? *J. Natl. Cancer Inst.* **65**, 671–674.

Shamberger, R. J. (1971). Inhibitory effect of vitamin A on carcinogenesis. *J. Natl. Cancer Inst.* **47**, 667–673.

Shekelle, R. B., Liu, S., Raynor, W. J., Lepper, M., Maliza, C., and Rossof, A. H. (1981). Dietary vitamin A and risk of cancer in the Western Electric study. *Lancet* **2**, 1185–1189.

Shklar, G., Flynn, E., Szbo, G., and Marefat, P. (1980). Retinoid inhibition of experimental lingual carcinogenesis: Ultrastructural observations. *J. Natl. Cancer Inst.* **65**, 1307–1316.

Silverman, J., Katayama, S., Zelenakas, K., Lauber, J., Musser, T. K., Reddy, M., Levenstein, M. J., and Weisburger, J. H. (1981). Effect of retinoids on the induction of colon cancer in F344 rats by N-methyl-N-nitrosourea or by 1,2-dimethylhydrazine. *Carcinogenesis* **2**, 1167–1172.

Smith, D. M., Rogers, A. E., Herndon, B. J., and Newberne, P. M. (1975a). Vitamin A (retinyl acetate) and benzo(a)pyrene-induced respiratory tract carcinogenesis in hamster fed a commercial diet. *Cancer Res.* **35**, 11–16.

Smith, D. M., Rogers, A. E., and Newberne, P. M. (1975b). Vitamin A and benzo(a)pyrene carcinogenesis in the respiratory tract of hamster fed a semi-synthetic diet. *Cancer Res.* **35**, 1485–1488.

Smith, J. E., and Goodman, D. S. (1979). Retinol-binding and the regulation of vitamin A transport. *Fed. Proc. Fed. Am. Soc. Exp. Biol.* **38**, 2504–2509.

Smith, J. E., Milch, P. O., Muto, Y., and Goodman, D. W. (1973). The plasma transport and metabolism of retinoic acid in the rat. *Biochem. J.* **132**, 821–827.

Smith, P. G., and Jick, H. (1978). Cancers among users of preparations containing vitamin A. A case-control investigation. *Cancer* **42**, 808–811.

Smith, W. E., Yazdi, E., and Miller, L. (1972). Carcinogenesis in pulmonary epithelia in mice on different levels of vitamin A. *Environ. Res.* **5**, 152–163.

Soprano, D. R., Smith, J. E., and Goodman, D. S. (1982). Effect of retinol status on retinol-binding protein biosynthesis rate and translatable messenger RNA level in rat liver. *J. Biol. Chem.* **257**, 7693–7697.

Sporn, M. B. (1976). Approaches to prevention of epithelial cancer during the preneoplastic period. *Cancer Res.* **36**, 2699–2702.

Sporn, M. B. (1977). Retinoids and carcinogenesis. *Nutr. Rev.* **35**, 65–69.

Sporn, M. B. (1978a). Chemoprevention of cancer. *Nature (London)* **272**, 402–403.

Sporn, M. B. (1978b). Pharmacological prevention of carcinogenesis by retinoids. In "Carcinogenesis," Vol. 2 "Mechanisms of Tumor Promotion and Carcinogenesis" (T. J. Slaga, A. Sivak, and R. K. Boutwell, eds.), pp. 545–564. Raven, New York.

Sporn, M. B. (1980). Retinoids and cancer prevention. In "Carcinogenesis," Vol. 5 "Modifiers of Chemical Carcinogenesis" (T. J. Slaga, ed.), pp. 99–109. Raven, New York.

Sporn, M. B., and Newton, D. L. (1979). Chemoprevention of cancer with retinoids. *Fed. Proc. Fed. Am. Soc. Exp. Biol.* **38**, 2528–2534.

Sporn, M. B., Dunlop, N. M., Newton, D. L., and Smith, J. M. (1976a). Prevention of chemical carcinogenesis by vitamin A and its synthetic analogs (retinoids). *Fed. Proc. Fed. Am. Soc. Exp. Biol.* **35**, 1332–1338.

Sporn, M. B., Dunlop, N. M., Newton, D. L., and Henderson, W. R. (1976b). Relationship between structure and activity of retinoids. *Nature (London)* **263**, 110–113.

Sporn, M. B., Squire, R. A., Brown, C. C. Smith, J. M., Wenk, M. L., and Springer, S. (1977). 13-cis Retinoic acid: Inhibition of bladder carcinogenesis in the rat. *Science* **195**, 487–489.

Squire, R. A., Sporn, M. B., Brown, C. C., Smith, J. M., Wenk, M. L., and Springer, S. (1977). Histopathological evaluation of the inhibition of rat bladder carcinogenesis by 13-cis-retinoic acid. *Cancer Res.* **37**, 2930–2936.

Staehelin, H. B., Buess, E., Roesel, F., and Widmer, L. K. (1982). Vitamin A cardiovascular risk factors, and mortality. *Lancet* **1**, 394–395.

Stewart, D. P., Speer, R. J., Ridgway, H. J., and Hill, J. M. (1979). Combination chemotherapy of leukemia L1210 with platinum compounds and vitamins. *J. Clin. Hematol. Or. col.* **9**, 235–239.

Stinson, S. F., Reznick, G., and Donahoe, R. (1981). Effect of three retinoids on tracheal carcinogenesis with N-methyl-N-nitrosourea in hamster. *J. Natl. Cancer Inst.* **66**, 947–951.

Sugiura, K., and Benedict, S. R. (1930a). The influence of high fat diets on the growth of carcinoma and sarcoma in rats. *J. Cancer Res.* **14**, 311–318.

Sugiura, K., and Benedict, S. R. (1930b). A critical study of vitamin A and carcinogenesis. *J. Cancer Res.* **14**, 306–310.

Surwit, E. A., Graham, V., Droegemueller, W., Alberts, D., Chvapil, M., Dorr, R. T., Davis, J. R., and Meyskens, F. L. (1982). Evaluation of topically applied transretinoic acid in the treatment of cervical intraepithelial lesions. *Am. J. Obstet. Gynecol.* **143**, 821–823.

Takase, S., Ong, D. E., and Chytil, F. (1979). Cellular retinol-binding protein allows specific interaction of retinol with the nucleus in vitro. *Proc. Natl. Acad. Sci. U.S.A.* **76**, 2204–2208.

Thatcher, N., Blackledge, G., and Crowther, D. (1980). Advanced recurrent squamous cell carcinoma of the head and neck. *Cancer* **46,** 1324–1328.

Thompson, H. J., Becci, P. J., Brown, C. C., and Moon, R. C. (1979). Effect of the duration of retinyl acetate feeding on inhibition of 1-methyl-1-nitroso-urea-induced mammary carcinogenesis in the rat. *Cancer Res.* **39,** 3977–3980.

Thompson, H. J., Becci, P. J., Grubbs, C. J., Shealy, Y. F., Stanek, E. J., Brown, C. C., Sporn, M. B., and Moon, R. C. (1981a). Inhibition of urinary bladder cancer by N-ethyl-all-trans retinamide and N-(2-hydroxyethyl)-all-trans-retinamide in rats and mice. *Cancer Res.* **41,** 933–936.

Thompson, H. J., Meeker, L. D., and Becci, P. J. (1981b). Effect of combined selenium and retinyl acetate treatment on mammary carcinogenesis. *Cancer Res.* **41,** 1413–1416.

Thompson, H. J., Meeker, L. D., Tagliaferro, A. R., and Becci, P. J. (1982). Effect of retinyl acetate on the occurrence of ovarian hormone-responsive and nonresponsive mammary cancers in the rat. *Cancer Res.* **42,** 903–905.

Thompson, J. N., Howell, J. McC., and Pitt, G. A. (1964). Vitamin A and reproduction in rats. *Proc. R. Soc. London Ser. B* **159,** 510–535.

Thompson, S. Y., Braude, R., Coates, M. E., Cowie, A. T., Ganguly, J., and Kon, S. K. (1950). Further studies of the conversion of β-carotene to vitamin A in the intestines. *Br. J. Nutr.* **4,** 398–420.

Trown, P. W., Buck, M. J., and Hansen, R. (1976). Inhibition of growth and regression of a transplantable rat chondrosarcoma by three retinoids. *Cancer Treat. Rep.* **60,** 1647–1653.

Trown, P. W., Palleroni, A. V., Bohoslawec, O., Richelo, B. N., Halpern, J. M., Gizzi, N., Geiger, R., Lewinski, C., Machlin, L. J., Jetten, A., and Jetten, M. E. R. (1980). Relationship between binding affinities to cellular retinoic acid-binding protein and in vivo and in vitro properties for 18 retinoids. *Cancer Res.* **40,** 212–220.

Verma, A. K., and Boutwell, R. K. (1977). Vitamin A acid (retinoic acid) a potent inhibitor of 12-O-tetradecanoyl-phorbol-13-acetate-induced ornithine decarboxylase activity in mouse epidermis. *Cancer Res.* **37,** 2196–2201.

Verma, A. K., Rice, H. M., Shapas, B. G., and Boutwell, R. K. (1978). Inhibition of 12-O-tetradecanoylphorbol-13-acetate-induced ornithine decarboxylase activity in mouse epidermis by vitamin A analogs (retinoids). *Cancer Res.* **38,** 793–801.

Verma, A. K., Slaga, T. J., Wertz, P. W., Mueller, G. C., and Boutwell, R. K. (1980). Inhibition of skin tumor promotion by retinoic acid and its metabolite 5,6-epoxyretinoic acid. *Cancer Res.* **40,** 2367–2371.

Visek, W. J., Clinton, S. K., and Truex, C. R. (1978). Nutrition and experimental carcinogenesis. *Cornell Vet.* **68,** 3–39.

Vollmar, H. (1939). Ueber den Einfluss von Vitaminen auf Gewebekulturen von Normal-und Tumorgewebe. *Arch. Exp. Zellforsch. Besonders Gewebezuecht.* **23,** 42–60.

Wahi, P. N., Kehar, U., and Lahiri, B. (1965). Factors influencing oral and oropharyngeal cancers in India. *Br. J. Cancer* **19,** 642–660.

Wald, N., Idle, M., Boreham, J., and Bailey, A. (1980). Low serum vitamin A and subsequent risk of cancer. *Lancet* **2,** 813–815.

Wang, C. C., Campbell, S., Furner, R. L., and Hill, D. L. (1980). Disposition of all-trans and 13-cis-retinoic acids and N-hydroxyethylretinamide in mice after intravenous administration. *Drug Metab. Dispos.* **8,** 8–11.

Ward, J. M., Sporn, M. B., Wenk, M. L., Smith, J. M., Feeser, D., and Dean, R. J. (1978). Dose response to intrarectal administration of N-methyl-N-nitrosourea and histopathologic evaluation of the effect of two retinoids on colon lesions induced in rats. *J. Natl. Cancer Inst.* **60,** 1489–1493.

Weeks, C. E., Slaga, T. J., Hennings, H., Gleason, G. L., and Bracken, W. M. (1979). Inhibition of phorbol ester-induced tumor promotion in mice by vitamin A analog and anti-inflammatory steroid. *J. Natl. Cancer Inst.* **63,** 401–406.

Welsch, C. W., Brown, C. K., Goodrich-Smith, M., Chiusano, J., and Moon, R. C. (1980). Synergistic effect of chronic prolactin suppression and retinoid treatment in the prophylaxis of N-methyl-N-nitrosourea-induced mammary tumorigenesis in female Sprague-Dawley rats. *Cancer Res.* **40,** 3095–3098.

Welsch, C. W., Goodrich-Smith, M., Brown, C. K., and Crowe, N. (1981). Enhancement by retinyl acetate of hormone-induced mammary tumorigenesis in female GR/A mice. *J. Natl. Cancer Inst.* **67,** 935–938.

Wenk, M. L., Ward, J. M., Reznik, G., and Dean, J. (1981). Effects of three retinoids on colon adenocarcinomas, sarcomas and hyperplastic polyps induced by intrarectal N-methyl-N-nitrosourea administration in male F344 rats. *Carcinogenesis* **2,** 1161–1166.

Wiggert, B., Russel, P., Lewis, M., and Chader, G. (1977). Differential binding to soluble nuclear receptors and effects on cell viability of retinol and retinoic acid in cultured retinoblastoma cells. *Biochem. Biophys. Res. Commun.* **79,** 218–226.

Wolbach, S. B., and Howe, P. R. (1925). Tissue changes following deprivation of fat-soluble A vitamin. *J. Exp. Med.* **42,** 753–777.

Wolbach, S. B., and Howe, P. R. (1933). Epihtelial repair in recovery from vitamin A deficiency. *J. Exp. Med.* **57,** 511–526.

Wong, Y. C., and Buck, R. C. (1971). An electron microscopic study of metaplasia on the rat tracheal epithelium in vitamin A deficiency. *Lab. Invest.* **24,** 55–66.

Wyard, S. (1922). The treatment of malignant disease by a diet free from fat soluble vitamin A. *Lancet* **202,** 840.

Young, V. R., and Newberne, P. M. (1981). Vitamins and cancer prevention: Issues and dilemmas. *Cancer* **47,** 1226–1240.

Zile, M., and DeLuca, H. F. (1968). Retinoic acid: Some aspects of growth promoting activity in the albino rat. *J. Nutr.* **94,** 302–308.

Hypothalamic–Hypophysial Vasculature and Its Relationship to Secretory Cells of the Hypothalamus and Pituitary Gland

JOHN C. PORTER, JANICE F. SISSOM, JUN ARITA, AND MARIANNE J. REYMOND

Cecil H. and Ida Green Center for Reproductive Biology Sciences,
Departments of Obstetrics and Gynecology and Physiology,
The University of Texas Health Science Center at Dallas,
Southwestern Medical School,
Dallas, Texas

I. Introduction

The documented beginning of scientific inquiry into the role of the pituitary gland in homeostasis can be rightly attributed to the publication of Marie in 1886. In his now classic treatise, this French physician convincingly presented evidence for the view that the occurrence in man of acromegaly—a disease attributed in our time to excessive secretion and/or activity of growth hormone—is strongly correlated with the presence of pituitary tumors in persons afflicted with this aberration.

Early in the development of our understanding of pituitary function, a distinction was made between two major divisions of the gland. This distinction evolved in part from the recognition of the fact that one component of the pituitary gland, the adenohypophysis, arises embryo-

145

logically from Rathke's pouch and the other component, the neurohypophysis, from the diencephalon of the brain. In many, if not most,
mammals, these two regions of the pituitary gland can be distinguished one from the other with sufficient ease to allow the development of certain operational views, especially views concerning the role
of a pituitary hormone as a trophic substance, as a regulator of water
excretion, or as a stimulator of smooth muscle contraction.

But, as our knowledge of the hypophysis has expanded, we have
come to realize that, in a functional sense, separation of the neurohypophysis and adenohypophysis is less easily justified than was
initially supposed. The blurring of the distinction between these two
glands is in large measure a consequence of the conjointed vasculature
of the components of the neurohypophysis and adenohypophysis. It is
the purpose of this article to delineate the development of our present
understanding of this vasculature, to discuss its relationship to hypophysial and hypothalamic cells that secrete hormones, and to identify
areas in our understanding that remain ambiguous and are in need of
further study.

II. HYPOTHALAMIC–HYPOPHYSIAL VASCULATURE

The particular components of the hypophysial vasculature that we
now know as the hypophysial portal vessels were independently described in man by Popa and Fielding (1930) and by Pietsch (1930).
They observed that the sinusoids of the pars distalis of the pituitary
gland and the capillaries in the floor of the ventricular recess of the
third ventricle (the median eminence of the hypothalamus) are con-
nected through veins that lie on the surface of the pituitary stalk.

The work of Popa and Fielding (1930, 1933) is distinguished from
that described by earlier investigators in that Popa and Fielding assigned a role to certain vessels that they called "hypophysio-portal
vessels." On the basis of the presence in the "hypophysio-portal vessels" of colloidal material, which they believed originated in the pars
distalis, Popa and Fielding concluded that the direction of blood flow in
the hypophysial portal vessels was toward the brain. (It is interesting
to speculate that their opinion may have been influenced by their
failure to identify clearly a venous drainage for the pars distalis. As we
shall see, the issue of the venous drainage of the pars distalis is not
fully resolved even today.) Although subsequent research has led to
the rejection of their claim concerning the direction of blood flow in the
portal vessels, the conclusion of Popa and Fielding regarding the portal

function of the veins connecting the ventromedial hypothalamus and pars distalis was correct.

In 1936, Wislocki and King conducted an extensive analysis of the direction of blood flow in the hypophysial portal vessels of the monkey. On the basis of their findings, they concluded that blood in the portal vessels flowed from the hypothalamus to the pars distalis. Although their examination of the human hypothalamic–hypophysial vasculature was less extensive than the one they conducted in the monkey, their findings, nevertheless, led them to conclude that flow in the hypophysial portal vessels of the human was similar to that in the monkey, thus disputing the conclusion of Popa and Fielding (1930, 1933) that blood in the portal vessels of the human flowed from the pars distalis toward the hypothalamus.

Wislocki and King (1936) also concluded that the pars distalis of the monkey received arterial blood as well as portal blood. In all instances, with the possible exception of the rabbit (Harris, 1947), there is no evidence that the secretory cells of the pars distalis of mammals are ordinarily exposed to arterial blood (Adams et al., 1965). To this extent, Wislocki and King may have erred in their conclusion. Despite the absence of supporting data, it is still tempting to speculate that an arterial blood supply to the pars distalis may be established under certain extraordinary circumstances. A consequence of such a vascularization would be the establishment of a circumscribed region of cells in the pituitary gland that is not perfused with portal blood, thus rendering such cells independent of hypothalamic regulation (Porter et al., 1978). In subsequent studies on the vascular supply of the hypophysis of the cat, man, and monkey, Wislocki (1937, 1938) confirmed the generality of his earlier conclusions regarding blood flow in the portal vessels (Wislocki and King, 1936).

The hypophysial portal vasculature of several species of mammals has been studied extensively by Adams, Daniel, Prichard, and associates. Their studies have included observations on man (Xuereb et al., 1954a,b; Daniel et al., 1958; Adams et al., 1963d), monkey (Adams et al., 1963a; Daniel et al., 1959, 1964a), sheep (Daniel and Prichard, 1957a,b; Adams et al., 1963b), goat (Daniel and Prichard, 1958; Adams et al., 1964, 1966), and rat (Daniel and Prichard, 1956; Adams et al., 1963c; Daniel et al., 1964b). These workers have emphasized the distribution in the pars distalis of blood from various portal vessels. On the basis of their findings, it seems clear that a given portal vessel supplies blood to a limited zone of the pars distalis.

It is of interest that in 1935 Houssay et al. observed in the toad that blood flowed from the hypothalamus to the pars distalis. For reasons that remain obscure, this direct observation on hypophysial blood flow appears to have gone unnoticed at the time by most workers in the field and therefore had little influence on the subsequent development of the concepts of neurosecretion and pituitary regulation. Later, Green (1947) examined the living bullfrog and found that the direction of blood flow in the portal vessels of this species was similar to that described by Wislocki for mammals. In 1949, Green and Harris observed that the direction of blood flow in the portal vessels of the living rat was from the hypothalamus to the pars distalis. Their observation was confirmed in the dog by Török (1954) and in the mouse by Worthington (1955).

We, too, have made many similar observations in the rat under several different conditions using a variety of experimental paradigms. One of these included an occasion when we inserted a fine glass microcannula into a portal vessel and instilled a solution of the dye, lissamine green, through the cannula into the vessel. Inasmuch as the diameter of the microcannula in this case was much less than that of the portal vessel, the cannula interfered little, if any, with the flow of blood in the vessel. One could simultaneously observe through a microscope the portal vessel and the cannula tip while slowly infusing the solution of dye into the bloodstream. In this preparation, one could see the dye flow as a laminated stream in the blood of the portal vessel going to the pars distalis. There was no doubt about the direction of blood flow in this portal vessel: flow was from the hypothalamus to the pars distalis. As noted earlier (Porter et al., 1971), once the dye reached the pars distalis, it was not homogeneously distributed within the pars distalis. A possible consequence of this fact will be discussed subsequently.

The blood supply of the hypophysis is illustrated in Fig. 1. The neurohypophysis, i.e., the median eminence, infundibular stem (hereafter called the pituitary stalk), and pars neuralis (also called the neural lobe), receives arterial blood through two and sometimes three sets of arteries: the superior hypophysial arteries, inferior hypophysial arteries, and, occasionally in some species, a middle hypophysial artery(s). The superior hypophysial arteries join capillaries of the median eminence; the inferior hypophysial arteries join capillaries of the neural lobe; and the middle hypophysial artery(s), when present, join capillaries of the lower pituitary stalk and/or upper neural lobe. Thus, the neurohypophysis receives arterial blood throughout its entirety, i.e., the median eminence, the pituitary stalk, and the neural lobe. As shown by Page et al. (1976) and Page and Bergland (1977), blood from these arteries flows into a continuum of capillaries that lie in the neurohypophysis.

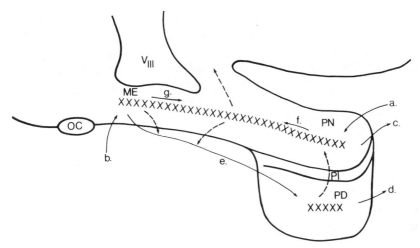

Fig. 1. Diagrammatic representation of the hypophysial vasculature of the rat. Solid arrows denote direction of blood flow. Broken arrows denote direction of net diffusion of hormonal substances. Crosses signify capillary plexuses. V_{III}, Third ventricle; OC, optic chiasma; ME, median eminence; PN, pars neuralis; PI, pars intermedia; PD, pars distalis; a., inferior hypophysial artery; b., superior hypophysial artery; c., vein; d., vein; e., portal vessel; f. and g., flows in the neurohypophysial capillary plexus.

Blood from capillaries of the median eminence and upper pituitary stalk enters the hypophysial portal vessels and is thereby transported to the pars distalis (Fig. 1). Thus, the pars distalis receives venous blood that has passed through part of the neurohypophysis.

III. BLOOD FLOW OF THE HYPOPHYSIAL COMPLEX

A. NEUROHYPOPHYSIS

Goldman and Sapirstein (1962) confirmed in an elegant manner that the neurohypophysis receives its affluent blood by way of an arterial vasculature and that the pars distalis receives blood by way of a portal vasculature. They injected into the right common carotid artery of young adult rats radiolabeled microspheres having a nominal diameter of 29 or 35 μm and analyzed the hypothalamic–hypophysial complex for these microspheres. The microspheres were trapped in the first capillary bed that was encountered, since they were too large to traverse the capillaries.

Several important findings evolved from this experiment. First, no microspheres were present in the pars distalis, indicating that all the microspheres in the affluent blood of the pars distalis had been trapped by an intervening capillary bed and that the pars distalis received no arterial blood. Second, a high concentration of microspheres was present in the neurohypophysis, viz. the median eminence and, as they stated, the posterior lobe of the pituitary gland. (In common parlance, the posterior lobe of the pituitary gland of the rat includes the pars nervosa and pars intermedia. Inasmuch as the pars intermedia is essentially avascular, it is reasonable to assume that the microspheres in the posterior lobe of the pituitary gland were only present in the pars nervosa.) Third, on a weight basis, the uptake of microspheres by the median eminence and the uptake by the posterior lobe of the pituitary gland were the same, indicative of equal rates of blood flow through these two parts of the neurohypophysis.

Recently, Page and associates (1981) reported similar findings in adult sheep. They calculated that the mean blood flows of the neural lobe and median eminence of the sheep were the same, being 4.4 and 4.6 μl/mg tissue/minute, respectively—flows that were 8 times that of cerebrocortical tissue and 16 times that of the white matter of the brain. These findings are supportive of the hypothesis that the neurohypophysis contains a vascular continuum in the form of a capillary plexus and that the flow of blood through one extremity of the plexus is equal to that of the other, viz. the median eminence and pars neuralis.

Page (1983), using microcinephotography, has provided further documentation for the functional existence of this continuum of capillaries (Fig. 1). When the dye, lissamine green, was injected intraarterially into young pigs, the neurohypophysis was seen to fill simultaneously from the central end and from the distal end of the neurohypophysis, i.e., the median eminence and pars neuralis, with the dye front meeting in the pituitary stalk.

Although the sources of arterial blood of the capillary plexus of the neurohypophysis are well documented, the egress of blood from this portion of the brain is not as well understood. This is because the egress of blood from the neurohypophysis is more complex than is its arterial supply, and the various regions of the neurohypophysis do not possess a common venous drainage.

The pars neuralis, which constitutes the most distal portion of the neurohypophysis, possesses large veins that pass to the cavernous sinus. It seems likely that a significant part of the venous blood of the neurohypophysis, especially the pars neuralis, leaves the pituitary gland by this route and thereby carries with it hormones secreted by cells of the pars neuralis, e.g., vasopressin and oxytocin. It must be acknowledged, however, that demonstration of this fact has not thus far been forthcoming. Until such time, it should be borne in mind that the means of transferral of hormones from the neurohypophysis to the general circulation, described previously, is a conclusion evolving from reasonable deductions.

In certain ways, the venous drainage of the rostral neurohypophysis is better understood than is that of the caudal neurohypophysis. The rostral neurohypophysis is identified as the median eminence and upper pituitary stalk. This portion of the neurohypophysis is, to an appreciable extent, drained by hypophysial portal vessels which supply blood to the pars distalis. This has been repeatedly documented.

B. Adenohypophysis

The rate of blood flow of the pars distalis of the rat has been evaluated by several investigators using a variety of techniques (Goldman, 1963; Dávid et al., 1965; Yates et al., 1966; Porter et al., 1967). On the basis of their findings, it would appear that the blood flow of the pars distalis of normotensive rats is 0.6–0.8 µl/mg tissue/minute. This slow rate of blood flow of the pars distalis, compared to that of the neurohypophysis, is in keeping with the fact that the volume of the pars distalis is much larger than that of the neurohypophysis. Since the venous drainage of the upper neurohypophysis is the blood supply of the pars distalis, it follows that the blood flow per unit volume of the pars distalis is less than that of the upper neurohypophysis.

The venous drainage of the pars distalis of the rabbit is believed to be in part through Y-shaped veins that also drain the pars nervosa (Page et al., 1976). Part of the venous drainage of the pars distalis is probably by way of small veins that connect the gland to surrounding sinuses. However, in the absence of meaningful quantitative data, these suggestions should be accepted with reservation.

IV. Neurohormones in Hypophysial Portal Blood

A. Peptide Hormones

It is thought that cells having cytoplasmic extensions, such as neurons, that protrude into the upper neurohypophysis release hormones that diffuse into the blood of the primary capillary plexus of the hypophysial portal vessels; these hormones in turn are conveyed in portal blood to the pars distalis. Evidence for this view has been provided by direct measurement of several hypothalamic hormones in portal blood. The first such evidence was obtained for a corticotropin-releasing factor (CRF) in pituitary stalk blood of dogs (Porter and Jones, 1956). CRF activity in these studies was evaluated by bioassay using an adrenal ascorbic acid depletion technique in cortisol-depressed rats.

Recently, a peptide having CRF activity was isolated from ovine hypothalami and fully characterized by Vale *et al.* (1981) and by Rivier *et al.* (1982). Utilizing a radioimmunoassay, Gibbs and Vale (1982) demonstrated the presence of CRF in hypophysial portal blood of rats. Whether the peptide isolated by Vale *et al.* (1981) represents the only CRF in hypothalamic tissue and in portal blood remains to be established. There is evidence to suggest that other substances having CRF activity are present in the hypothalamus, some of which may represent biologically active metabolites and/or precursors of CRF (Mathew *et al.*, 1982). In addition, vasopressin markedly potentiates the activity of synthetic CRF (Linton *et al.*, 1982).

Luteinizing hormone-releasing hormone (LHRH) has been shown to be present in hypophysial portal blood of rats (Eskay *et al.*, 1975, 1977; Fink and Jamieson, 1976), monkeys (Carmel *et al.*, 1976; Neill *et al.*, 1977), and rabbits (Tsou *et al.*, 1977). A relationship between the concentration of LHRH in hypophysial portal blood and the rate of release of luteinizing hormone (LH) has been demonstrated by Eskay *et al.* (1977). Using female rats on the day of proestrus, these workers found that the concentration of LHRH in portal blood rose severalfold following electrochemical stimulation of the preoptic region of the brain. Such stimulation also resulted in a marked increase in the release of LH. If, immediately before electrochemical stimulation, the animals were passively immunized with antiserum against LHRH to neutralize LHRH in the circulation, stimulation of the preoptic area had no effect on the release of LH. These findings are supportive of the view that (1) stimulation of neurons in the preoptic area of the hypothalamus causes the release of LHRH, resulting in an increase in the concentration of LHRH in portal blood and (2) there is a cause-and-effect relationship between the concentration of LHRH in portal blood and the rate of release of LH.

The results of other experimental paradigms also provide support for the view that the release of LH is a function of LHRH. Arimura *et al.* (1973) were first to show that the testes of a rabbit that had been actively immunized against LHRH were highly atrophic. The intravenous administration of antiserum to LHRH to female rats on the morning of proestrus prevented the release of LH during the subsequent early evening and thereby prevented ovulation (Eskay *et al.*, 1977). The administration of LHRH antiserum to chronically ovariectomized rats (Koch *et al.*, 1973; Porter *et al.*, 1980) or monkeys (McCormack *et al.*, 1977) resulted in a prolonged reduction in the concentration of LH and follicle-stimulating hormone (FSH) in the circulation, due presumably to a reduction in the release of the gonadotropins. Such observations support the view that, once antibodies bind LHRH in the circulation, the peptide is unable to interact with gonadotropin-secreting cells of the pituitary gland in such a way as to cause the release of LH and FSH.

Although thyrotropin-releasing hormone (TRH) was shown by Eskay *et al.* (1975) to be present in hypophysial portal blood, a relationship between the concentration of TRH in portal blood and the release of thyroid-stimulating hormone (TSH) by pituitary cells was not established. These workers found no significant difference in the concentration of TRH in portal blood of rats that were euthyroid, hypothyroid, or hyperthyroid, despite the fact that the rates of release of TSH in these animals were markedly different. On the other hand, the concentration of TRH in hypophysial portal blood of rats was shown by de Greef and Visser (1981) to increase significantly following electrochemical stimulation of the mammary nerve of the donor.

The results of studies using animals that had been passively immunized against TRH support the view that TRH has a role in the control of the release of TSH. Koch *et al.* (1977) found that male as well as female rats that had been treated with antiserum against TRH had circulating TSH levels that were markedly less than those of control animals treated with nonspecific serum. Harris *et al.* (1978) also found in rats treated with antiserum to TRH that cold-induced release of TSH was suppressed compared to that of control animals treated with nonspecific serum. They also observed in rats passively immunized against TRH that prolactin was still released when the animals were exposed to cold, suggesting that cold-induced release of prolactin is not solely a function of TRH release. Koch *et al.* (1977), however, found that the release of prolactin in rats treated with antiserum to TRH was less than that in the controls. If the release of TRH into hypophysial blood is an event that occurs under physiological stress, the release of prolactin should be a consequence of its action, since TRH can unequivocally cause the release of prolactin from pituitary cells in culture (Tashjian *et al.*, 1971). Recently, Fink *et al.* (1982) reported that the concentration of TRH in hypophysial portal plasma of rats rose in the afternoon of proestrus, and the authors suggested that the increase in TRH release might be related to the proestrous surge of prolactin.

β-Endorphin has been shown to be present in high concentrations in hypophysial portal blood of pig-tailed monkeys (Wardlaw *et al.*, 1980a) as well as rhesus monkeys (Wehrenberg *et al.*, 1982). Vasoactive intestinal peptide (VIP) has been demonstrated in pituitary stalk blood of rats (Said and Porter, 1979; Shimatsu et al., 1981). Recently, Shimatsu et al. (1982) demonstrated that serotonin, when administered intracerebroventricularly to rats, resulted in a marked increase in the concentration of VIP in portal blood. Their finding is noteworthy in view of the fact that VIP may be a prolactin-releasing factor (Kato et al., 1978; Ruberg et al., 1978; Clemens and Shaar, 1980). These observations lead to speculation that serotonin may act as a neurotransmitter that stimulates the release of VIP into hypophysial portal blood and thereby causes the release of prolactin.

Somatostatin, a hypothalamic peptide, was identified in the hypophysial portal blood of rats (Gillioz et al., 1979; Chihara et al., 1979a,b). Chihara et al. (1981) found that the intracerebroventricular administration of growth hormone to rats caused a prompt increase in the release of somatostatin into portal blood without affecting blood flow through the portal vessels.

B. CATECHOLAMINES

Dopamine is released by hypothalamic neurons into hypophysial portal blood of rats (Ben-Jonathan et al., 1977; Plotsky et al., 1978; de Greef and Visser, 1981) and monkeys (Neill et al., 1981). The concentration of dopamine in plasma of arterial blood is low, often less than the sensitivity of the radioenzymatic assay we employ, whereas the concentration of dopamine in plasma of hypophysial portal blood is nearly always measurable and is greater than that of plasma of the arterial blood of the same animal. This fact is a consequence of the secretion of dopamine by hypothalamic neurons into hypophysial portal blood.

The concentrations of norepinephrine and epinephrine in arterial plasma are always sufficiently great to allow easy quantification. A comparison of the concentrations of these two catecholamines in arterial plasma with those in hypophysial portal plasma shows that the concentrations of norepinephrine and epinephrine in portal plasma are never greater than those in arterial plasma, indicating that release into portal blood of these two catecholamines does not occur.

This finding is particularly surprising for norepinephrine which shows a concentration in the median eminence that is appreciable, one-fifth to one-half that of dopamine (Palkovits et al., 1974; Selmanoff et al., 1976; Kizer et al., 1978; Demarest et al., 1979; Selmanoff, 1981). The concentration of norepinephrine and epinephrine in the plasma of blood from a single hypophysial portal vessel is appreciably less than that in arterial plasma (Reymond and Porter, 1982). This finding is consistent with the view that norepinephrine and epinephrine may be extracted from arterial blood by the median eminence. The effect, if any, of norepinephrine and epinephrine on the function of the median eminence is not known.

V. Dopamine Concentration in Blood of Individual Portal Vessels

It has long been recognized that blood of a given hypophysial portal vessel is not homogeneously distributed throughout the pars distalis (Adams *et al.*, 1965; Porter *et al.*, 1971). We have observed that blood from a portal vessel located centrally on the pituitary stalk often goes to the central portion of the gland, whereas blood from a lateral portal vessel goes to a lateral region of the gland (Fig. 2). However, on occasion, blood from a portal vessel on one side of the pituitary stalk will go

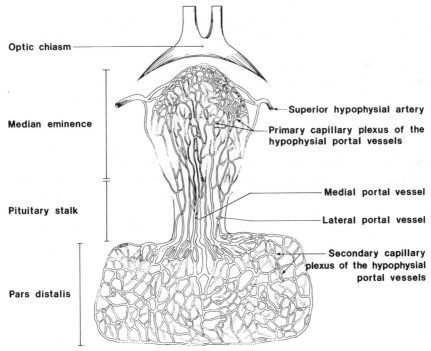

FIG. 2. Schematic representation of the hypothalamic–hypophysial portal vasculature of the rat.

to the contralateral side of the pars distalis. Despite such variance, however, it seems clear that blood from a single portal vessel is rarely distributed throughout the pars distalis.

Thus, the restricted distribution of blood from a given portal vessel within the pars distalis makes important the question of whether the concentration of a given hypothalamic hormone in blood of one portal vessel differs from that of another vessel. If variation does exist, then cells in one part of the pars distalis would be affected differently from those in another, depending upon the concentration of the hypothalamic hormone in the blood perfusing those particular pituitary cells.

Of all the hypothalamic hormones known to be released into hypophysial portal blood, dopamine appears to be present in highest concentration and therefore is among the easiest to quantify. In portal plasma of rats, the concentration of dopamine may be as great as 10 nM (Ben-Jonathan et al., 1977), whereas LHRH and CRF are present in concentrations of 0.1 nM (Eskay et al., 1977; Gibbs and Vale, 1982). Thus, we asked the question: Is the concentration of dopamine in blood of a portal vessel that is located laterally on the pituitary stalk and drains capillaries in the lateral region of the median eminence different from the concentration of dopamine in blood of a portal vessel that is located centrally on the pituitary stalk and drains capillaries in the central region of the median eminence (Fig. 2)?

To address this question, we collected blood from a lateral portal vessel or a central portal vessel of female rats that were in the diestrous phase of their ovulatory cycle. The blood was collected through a microcannula—the tip of which was directed toward the hypothalamus—to enable us to collect the venous effluent of a circumscribed part of the median eminence draining into one portal vessel. We (unpublished observations) found that the concentration of dopamine in blood from a centrally located portal vessel was two times that in blood from a portal vessel located on the right or left side of the pituitary stalk. There was no difference in the concentration of dopamine in blood from vessels located on the right or left side of the stalk. When the rates of release were calculated, it was found that the rate of release of dopamine into a central portal vessel was more than two times that into a lateral portal vessel.

In order to ascertain whether the reduced rate of dopamine release into a lateral portal vessel compared to a central vessel was due to a reduced rate of biosynthesis of dopamine in the lateral regions of the median eminence compared to that in the central region of the median eminence, we measured the rate of accumulation of L-dihydroxyphenylalanine (DOPA) in these regions of the brains of rats treated with NSD 1015 (3-hydroxybenzylhydrazine), an inhibitor of the activity of aromatic L-amino acid decarboxylase in the brain (Carlsson *et al.*, 1972; Carlsson and Lindqvist, 1973) and in particular the median eminence (Demarest and Moore, 1980; Reymond and Porter, 1982). Surprisingly, the rate of accumulation of DOPA in the lateral median eminence was not different from that in the medial median eminence. If it be true that the rate of biosynthesis of DOPA in the median eminence reflects the rate of biosynthesis of dopamine, it follows that the rate of biosynthesis of dopamine in the lateral median eminence is the same as that in the medial median eminence.

Thus, it seems paradoxical that the rate of release of dopamine into blood of a lateral portal vessel is less than that into blood of a medial portal vessel. It is possible that dopamine in the lateral median eminence is metabolized faster than that in the medial median eminence. However, the appropriateness of this last possibility seems suspect since Selmanoff (1981) failed to demonstrate a difference in the turnover of dopamine in the lateral median eminence and medial median eminence. Indeed, Löfström *et al.* (1976) observed a slower turnover of dopamine in the lateral median eminence than in the medial median eminence. After an analysis of this issue, we are led to suggest that dopamine released in the lateral zone of the median eminence may be more likely to enter such spaces as neurons, glial cells, cerebrospinal fluid (CSF), etc., than is dopamine released from neuronal endings in the medial median eminence.

On the basis of these observations, it follows that the location of dopaminergic neuronal endings in the median eminence is an important determinant in the establishment of the concentration of dopamine in blood going to a specific zone of the pars distalis. Although unproven, such a consideration may be important for other hypothalamic hormones as well.

It is interesting to speculate that certain anomalous functions of the pars distalis may be consequences of a heterogeneous composition of the affluent blood of this gland. Is it possible that in some instances the concentration of dopamine in portal blood perfusing a particular group of prolactin-secreting cells is sufficiently low that the lactotrophs are not suppressed, resulting in hypersecretion of prolactin by these cells and perhaps hypertrophy of the cells as well? If so, and if the hypertrophy were extensive, a localized tumor of the pars distalis would occur. This may be the reason why some prolactin-secreting pituitary tumors respond to treatment with a dopamine agonist, e.g., bromoergocryptine, not only by a reduction in the rate of release of prolactin but also by a reduction in the apparent mass of the tumor.

It is interesting that prolactin-secreting tumors of the pituitary gland often possess a cyanotic appearance. We speculate that the cyanosis is a consequence of the fact that the rate of blood flow through the pars distalis, including a tumor, is determined at the level of the arterioles of the neurohypophysis and not at the level of the pars distalis. Thus, as a tumor enlarges, its rate of perfusion, i.e., volume of blood per unit volume of tissue per unit time, becomes less. When the tumor becomes sufficiently large that its blood flow is inadequate to meet the metabolic requirements of the tissue, cyanosis of the tumor tissue occurs.

A consequence of an inadequate perfusion would be an accumulation of acidic metabolites and an increase in the hydrogen ion concentration in the vicinity of the tumor. Inasmuch as bone tissue is never far from the pituitary gland, an adjacent acidic zone would result in dissolution of the sphenoid bone and distortion of the sella turcica as a consequence of weakened, decalcified bone. Indeed, distortion of the sella turcica, when documented, is an important means of verifying the presence of a pituitary tumor (Ezrin *et al.*, 1980). After successful therapy with a dopamine agonist has resulted in a reduction of the mass of the tumor, reossification of the sphenoid bone of the sella turcica occurs. In light of the above argument, reossification would be expected. As the tumor shrinks, its rate of perfusion should increase, the accumulation of acidic metabolites within and around the tumor should diminish, dissolution of the bone of the sella turcica should cease, and remodeling of the floor of the sella turcica should occur as a consequence of the deposition of new bone.

VI. Transport of Pituitary Hormones to the Brain

A. Systemic Circulation

The observation that certain pituitary hormones can, under appropriate experimental conditions, affect the activity of neurons of the brain has raised the question of whether such hormones normally exercise such a role and, if so, of the mechanism whereby peptide and protein hormones of pituitary origin reach the brain. Broadwell and Brightman (1976), using an immunocytochemical procedure, demonstrated that horseradish peroxidase injected into the general circulation could enter the brain, especially the ventral hypothalamus. If this finding is indicative of a general phenomenon and not an event peculiar to horseradish peroxidase, it would appear that pituitary hormones in the systemic circulation could serve as a significant source of hormones that affect brain function.

Although unequivocal evidence for a significant transport of pituitary hormones from the circulation into cerebrospinal fluid is sparse (Clemens and Sawyer, 1974; Login and MacLeod, 1977; Perlow, 1982), there is evidence showing that prolactin, when injected systemically, leads to an increase in the turnover of dopamine in some neurons of the brain (Hökfelt and Fuxe, 1972; Gudelsky *et al.*, 1976; Andersson *et al.*, 1981), suggesting that circulating prolactin does enter the brain. At present, however, the precise relationship of the concentration of prolactin in the circulation to the transport of prolactin into the brain is not clearly defined.

It is of interest that, in certain pathological conditions, the concentration of prolactin in cerebrospinal fluid of women appears to be increased over that of healthy women. Bates *et al.* (1982a) observed that the concentration of prolactin in cerebrospinal fluid of young women diagnosed as having pseudotumor cerebri—a condition characterized by elevated intracranial pressure in the absence of a space-occupying lesion, an acute ventricular enlargement, or a sudden occlusion of a venous sinus (Raichle *et al.*, 1978)—was twice that of subjects without the disease. Bates *et al.* (1982b) found that treatment of subjects having pseudotumor cerebri with bromoergocryptine for 5 days resulted in a 60% reduction in the concentration of prolactin in cerebrospinal fluid. Inasmuch as the circulating concentration of prolactin in these young women with pseudotumor cerebri was not appreciably different before treatment from that of healthy young women, it is reasonable to suspect that the process leading to the entry of prolactin into the brain may be accentuated in persons with this disease.

In subjects with pseudotumor cerebri, Bates *et al.* (1982a) advanced the view that a cause-and-effect relationship may exist between the elevated concentration of prolactin in cerebrospinal fluid and the rate of formation of this fluid. Their suggestion is interesting in view of reports on the presence of prolactin receptors in the brain, viz. ependymal cells of the choroid plexus of the rat (Walsh *et al.*, 1978) and hypothalamus of the rabbit (Di Carlo and Muccioli, 1981).

B. Retrograde Transport by Way of the Pituitary Stalk

1. *Neurohypophysial Vasculature*

In addition to the general circulation, other mechanisms have been proposed as a means of deliverance of pituitary hormones to the brain. These include the transport of pituitary hormones to the brain by way of the vasculature of the neurohypophysis. (This vasculature is not to be confused with the hypophysial portal vessels.)

As noted earlier, Page (1983) observed in the pig that the direction of blood flow in the neurohypophysis is simultaneously from the median eminence toward the pars neuralis and from the pars neuralis toward the median eminence with the two flows meeting along a variable front in the pituitary stalk. Such an arrangement could provide a means for retrograde transport in the stalk of pituitary hormones. Hormones secreted by cells in the three major divisions of the pituitary gland, viz. the pars neuralis, pars intermedia, and pars distalis, could diffuse into the blood of the capillary plexus of the pars neuralis and be transported thereby up the stalk to the point where the interface is established with blood from the median eminence (Fig. 1).

The concentrations of pituitary hormones in the neurohypophysial capillary plexus are many times greater than in the peripheral circulation. This phenomenon should be conducive to further diffusion, along a concentration gradient, into regions of low pituitary hormone concentration. Such regions include the median eminence, ventromedial hypothalamus, as well as blood in the primary capillary plexus of the hypophysial portal vessels, whence the hormones could be returned to the pars distalis. This system would provide a countercurrent mechanism that would result in the establishment of high concentrations of pituitary hormones in the blood around the cells of both the neurohypophysis and adenohypophysis.

Retrograde transport of pituitary hormones involves first diffusion into the capillary plexus of the distal neurohypophysis, then transport up the stalk in the neurohypophysial capillaries, followed by diffusion into the upper neurohypophysis (Fig. 1). It is emphasized that net diffusion always occurs along a concentration gradient (Jacobs, 1967). In such a model as envisioned here, the concentration of pituitary hormones would be exceedingly high in the blood of the neurohypophysial capillary plexus compared to that in blood of the general circulation. Thus, the effect of pituitary hormones on brain cells that lie within diffusion distances of the neurohypophysial vasculature must be interpreted in light of high concentrations of such hormones.

It might be argued that the polypeptide and protein hormones of the pituitary gland would not be expected to diffuse through tissue so easily as envisioned here. We do not believe such an argument is valid. First, diffusion from the surface of any extravascular secretory cell (as opposed to an immunoglobulin-secreting lymphocyte within the circulation) into nearby capillaries or sinuses is part of the mechanism by which all secretory products of cells, protein and otherwise, reach the blood. Moreover, it is well known that pituitary glands, when incubated under *in vitro* conditions in the absence of blood flow, release polypeptide and protein hormones into the surrounding incubation medium. In addition, it has been shown that pituitary and hypothalamic hormones, when injected intracerebroventricularly into rats, readily diffuse through the median eminence into hypophysial portal blood (Ondo *et al.*, 1972, 1973; Oliver *et al.*, 1975).

There is other evidence to suggest validity of the thesis of retrograde transport of pituitary hormones to the brain by way of the pituitary stalk. Oliver *et al.* (1977) collected blood from a single hypophysial portal vessel through a microcannula, the tip of which was directed toward the median eminence. (It is worth repeating that the direction of blood flow in the portal vasculature is from the hypothalamus to the pars distalis. Moreover, we have found that the blood pressure in the portal vessels is equal to that of 20–25 cm of water. Therefore, flow of blood in the portal vessel from the pars distalis to the cannula was not a factor in these experiments.) The plasma of the portal blood was analyzed for the following hormones: LH, TSH, prolactin, ACTH, melanocyte-stimulating hormone (α-MSH), and vasopressin. It was found that the concentration of each of these hormones in the portal blood was 100–500 times that of the corresponding hormone in the general circulation. Hypophysectomy reduced markedly the concentration in portal blood of each hormone.

These findings are supportive of the view that hormones transported retrograde to the upper neurohypophysis in the neurohypophysial vasculature diffuse into the surrounding tissue, including blood in the hypophysial portal circulation (Fig. 1). Such diffusion is made possible by the fact that the blood entering the hypophysial portal vasculature contains low concentrations of pituitary hormones, being as it is an aliquot of the blood in the general circulation.

Additional support for the concept of retrograde transport of pituitary hormones to the brain was provided by Mezey *et al.* (1978) and Dorsa *et al.* (1979). Mezey *et al.* (1978) injected into the pars distalis a small volume of a solution containing radiolabeled ACTH 4–9. Within a short time, radioactivity was measurable in the brain, with the highest concentration being present in hypothalamic tissue. Dorsa *et al.* (1979) conducted a similar experiment in which neurotensin was injected into the pars distalis and obtained evidence for the transport of this peptide to the hypothalamus as well as evidence for an action of neurotensin on hypothalamic neurons.

2. Axonal Transport

The experiments of Mezey et al. (1978) and Dorsa et al. (1979) make it clear that ACTH 4–9 and neurotensin did not reach the hypothalamus by way of the general circulation; but it is possible, although not highly probable, that their molecular probes were transported to the hypothalamus by way of neuronal axons of the pituitary stalk. Fisher et al. (1978) found that when a solution of horseradish peroxidase is injected into the pituitary gland, the enzyme appears to be internalized by neuronal terminals in the pars neuralis and transported to the perikarya of these cells in the hypothalamus. Inasmuch as Fisher et al. (1978) examined the brain 18–24 hours after injection when transport had already occurred, it is uncertain how much time is required for the retrograde transport of a protein by nerve axons to their perikarya.

VII. HYPOTHALAMIC SECRETION OF DOPAMINE AND ITS REGULATION

The rate of release of dopamine into hypophysial portal blood of rats is influenced by a variety of hormones and drugs as well as age of the animals. Ben-Jonathan et al. (1977) observed that, during the estrous cycle, the concentration of dopamine in portal blood varies significantly, being highest on the day of estrus and lowest on proestrus. Although the concentration of dopamine in portal blood of female rats is consistently higher than that of male rats (Ben-Jonathan et al., 1977; Gudelsky and Porter, 1981), this sex difference is diminished by chronic treatment of male rats with estradiol. Moreover, the concentration of dopamine in portal blood of female rats can be markedly increased by treating them chronically with estradiol (Gudelsky et al., 1981a). The increase in the concentration of dopamine in portal blood is due to an increased release of dopamine by hypothalamic neurons and not to a change in hypophysial blood flow.

In rats treated with prolactin, Hökfelt and Fuxe (1972), Gudelsky et al. (1976), Annunziato and Moore (1978), Selmanoff (1981), and Andersson et al. (1981) observed that the turnover of dopamine in the median eminence was greater than that of rats not treated with prolactin. Hyperprolactinemia induced in rats by treatment with dopaminergic antagonists also results in increased turnover of dopamine in the median eminence (Gudelsky and Moore, 1977). Although the median eminence contains neuronal terminals of dopaminergic neurons as well as noradrenergic neurons, prolactin affects the turnover of dopamine but not norepinephrine (Selmanoff, 1981). Moreover, Selmanoff (1981) found that prolactin treatment results in a marked increase in the turnover of dopamine not only in the medial median eminence but also in the lateral median eminence.

Intracerebroventricular administration of prolactin to rats causes a marked increase in the release of hypothalamic dopamine into hypophysial portal blood (Gudelsky and Porter, 1980). Hyperprolactinemia also leads to an increase in the release of hypothalamic dopamine (Cramer et al., 1979; Gudelsky and Porter, 1980). As noted earlier, treatment of rats with estradiol for several days results in a simultaneous increase in the release of dopamine into hypophysial portal blood by the hypothalamus and of prolactin into the general circulation by the pituitary gland. Inasmuch as dopamine is an inhibitor of prolactin release, these two findings, when occurring simultaneously, appear paradoxical.

We suggest the following explanation for these findings. Although dopamine is an inhibitor of the release of prolactin, the efficacy of dopamine as such an inhibitor is readily impaired. Nansel et al. (1981) found that anterior pituitary tissue from estradiol-treated rats, when incubated in the presence of dopamine, released prolactin at a rate that was similar to that seen in the absence of dopamine. The release of prolactin from pituitary tissue from animals not treated with estradiol was markedly suppressed when incubated in the presence of the same concentration of dopamine. Thus, with respect to the prolactin-secreting cells of the pars distalis, estradiol appears to act as an antidopaminergic agent (Raymond et al., 1978; Ferland et al., 1979). If this explanation of this action of estradiol is correct, it would provide a basis for the hyperprolactinemia that occurs in animals treated with estrogen, in human newborns who are exposed in utero to high estrogen stimulation (Hauth et al., 1978), as well as in pregnant women (unpublished observations).

It seems likely that the high rate of release of dopamine by dopaminergic neurons of the hypothalamus following estrogen treatment is a consequence of stimulation of these neurons by prolactin. Evidence for this view is provided by the observation that the rate of dopamine release into portal blood by hyperprolactinemic rats can be significantly reduced by treatment of the animals with antiserum to prolactin (Gudelsky and Porter, 1980). Thus, the following conclusions seem warranted: estradiol inhibits the action of dopamine on prolactin-secreting cells, resulting in hyperprolactinemia, and hyperprolactinemia in turn results in an increase in the release of dopamine into hypophysial portal blood.

The release of hypothalamic dopamine into hypophysial portal blood is readily suppressed by certain agents. Morphine, β-endorphin, or the synthetic analog of enkephalin, [D-Ala²]-methionine-enkephalin-amide, administered intracerebroventricularly or systemically, suppresses the release of dopamine into portal blood of rats (Gudelsky and Porter, 1979a; Reymond et al., 1983). Morphine appears to inhibit the release of hypothalamic dopamine by acting on cells of the arcuate nuclei. When morphine is instilled into the arcuate nuclei by microiontophoresis, the release of dopamine is promptly suppressed (Haskins et al., 1981). Instillation of sodium chloride, as opposed to morphine, has no effect on the release of dopamine, and pretreatment of the animals with naloxone, a specific opiate antagonist, inhibits the action of morphine instilled into the arcuate nuclei. As one would expect, the suppression of dopamine release by instillation of morphine into the arcuate nuclei is associated with a marked increase in the release of prolactin.

Opiate-like peptides may act in monkeys in a manner similar to that seen for rats. When β-endorphin is administered to intact monkeys, a marked increase in the release of prolactin occurs. Yet, when this opiate-like peptide was given to monkeys in which the pituitary stalk had been transected, no effect on the release of prolactin was observed (Wardlaw et al., 1980b). This finding is consistent with the interpretation that β-endorphin suppresses dopamine release into hypophysial portal blood, resulting in a reduction of the concentration of dopamine in blood going to the pars distalis and, in turn, in an increase in the release of prolactin from the prolactin-secreting cells of the pars distalis.

The median eminence contains a high concentration of monoamines, especially dopamine, that are localized principally in the nerve endings (Carlsson et al., 1962; Fuxe, 1964; Fuxe and Hökfelt, 1966). Thus, the question arises: Is hypothalamic dopamine that is released into hypophysial portal blood derived primarily from the dopamine stores? Or, is it derived from newly synthesized dopamine?

The evidence available is supportive of the view that newly synthesized dopamine, and not stored dopamine, is preferentially released into portal blood. This conclusion is based on the following evidence. Treatment of rats with α-methyl-p-tyrosine, an inhibitor of the activity of tyrosine hydroxylase, results in an abrupt reduction in the release of dopamine (Gudelsky and Porter, 1979b). Similarly, inhibition of dopamine synthesis by the administration of 3-hydroxybenzylhydrazine (NSD 1015), an agent that inhibits the activity of the enzyme aromatic L-amino acid decarboxylase in the central nervous system (Carlsson et al., 1972; Carlsson and Linqvist, 1973), leads to an immediate inhibition of dopamine release into portal blood (Reymond and Porter, 1982). Within 30 minutes of the treatment with NSD 1015, the quantity of DOPA, the precursor of dopamine, increases manyfold in the median eminence (Demarest et al., 1979; Demarest and Moore, 1980). Approximately 18% of the newly synthesized dopamine in the median eminence is released into portal blood (Reymond and Porter, 1982). Such observations leave unanswered the function of the large quantity of dopamine stored in hypothalamic neurons. Although such stores do not constitute a static pool, the relationship, if any, of these stores to pituitary function is obscure.

In addition to hormones and various drugs that affect dopamine secretion, the release of dopamine into hypophysial portal blood by hypothalamic neurons is appreciably less in old rats of both sexes than in young, mature rats (Gudelsky et al., 1981b; Reymond and Porter, 1981). This reduced secretion of dopamine into portal blood in old rats appears to be due mostly, if not entirely, to an inability of hypothalamic neurons to synthesize sufficient DOPA from tyrosine. Increasing the availability of tyrosine, however, has no effect on the release of dopamine, indicating that availability of tyrosine does not ordinarily limit the rate of secretion of dopamine.

However, treatment of old rats with DOPA results in a marked increase (50-fold) in the concentration of dopamine in portal blood without an appreciable change in the concentration of dopamine in arterial blood (Reymond and Porter, 1981). Thus, it appears that the rate of release of dopamine into portal blood is influenced to a major extent by the availability of DOPA. Although it has not been determined unequivocally that systemically administered DOPA is converted to dopamine in hypothalamic dopaminergic neurons, it is clear that the synthesis of dopamine takes place in the median eminence; and, it is reasonable to suspect that the conversion occurs in the dopaminergic neurons.

Although the rate of release of dopamine into hypophysial portal blood is usually sufficient to account for hypothalamic control of prolactin release, there is evidence to suggest that a hypothalamic releasing factor(s) for prolactin (PRF) also exists (Clemens et al., 1977, 1978). In addition, it has long been known that serotonin, injected intracerebroventricularly into rats, results in a marked release of prolactin (Kamberi et al., 1971). Recently, Pilotte and Porter (1981) demonstrated that treatment of rats with serotonin can lead to the release of prolactin even though the concentration of dopamine in the circulation was maintained at a high concentration by an intravenous infusion of dopamine. Inasmuch as serotonin is not believed to affect the release of prolactin by a direct action on prolactin-secreting cells (Lamberts and MacLeod, 1978), it is reasonable to conclude that serotonin, administered intracerebroventricularly, causes the release of prolactin by stimulating the release of a PRF from the hypothalamus as well as by inhibiting the release of hypothalamic dopamine.

Although the identity of such a factor remains to be established, it is interesting to consider the vasoactive intestinal peptide (VIP) as a candidate for the role of PRF. Since the concentration of VIP in plasma of hypophysial portal blood is significantly increased following the intracerebroventricular injection of serotonin (Shimatsu et al., 1982) and since VIP stimulates the release of prolactin from the anterior pituitary gland (Kato et al., 1978; Ruberg et al., 1978; Shaar et al., 1979; Gourdji et al., 1979), it is reasonable to suspect that serotonin stimulates the release of prolactin through the intermediacy of VIP. Considerable strength would be added to this argument if it could be demonstrated that in vivo neutralization of VIP by the administration of antibodies to VIP prevented the release of prolactin following the administration of serotonin.

VIII. Summary

1. The neurohypophysis, which for operational purposes can be considered to consist of the median eminence, pituitary stalk, and pars neuralis, receives arterial blood that is distributed throughout the neurohypophysis by means of a capillary plexus that forms a vascular continuum throughout this portion of the brain.

2. The venous drainage of the neurohypophysis, by way of veins, connects the pars neuralis with the cavernous sinus and by way of portal vessels connects the median eminence and pituitary stalk with the pars distalis.

3. The pars distalis of the adenohypophysis receives only venous blood by way of hypophysial portal vessels. The primary capillary plexus of the portal vessels lies in the median eminence and pituitary stalk; the secondary capillary plexus of these vessels lies in the pars distalis.

4. Neurosecretory cells lying within diffusion distances of the primary capillary plexus of the portal vessels secrete products that diffuse into the blood of the portal vessels. Such products include CRF, LHRH, TRH, VIP, somatostatin, β-endorphin, and dopamine.

5. The concentration of dopamine in blood of the portal vessels draining the medial median eminence is twice the concentration of

dopamine in blood of the portal vessels draining the lateral median eminence. Inasmuch as blood from each portal vessel is not distributed homogeneously throughout the pars distalis, heterogeneity in the concentrations of dopamine in blood of various portal vessels could lead to dissimilar inhibitions of prolactin-secreting cells of the pars distalis. We speculate that prolactin cells perfused with portal blood containing a low concentration of dopamine may become hypersecretors of prolactin and possible foci for the development of pituitary tumors.

6. Pituitary hormones may reach the brain, especially the ventral diencephalon, by one of three routes: (1) the systemic circulation, (2) retrograde transport in the vasculature of the pituitary stalk, and (3) retrograde transport by way of neurohypophysial axons.

7. There is strong evidence to support the view that some pituitary hormones act on neurons of the hypothalamus to alter their activity. Prolactin acts on dopaminergic neurons to cause increased synthesis of dopamine as well as increased release of dopamine into hypophysial portal blood. Opiate-like peptides, e.g., β-endorphin, inhibit the release of dopamine into hypophysial portal blood. Inasmuch as morphine, when instilled by microiontophoresis into the arcuate nuclei, suppresses the release of hypothalamic dopamine, we speculate that the opiate-like peptides act in a similar manner.

ACKNOWLEDGMENT

The authors are most appreciative of the editorial assistance provided by Ms. Anita Crockett in the preparation of this manuscript.

REFERENCES

Adams, J. H., Daniel, P. M., and Prichard, M. M. L. (1963a). Volume of the infarct in the anterior lobe of the monkey's pituitary gland shortly after stalk section. *Nature (London)* **198**, 1205–1206.

Adams, J. H., Daniel, P. M., and Prichard, M. M. L. (1963b). The effect of stalk section on the volume of the pituitary gland of the sheep. *Acta Endocrinol. (Copenhagen)*, Suppl. **81**, 3–27.

Adams, J. H., Daniel, P. M., and Prichard, M. M. L. (1963c). The volumes of pars distalis, pars intermedia and infundibular process of the pituitary gland of the rat, with special reference to the effect of stalk section. *Q. J. Exp. Physiol.* **48**, 217–234.

Adams, J. H., Daniel, P. M., Prichard, M. M. L., and Schurr, P. H. (1963d). The volume of the infarct in pars distalis of a human pituitary gland, 30 hr after transection of the pituitary stalk. *J. Physiol. (London)* **166**, 39P–41P.

Adams, J. H., Daniel, P. M., and Prichard, M. M. L. (1964). Transection of the pituitary stalk in the goat, and its effect on the volume of the pituitary gland. *J. Pathol. Bacteriol.* **87**, 1–14.

Adams, J. H., Daniel, P. M., and Prichard, M. M. L. (1965). Observations on the portal circulation of the pituitary gland. *Neuroendocrinology* **1**, 193–213.

Adams, J. H., Daniel, P. M., and Prichard, M. M. L. (1966). The long-term effect of transection of the pituitary stalk on the volume of the pituitary gland of the adult goat. *Acta Endocrinol. (Copenhagen)* **51**, 377–390.

Andersson, K., Fuxe, K., Eneroth, P., Nyberg, F., and Roos, P. (1981). Rat prolactin and hypothalamic catecholamine nerve terminal systems. Evidence for rapid and discrete increases in dopamine and noradrenaline turnover in the hypophysectomized male rat. *Eur. J. Pharmacol.* **76**, 261–265.

Annunziato, L., and Moore, K. E. (1978). Prolactin in CSF selectively increases dopamine turnover in the median eminence. *Life Sci.* **22**, 2037–2042.

Arimura, A., Sato, H., Kumasaka, T., Worobec, R. B., Debeljuk, L., Dunn, V., and Schally, A. V. (1973). Production of antiserum to LH-releasing hormone (LH-RH) associated with gonadal atrophy in rabbits: Development of radioimmunoassays for LH-RH. *Endocrinology* **93**, 1092–1103.

Bates, G. W., Whitworth, N. S., Parker, J. L., and Johnson, M. P. (1982a). Elevated cerebrospinal fluid prolactin concentration in women with pseudotumor cerebri. *South. Med. J.* **75**, 807–808.

Bates, G. W., Whitworth, N. S., Parker, J. L., and Johnson, M. P. (1982b). Effect of bromocriptine on cerebral spinal fluid prolactin in women with pseudotumor cerebri. *Annu. Meet. Soc. Gynecol. Invest., 29th, Dallas, Texas,* p. 9.

Ben-Jonathan, N., Oliver, C., Weiner, H. J., Mical, R. S., and Porter, J. C. (1977). Dopamine in hypophysial portal plasma of the rat during the estrous cycle and throughout pregnancy. *Endocrinology* **100**, 452–458.

Broadwell, R. D., and Brightman, M. W. (1976). Entry of peroxidase into neurons of the central and peripheral nervous systems from extracerebral and cerebral blood. *J. Comp. Neurol.* **166**, 257–284.

Carlsson, A., and Lindqvist, M. (1973). In-vivo measurements of tryptophan and tyrosine hydroxylase activities in mouse brain. *J. Neural Transm.* **34**, 79–91.

Carlsson, A., Falck, B., and Hillarp, N. A. (1962). Cellular localization of brain monoamines. *Acta Physiol. Scand. Suppl.* **196**, 1–28.

Carlsson, A., Davis, J. N., Kehr, W., Lindqvist, M., and Atack, C. V. (1972). Simultaneous measurement of tyrosine and tryptophan hydroxylase activities in brain *in vivo* using an inhibitor of the aromatic amino acid decarboxylase. *Naunyn-Schmiedebergs Arch. Pharmacol.* **275**, 153–168.

Carmel, P. W., Araki, S., and Ferin, M. (1976). Pituitary stalk portal blood collection in rhesus monkeys: Evidence for pulsatile release of gonadotropin-releasing hormone (GnRH). *Endocrinology* **99**, 243–248.

Chihara, K., Arimura, A., and Schally, A. V. (1979a). Immunoreactive somatostatin in rat hypophyseal portal blood: Effects of anesthetics. *Endocrinology* **104**, 1434–1441.

Chihara, K., Arimura, A., Kubli-Garfias, C., and Schally, A. V. (1979b). Enhancement of immunoreactive somatostatin release into hypophysial portal blood by electrical stimulation of the preoptic area in the rat. *Endocrinology* **105**, 1416–1418.

Chihara, K., Minamitani, N., Kaji, H., Arimura, A., and Fujita, T. (1981). Intraventricularly injected growth hormone stimulates somatostatin release into rat hypophysial portal blood. *Endocrinology* **109**, 2279–2281.

Clemens, J. A., and Sawyer, B. D. (1974). Identification of prolactin in cerebrospinal fluid. *Exp. Brain Res.* **21**, 399–402.

Clemens, J. A., and Shaar, C. J. (1980). Control of prolactin secretion in mammals. *Fed. Proc. Fed. Am. Soc. Exp. Biol.* **39**, 2588–2592.

Clemens, J. A., Sawyer, B. D., and Cerimele, B. (1977). Further evidence that serotonin is a neurotransmitter involved in the control of prolactin secretion. *Endocrinology* **100**, 692–698.

Clemens, J. A., Roush, M. E., and Fuller, R. W. (1978). Evidence that serotonin neurons stimulate secretion of prolactin releasing factor. *Life Sci.* **22,** 2209–2214.

Cramer, O. M., Parker, C. R., Jr., and Porter, J. C. (1979). Secretion of dopamine into hypophysial portal blood by rats bearing prolactin-secreting tumors or ectopic pituitary glands. *Endocrinology* **105,** 636–640.

Daniel, P. M., and Prichard, M. M. L. (1956). Anterior pituitary necrosis. Infarction of the pars distalis produced experimentally in the rat. *Q. J. Exp. Physiol.* **41,** 215–229.

Daniel, P. M., and Prichard, M. M. L. (1957a). The vascular arrangements of the pituitary gland of the sheep. *Q. J. Exp. Physiol.* **42,** 237–248.

Daniel, P. M., and Prichard, M. M. L. (1957b). Anterior pituitary necrosis in the sheep produced by section of the pituitary stalk. *Q. J. Exp. Physiol.* **42,** 248–254.

Daniel, P. M., and Prichard, M. M. L. (1958). The effects of pituitary stalk section in the goat. *Am. J. Pathol.* **34,** 433–469.

Daniel, P. M., Prichard, M. M. L., and Schurr, P. H. (1958). Extent of the infarct in the anterior lobe of the human pituitary gland after stalk section. *Lancet* **1,** 1101–1103.

Daniel, P. M., Prichard, M. M. L., and Smith, B. (1959). The extent of the infarct in the anterior pituitary found soon after pituitary stalk section in the baboon and the rhesus monkey. *J. Physiol. (London)* **146,** 2P–3P.

Daniel, P. M., Duchen, L. W., and Prichard, M. M. L. (1964a). The cytology of the pituitary gland of the rhesus monkey: Changes in the gland and its target organs after section of the pituitary stalk. *J. Pathol. Bacteriol.* **87,** 385–393.

Daniel, P. M., Duchen, L. W., and Prichard, M. M. L. (1964b). The effect of transection of the pituitary stalk on the cytology of the pituitary gland of the rat. *Q. J. Exp. Physiol.* **49,** 235–242.

Dávid, M. A., Csernay, L., László, F. A., and Kovács, K. (1965). Hypophysial blood flow in rats after destruction of the pituitary stalk. *Endocrinology* **77,** 183–187.

de Greef, W. J., and Visser, T. J. (1981). Evidence for the involvement of hypothalamic dopamine and thyrotrophin-releasing hormone in suckling-induced release of prolactin. *J. Endocrinol.* **91,** 213–223.

Demarest, K. T., and Moore, K. E. (1980). Accumulation of L-dopa in the median eminence: An index of tuberoinfundibular dopaminergic nerve activity. *Endocrinology* **106,** 463–468.

Demarest, K. T., Alper, R. H., and Moore, K. E. (1979). Dopa accumulation is a measure of dopamine synthesis in the median eminence and posterior pituitary. *J. Neural Transm.* **46,** 183–193.

Di Carlo, R., and Muccioli, G. (1981). Presence of specific prolactin binding sites in the rabbit hypothalamus. *Life Sci.* **28,** 2299–2307.

Dorsa, D. M., de Kloet, E. R., Mezey, E., and de Wied, D. (1979). Pituitary-brain transport of neurotensin: Functional significance of retrograde transport. *Endocrinology* **104,** 1663–1666.

Eskay, R. L., Oliver, C., Ben-Jonathan, N., and Porter, J. C. (1975). Hypothalamic hormones in portal and systemic blood. *In* "Hypothalamic Hormones: Chemistry, Physiology, Pharmacology and Clinical Uses" (M. Motta, P. G. Crosignani, and L. Martini, eds.), pp. 125–137. Academic Press, New York.

Eskay, R. L., Mical, R. S., and Porter, J. C. (1977). Relationship between luteinizing hormone releasing hormone concentration in hypophysial portal blood and luteinizing hormone release in intact, castrated, and electrochemically-stimulated rats. *Endocrinology* **100,** 263–270.

Ezrin, C., Horvath, E., Kaufman, B., Kovacs, K., and Weiss, M. H. (eds.) (1980). "Pituitary Diseases." CRC Press, Boca Raton, Florida.

Ferland, L., Labrie, F., Euvrard, C., and Raynaud, J. P. (1979). Antidopaminergic activity of estrogens on prolactin release at the pituitary level in vivo. *Mol. Cell. Endocrinol.* **14**, 199–204.

Fink, G., and Jamieson, M. G. (1976). Immunoreactive luteinizing hormone releasing factor in rat pituitary stalk blood: Effects of electrical stimulation of the medial preoptic area. *J. Endocrinol.* **68**, 71–87.

Fink, G., Koch, Y., and Ben Aroya, N. (1982). Release of thyrotropin releasing hormone into hypophysial portal blood is high relative to other neuropeptides and may be related to prolactin secretion. *Brain Res.* **243**, 186–189.

Fisher, A. W. F., Price, P. G., Burford, G. D., and Lederis, K. (1978). A reappraisal of the topography of the rat's hypothalamo-neurohypophysial system. *In* "Current Studies of Hypothalamic Function; Vol. 1. Hormones" (K. Lederis and W. L. Veale, eds.), pp. 1–14. Karger, Basel.

Fuxe, K. (1964). Cellular localization of monoamines in the median eminence and the infundibular stem of some mammals. *Z. Zellforsch. Mikrosk. Anat.* **61**, 710–724.

Fuxe, K., and Hökfelt, T. (1966). Further evidence for the existence of tubero-infundibular dopamine neurons. *Acta Physiol. Scand.* **66**, 245–246.

Gibbs, D. M., and Vale, W. (1982). Presence of corticotropin releasing factor-like immunoreactivity in hypophysial portal blood. *Endocrinology* **111**, 1418–1420.

Gillioz, P., Giraud, P., Conte-Devolx, B., Jaquet, P., Codaccioni, J. L., and Oliver, C. (1979). Immunoreactive somatostatin in rat hypophysial portal blood. *Endocrinology* **104**, 1407–1410.

Goldman, H. (1963). Effect of acute stress on the pituitary gland: Endocrine gland blood flow. *Endocrinology* **72**, 588–591.

Goldman, H., and Sapirstein, L. A. (1962). Nature of the hypophysial blood supply in the rat. *Endocrinology* **71**, 857–858.

Gourdji, D., Bataille, D., Vauclin, N., Grouselle, D., Rosselin, G., and Tixier-Vidal, A. (1979). Vasoactive intestinal peptide (VIP) stimulates prolactin (PRL) release and cAMP production in a rat pituitary cell line (GH3/B6). Additive effects of VIP and TRH on PRL release. *FEBS Lett.* **104**, 165–168.

Green, J. D. (1947). Vessels and nerves of amphibian hypophyses. *Anat. Rec.* **99**, 21–53.

Green, J. D., and Harris, G. W. (1949). Observation of the hypophysio-portal vessels of the living rat. *J. Physiol. (London)* **108**, 359–361.

Gudelsky, G. A., and Moore, K. E. (1977). A comparison of the effects of haloperidol on dopamine turnover in the striatum, olfactory tubercle and median eminence. *J. Pharmacol. Exp. Ther.* **202**, 149–156.

Gudelsky, G. A., and Porter, J. C. (1979a). Morphine- and opioid peptide-induced inhibition of the release of dopamine from tuberoinfundibular neurons. *Life Sci.* **25**, 1697–1702.

Gudelsky, G. A., and Porter, J. C. (1979b). Release of newly synthesized dopamine into the hypophysial portal vasculature of the rat. *Endocrinology* **104**, 583–587.

Gudelsky, G. A., and Porter, J. C. (1980). Release of dopamine from tuberoinfundibular neurons into pituitary stalk blood following prolactin or haloperidol administration. *Endocrinology* **106**, 526–529.

Gudelsky, G. A., and Porter, J. C. (1981). Sex-related difference in the release of dopamine into hypophysial portal blood. *Endocrinology* **109**, 1394–1398.

Gudelsky, G. A., Simpkins, J., Mueller, G. P., Meites, J., and Moore, K. E. (1976). Selective actions of prolactin on catecholamine turnover in the hypothalamus and on serum LH and FSH. *Neuroendocrinology* **22**, 206–215.

Gudelsky, G. A., Nansel, D. D., and Porter, J. C. (1981a). Role of estrogen in the dopaminergic control of prolactin secretion. *Endocrinology* **108**, 440–444.

Gudelsky, G. A., Nansel, D. D., and Porter, J. C. (1981b). Dopaminergic control of prolactin secretion in the aging male rat. *Brain Res.* **204**, 446–450.

Harris, A. R. C., Christianson, D., Smith, M. S., Fang, S. L., Braverman, L. E., and Vagenakis, A. G. (1978). The physiological role of thyrotropin-releasing hormone in the regulation of thyroid-stimulating hormone and prolactin secretion in the rat. *J. Clin. Invest.* **61**, 441–448.

Harris, G. W. (1947). The blood vessels of the rabbit's pituitary gland, and the significance of the pars and zona tuberalis. *J. Anat.* **81**, 343–351.

Haskins, J. T., Gudelsky, G. A., Moss, R. L., and Porter, J. C. (1981). Iontophoresis of morphine into the arcuate nucleus: Effects on dopamine concentrations in hypophysial portal plasma and serum prolactin concentrations. *Endocrinology* **108**, 767–771.

Hauth, J. C., Parker, C. R., Jr., MacDonald, P. C., Porter, J. C., and Johnston, J. M. (1978). A role of fetal prolactin in lung maturation. *Obstet. Gynecol.* **51**, 81–88.

Hökfelt, T., and Fuxe, K. (1972). Effects of prolactin and ergot alkaloids on the tuberoinfundibular dopamine (DA) neurons. *Neuroendocrinology* **9**, 100–122.

Houssay, B. A., Biasotti, A., and Sammartino, R. (1935). Modifications fonctionnelles de l'hypophyse après les lésions infundibulo-tubériennes chez le crapaud. *C. R. Soc. Biol. Paris* **120**, 725–727.

Jacobs, M. H. (1967). "Diffusion Processes." Springer-Verlag, Berlin and New York.

Kamberi, I. A., Mical, R. S., and Porter, J. C. (1971). Effects of melatonin and serotonin on the release of FSH and prolactin. *Endocrinology* **88**, 1288–1293.

Kato, Y., Iwasaki, Y., Iwasaki, J., Abe, H., Yanaihara, N., and Imura, H. (1978). Prolactin release by vasoactive intestinal polypeptide in rats. *Endocrinology* **103**, 554–558.

Kizer, J. S., Humm, J., Nicholson, G., Greeley, G., and Youngblood, W. (1978). The effect of castration, thyroidectomy and haloperidol upon the turnover rates of dopamine and norepinephrine and the kinetic properties of tyrosine hydroxylase in discrete hypothalamic nuclei of the male rat. *Brain Res.* **146**, 95–107.

Koch, Y., Chobsieng, P., Zor, U., Fridkin, M., and Lindner, H. R. (1973). Suppression of gonadotropin secretion and prevention of ovulation in the rat by antiserum to synthetic gonadotropin-releasing hormone. *Biochem. Biophys. Res. Commun.* **55**, 623–629.

Koch, Y., Goldhaber, G., Fireman, I., Zor, U., Shani, J., and Tal, E. (1977). Suppression of prolactin and thyrotropin secretion in the rat by antiserum to thyrotropin-releasing hormone. *Endocrinology* **100**, 1476–1478.

Lamberts, S. W. J., and MacLeod, R. M. (1978). The interaction of the serotonergic and dopaminergic systems on prolactin secretion in the rat: The mechanism of action of the "specific" serotonin receptor antagonist, methysergide. *Endocrinology* **103**, 287–295.

Linton, E. A., Gillies, G. E., and Lowry, P. J. (1982). Synergism between vasopressin and the new 41 residue corticotrophin-releasing factor. *Annu. Meet. Endocr. Soc., 64th, San Francisco, California,* p. 83.

Löfström, A., Jonsson, G., Wiesel, F. A., and Fuxe, K. (1976). Microfluorimetric quantitation of catecholamine fluorescence in rat median eminence. II. Turnover changes in hormonal states. *J. Histochem. Cytochem.* **24**, 430–442.

Login, I. S., and MacLeod, R. M. (1977). Prolactin in human and rat serum and cerebrospinal fluid. *Brain Res.* **132**, 477–483.

172   JOHN C. PORTER ET AL.

McCormack, J. T., Plant, T. M., Hess, D. L., and Knobil, E. (1977). The effect of luteinizing hormone releasing hormone (LHRH) antiserum administration on gonadotropin secretion in the rhesus monkey. *Endocrinology* **100**, 663–667.

Marie, P. (1886). Sur deux cas d'acromégalie: Hypertrophie singulière, non congénitale, des extremités supérieures, inférieures et céphalique. *Rev. Med. (Paris)* **6**, 297–333.

Mathew, J. K., Glenn, T. C., and Sayers, G. (1982). Hypothalamic CRF's. *Annu. Meet. Endocr. Soc., 64th, San Francisco, California,* p. 83.

Mezey, E., Palkovits, M., de Kloet, E. R., Verhoef, J., and de Wied, D. (1978). Evidence for pituitary-brain transport of a behaviorally potent ACTH analog. *Life Sci.* **22**, 831–838.

Nansel, D. D., Gudelsky, G. A., Reymond, M. J., and Porter, J. C. (1981). Estrogen alters the responsiveness of the anterior pituitary gland to the actions of dopamine on lysosomal enzyme activity and prolactin release. *Endocrinology* **108**, 903–907.

Neill, J. D., Patton, J. M., Dailey, R. A., Tsou, R. C., and Tindall, G. T. (1977). Luteinizing hormone releasing hormone (LHRH) in pituitary stalk blood of rhesus monkeys: Relationship to level of LH release. *Endocrinology* **101**, 430–434.

Neill, J. D., Frawley, L. S., Plotsky, P. M., and Tindall, G. T. (1981). Dopamine in hypophysial stalk blood of the rhesus monkey and its role in regulating prolactin secretion. *Endocrinology* **108**, 489–494.

Oliver, C., Ben-Jonathan, N., Mical, R. S., and Porter, J. C. (1975). Transport of thyrotropin-releasing hormone from cerebrospinal fluid to hypophysial portal blood and the release of thyrotropin. *Endocrinology* **97**, 1138–1143.

Oliver, C., Mical, R. S., and Porter, J. C. (1977). Hypothalamic-pituitary vasculature: Evidence for retrograde blood flow in the pituitary stalk. *Endocrinology* **101**, 598–604.

Ondo, J. G., Mical, R. S., and Porter, J. C. (1972). Passage of radioactive substances from CSF to hypophysial portal blood. *Endocrinology* **91**, 1239–1246.

Ondo, J. G., Eskay, R. L., Mical, R. S., and Porter, J. C. (1973). Release of LH by LRF injected into the CSF: A transport role for the median eminence. *Endocrinology* **93**, 231–237.

Page, R. B. (1983). Directional pituitary blood flow: A microcinephotographic study. *Endocrinology* **112**, 157–165.

Page, R. B., and Bergland, R. M. (1977). The neurohypophyseal capillary bed. I. Anatomy and arterial supply. *Am. J. Anat.* **148**, 345–358.

Page, R. B., Munger, B. L., and Bergland, R. M. (1976). Scanning microscopy of pituitary vascular casts. *Am. J. Anat.* **146**, 273–302.

Page, R. B., Funsch, D. J., Brennan, R. W., and Hernandez, M. J. (1981). Regional neurohypophyseal blood flow and its control in adult sheep. *Am. J. Physiol.* **241**, R36–R43.

Palkovits, M., Brownstein, M., Saavedra, J. M., and Axelrod, J. (1974). Norepinephrine and dopamine content of hypothalamic nuclei of the rat. *Brain Res.* **77**, 137–149.

Perlow, M. J. (1982). Cerebrospinal fluid prolactin: A daily rhythm and response to an acute perturbation. *Brain Res.* **243**, 382–385.

Pietsch, K. (1930). Aufbau und Entwicklung der Pars Tuberalis des menschlichen Hirnanhangs in ihren Beziehungen zu den übrigen Hypophysenteilen. *Z. Mikrosk. Anat. Forsch.* **22**, 227–256.

Pilotte, N. S., and Porter, J. C. (1981). Dopamine in hypophysial portal plasma and prolactin in systemic plasma of rats treated with 5-hydroxytryptamine. *Endocrinology* **108**, 2137–2141.

Plotsky, P. M., Gibbs, D. M., and Neill, J. D. (1978). Liquid chromatographic-electrochemical measurement of dopamine in hypophysial stalk blood of rats. *Endocrinology* **102**, 1887–1894.

Popa, G., and Fielding, U. (1930). A portal circulation from the pituitary to the hypothalamic region. *J. Anat.* **65**, 88–91.

Popa, G. T., and Fielding, U. (1933). Hypophysio-portal vessels and their colloid accompaniment. *J. Anat.* **67**, 227–232.

Porter, J. C., and Jones, J. C. (1956). Effect of plasma from hypophyseal-portal vessel blood on adrenal ascorbic acid. *Endocrinology* **58**, 62–67.

Porter, J. C., Hines, M. F. M., Smith, K. R., Repass, R. L., and Smith, A. J. K. (1967). Quantitative evaluation of local blood flow of the adenohypophysis in rats. *Endocrinology* **80**, 583–598.

Porter, J. C., Mical, R. S., Ondo, J. G., and Kamberi, I. A. (1971). Perfusion of the rat anterior pituitary via a cannulated portal vessel. *Acta Endocrinol. (Copenhagen) Suppl.* **158**, 249–269.

Porter, J. C., Barnea, A., Cramer, O. M., and Parker, C. R., Jr., (1978). Hypothalamic peptide and catecholamine secretion: Roles for portal and retrograde blood flow in the pituitary stalk in the release of hypothalamic dopamine and pituitary prolactin and LH. *Clin. Obstet. Gynaecol.* **5**, 271–282.

Porter, J. C., Nansel, D. D., Gudelsky, G. A., Foreman, M. M., Pilotte, N. S., Parker, C. R., Jr., Burrows, G. H., Bates, G. W., and Madden, J. D. (1980). Neuroendocrine control of gonadotropin secretion. *Fed. Proc. Fed. Am. Soc. Exp. Biol.* **39**, 2896–2901.

Raichle, M. E., Grubb, R. L., Jr., Phelps, M. E., Gado, M. H., and Caronna, J. J. (1978). Cerebral hemodynamics and metabolism in pseudotumor cerebri. *Ann. Neurol.* **4**, 104–111.

Raymond, V., Beaulieu, M., Labrie, F., and Boissier, J. (1978). Potent antidopaminergic activity of estradiol at the pituitary level on prolactin release. *Science* **200**, 1173–1175.

Reymond, M. J., and Porter, J. C. (1981). Secretion of hypothalamic dopamine into pituitary stalk blood of aged female rats. *Brain Res. Bull.* **7**, 69–73.

Reymond, M. J., and Porter, J. C. (1982). Hypothalamic secretion of dopamine after inhibition of aromatic L-amino acid decarboxylase activity. *Endocrinology* **111**, 1051–1056.

Reymond, M. J., Kaur, C., and Porter, J. C. (1983). An inhibitory role for morphine on the release of dopamine into hypophysial portal blood and on the synthesis of dopamine in tuberoinfundibular neurons. *Brain Res.* **262**, 253–258.

Rivier, C., Brownstein, M., Spiess, J., Rivier, J., and Vale, W. (1982). In vivo corticotropin-releasing factor-induced secretion of adrenocorticotropin, β-endorphin, and corticosterone. *Endocrinology* **110**, 272–278.

Ruberg, M., Rotsztejn, W. H., Arancibia, S., Besson, J., and Enjalbert, A. (1978). Stimulation of prolactin release by vasoactive intestinal peptide (VIP). *Eur. J. Pharmacol.* **51**, 319–320.

Said, S. I., and Porter, J. C. (1979). Vasoactive intestinal polypeptide: Release into hypophyseal portal blood. *Life Sci.* **24**, 227–230.

Selmanoff, M. (1981). The lateral and medial median eminence: Distribution of dopamine, norepinephrine, and luteinizing hormone-releasing hormone and the effect of prolactin on catecholamine turnover. *Endocrinology* **108**, 1716–1722.

Selmanoff, M. K., Pramik-Holdaway, M. J., and Weiner, R. I. (1976). Concentrations of dopamine and norepinephrine in discrete hypothalamic nuclei during the rat estrous cycle. *Endocrinology* **99**, 326–329.

Shaar, C. J., Clemens, J. A., and Dininger, N. B. (1979). Effect of vasoactive intestinal polypeptide on prolactin release in vitro. *Life Sci.* **25,** 2071–2074.

Shimatsu, A., Kato, Y., Matsushita, N., Katakami, H., Yanaihara, N., and Imura, H. (1981). Immunoreactive vasoactive intestinal polypeptide in rat hypophysial portal blood. *Endocrinology* **108,** 395–398.

Shimatsu, A., Kato, Y., Matsushita, N., Katakami, H., Yanaihara, N., and Imura, H. (1982). Stimulation by serotonin of vasoactive intestinal polypeptide release into rat hypophysial portal blood. *Endocrinology* **111,** 338–340.

Tashjian, A. H., Jr., Barowsky, N. J., and Jensen, D. K. (1971). Thyrotropin releasing hormone: Direct evidence for stimulation of prolactin production by pituitary cells in culture. *Biochem. Biophys. Res. Commun.* **43,** 516–523.

Török, B. (1954). Lebendbeobachtung des Hypophysenkreislaufes an Hunden. *Acta Morphol. Acad. Sci. Hung.* **4,** 83–89.

Tsou, R. C., Dailey, R. A., McLanahan, C. S., Parent, A. D., Tindall, G. T., and Neill, J. D. (1977). Luteinizing hormone releasing hormone (LHRH) levels in pituitary stalk plasma during the preovulatory gonadotropin surge of rabbits. *Endocrinology* **101,** 534–539.

Vale, W., Spiess, J., Rivier, C., and Rivier, J. (1981). Characterization of a 41-residue ovine hypothalamic peptide that stimulates secretion of corticotropin and β-endorphin. *Science* **213,** 1394–1397.

Walsh, R. J., Posner, B. I., Kopriwa, B. M., and Brawer, J. R. (1978). Prolactin binding sites in the rat brain. *Science* **201,** 1041–1043.

Wardlaw, S. L., Wehrenberg, W. B., Ferin, M., Carmel, P. W., and Frantz, A. G. (1980a). High levels of β-endorphin in hypophyseal portal blood. *Endocrinology* **106,** 1323–1326.

Wardlaw, S. L., Wehrenberg, W. B., Ferin, M., and Frantz, A. G. (1980b). Failure of β-endorphin to stimulate prolactin release in the pituitary stalk-sectioned monkey. *Endocrinology* **107,** 1663–1666.

Wehrenberg, W. B., Wardlaw, S. L., Frantz, A. G., and Ferin, M. (1982). β-Endorphin in hypophyseal portal blood: Variations throughout the menstrual cycle. *Endocrinology* **111,** 879–881.

Wislocki, G. B. (1937). The vascular supply of the hypophysis cerebri of the cat. *Anat. Rec.* **69,** 361–387.

Wislocki, G. B. (1938). The vascular supply of the hypophysis cerebri of the rhesus monkey and man. *Res. Publ. Assoc. Res. Nerv. Ment. Dis.* **17,** 48–68.

Wislocki, G. B., and King, L. S. (1936). The permeability of the hypophysis and hypothalamus to vital dyes, with a study of the hypophyseal vascular supply. *Am. J. Anat.* **58,** 421–472.

Worthington, W. C., Jr. (1955). Some observations on the hypophyseal portal system in the living mouse. *Bull. Johns Hopkins Hosp.* **97,** 343–357.

Xuereb, G. P., Prichard, M. M. L., and Daniel, P. M. (1954a). The arterial supply and venous drainage of the human hypophysis cerebri. *Q. J. Exp. Physiol.* **39,** 199–217.

Xuereb, G. P., Prichard, M. M. L., and Daniel, P. M. (1954b). The hypophysial portal system of vessels in man. *Q. J. Exp. Physiol.* **39,** 219–230.

Yates, F. E., Kirschman, R., and Olshen, B. (1966). Analysis of adenohypophysial blood flow in the rat by radioisotope washout: Estimate of the vasomotor activity of vasopressin in the anterior pituitary. *Endocrinology* **79,** 341–351.

Growth and Somatomedins

K. HALL

Department of Endocrinology, Karolinska Hospital,
Stockholm, Sweden

V. R. SARA

Karolinska Institute's Department of Psychiatry, St Göran's Hospital,
Stockholm, Sweden

This article presents a personal approach to the somatomedins, from their beginnings as operationally defined activities to their emergence, in the last decade, as structural entities. In presenting such a personal viewpoint, we have not covered the entire field of somatomedin research but have attempted to give an overall concept of their integrated biological role. Additionally, we recognize the existence of other

175

growth factors isolated from serum and tissue such as epidermal growth factor and platelet-derived growth factor. However, discussion of these peptides is beyond the scope of the present article. To compensate, we direct the interested reader to several excellent reviews (van Wyk and Underwood, 1978; Carpenter and Cohen, 1979; Levi-Montalcini and Calissana, 1979; Phillips and Vassilopoulou-Sellin, 1980a,b; Hintz, 1981; Rechler *et al.*, 1981; Zapf *et al.*, 1981a; Rothstein, 1982; Preece and Holder, 1982; Heldin *et al.*, 1983).

I. Growth

The term growth is used to designate an increase in the number or size of cells. Growth occurs first as rapid proliferation, then hypertrophy and differentiation into the mature state. This pattern of growth is common to all cells but the time course is unique for each cell type. For example, the period of rapid proliferation in the brain occurs during fetal and early postnatal life, whereas in the gonads the maximum proliferative period occurs during puberty (Winick, 1968; Dobbing and Sands, 1973; Brasel and Gruen, 1978; Widdowson, 1981). Cells also differ in other characteristics such as life span and renewal ability. Blood cells such as erythrocytes have a short life span and are constantly renewed from their stem cells. The fully differentiated neuron does not normally divide during its long life span (Sara *et al.*, 1981b). Fibroblasts and hepatocytes have maintained the ability to divide. In these cells, marked proliferation can be evoked as a repair response. Thus, although statural growth is complete after puberty, it is clear that cellular growth is a continual process throughout life.

A basis for understanding this growth process and its regulation can be derived from considering the terms anabolism and catabolism in their most elementary sense. We use the term "anabolism" to refer to a building up of materials and "catabolism" to refer to a breaking down of materials. Growth results when anabolism is greater than catabolism. When both these processes are equal, the cell and organ are maintained in a steady integrated state. Aging results when anabolism is less than catabolism. Thus, according to this simplified view, growth, maintenance, and aging all depend on the relationship between cell anabolism and catabolism. It is most likely that these processes are all regulated by similar mechanisms but that the response depends upon the unique characteristics of each cell type. In this article we will discuss regulatory substances belonging to the somatomedin family and their role in growth, maintenance, and aging.

II. Anabolic Factors in Serum

The presence of growth-promoting factors in serum has been recognized since the beginning of this century. Serum has been regularly used as a constituent of cell culture media to stimulate the proliferation of cells *in vitro*. Many early attempts were made to isolate this serum-derived activity but its chemical nature remained unresolved until 1978, when Rinderknecht and Humbel sequenced insulin-like growth factor I (IGF-I), the first growth factor that was identified definitively (Rinderknecht and Humbel, 1978a). IGF-I is a member of a family of polypeptides with growth-promoting and insulin-like properties. In this article, these polypeptide hormones are termed somatomedins. They were first discovered as three different biological activities in serum, namely multiplication-stimulating activity (MSA), insulin-like activity (ILA), and sulfation factor activity (SFA).

A. Multiplication-Stimulating Activity (MSA)

Since the inception of cell culture techniques with the routine use of serum-saturated plasma clots, it has been recognized that serum is a necessary constituent of the incubation medium in order for cells to proliferate. However, the mechanism of serum action was not fully investigated until the 1960s when studies by Temin and others indicated that serum contained specific factors necessary for cell proliferation (Temin, 1971; Temin *et al.*, 1972). Some established cell lines proliferate in the absence of serum and it soon became apparent that these cells synthesize substances that could replace the serum factors necessary for cell proliferation. With one such cell line, a clone from rat liver (BRL-3A cells), Temin showed that conditioned media, from these cells added to cultures of stationary rat embryo fibroblasts stimulated DNA synthesis. Dulak and Temin (1973a,b) then partially purified the active stimulatory components from the conditioned media. This activity, called multiplication-stimulating activity (MSA), was shown to consist of several peptides (Nissley and Rechler, 1978; Moses *et al.*, 1980b).

MSA, however, cannot explain the complete growth-promoting activity of serum. The observation that platelet-poor plasma is less efficient than serum in stimulating the growth of cultured fibroblasts led to the discovery of platelet-derived growth factor (PDGF). PDGF is a cationic polypeptide with a molecular size of 33,000 (Heldin *et al.*, 1983). It does not belong to the somatomedin family of growth factors.

It seems to have specificity for connective tissue-derived cells and is proposed to be a competence factor (Clemmons and van Wyk, 1981). PDGF is proposed to play a physiological role *in vivo* as a repair factor (Ross and Glomset, 1976).

B. INSULIN-LIKE ACTIVITY (ILA)

As early as 1945, Young, in considering the anabolic actions of growth hormone and insulin, postulated the existence of an additional insulin-like hormone which promoted growth but was devoid of hypoglycemic activity. Before the development of the radioimmunoassay, insulin was determined by a bioassay measuring glucose uptake in either rat adipose or diaphragm tissue. As soon as the radioimmunoassay for insulin was developed it became apparent that human serum contained far more insulin-like activity (ILA) than could be attributed to its content of immunoreactive insulin. The portion of ILA that was not inhibited by insulin antibodies was designated "bound insulin" by Antoniades, "atypical insulin" by Samaan, and "nonsuppressible insulin-like activity" (NSILA) by Froesch (Antoniades, 1961; Samaan *et al.*, 1962; Froesch *et al.*, 1963). Successful purification was achieved by the group working with NSILA. Starting with a Cohn fraction from human plasma they found that a portion of NSILA was soluble in acid ethanol and was called NSILA-S (Froesch *et al.*, 1963; Bürgi *et al.*, 1966). An acid-stable high molecular form of ILA has also been purified from human plasma and is termed NSILP (Poffenbarger, 1975). So far, there is no evidence that it is a precursor of IGF. The purified NSILA-S was later shown to consist of two biologically active peptides, insulin-like growth factors I and II (IGF-I and IGF-II) (Rinderknecht and Humbel, 1976a).

C. SULFATION FACTOR ACTIVITY (SFA)

The significance of pituitary growth hormone (GH) for regulation of postnatal skeletal growth is uniformly accepted. A century ago the coincidence of an enlarged pituitary and enhanced growth was recognized in patients with acromegaly (Marie, 1889). Evans and Long (1921) demonstrated that crude extracts from the anterior lobe of bovine pituitary glands produced gigantism in rats. Smith (1927) produced dwarfism in rats by hypophysectomy and restored growth after administration of pituitary extracts. The width of the rat epiphyseal plate declined after hypophysectomy and increased after treatment with pituitary extract (Evans *et al.*, 1943). This bioassay guided the purification of GH. Only GH purified from human pituitary was found to restore growth in patients with pituitary dwarfism (Raben, 1958). Long-term treatment with human GH normalized growth in children with GH deficiency.

Even though the growth-promoting effect of GH *in vivo* was generally observed, few investigators were able to show a direct effect of GH on cell proliferation *in vitro*. One of the most useful measurements of the biological effects of GH has been its stimulation of the incorporation of radioactive sulfate into rat cartilage after its administration *in vivo* (Ellis *et al.*, 1953). Physiological amounts of GH added *in vitro* to rat costal cartilage, however, caused little effect on sulfate uptake. Salmon and Daughaday (1957) made the important discovery that the sulfate uptake into the rat costal cartilage was enhanced by serum from normal rats, but not from hypophysectomized rats. Pretreatment of the hypophysectomized rats with GH restored the capacity of the serum to stimulate sulfate uptake into cartilage. These observations led the authors to propose that the action of GH on skeletal tissue was mediated by a secondary substance which they termed sulfation factor activity (SFA). Similarly, the thymidine factor activity of serum, measured by the incorporation of tritiated thymidine into cartilage DNA, was shown to be regulated by GH (Daughaday and Reeder, 1966).

When it became apparent that partially purified SFA showed biological activities beyond that of sulfate uptake alone, the term SFA became obsolete. Due consideration of many suggested names led workers in the field to substitute the term somatomedin for SFA (Daughaday *et al.*, 1972). The prefix "somato" denoted both the hormonal relationship to somatotropin and also to the soma which is the target tissue. "Medin" was included in the name to indicate that it was an intermediary in somatotropin action.

Since somatomedin, like GH, may prove to be species-specific, plasma from human beings was chosen as the starting material for the purification. Acid–ethanol extraction was used as the initial step in the purification because a relationship was suspected between the somatomedins and NSILA (Hall and Uthne, 1971). Two peptides with similar molecular size but different charge were purified. The neutral peptide and the basic peptide were termed somatomedin A (SMA) and somatomedin C (SMC), respectively (Hall, 1972; van Wyk *et al.*, 1978). The peptide somatomedin B is no longer considered part of the somatomedin family (Uthne, 1973; Fryklund and Sievertsson, 1978).

III. Chemical Characterization of the Somatomedins

A. Human Somatomedins

Human plasma has been used as the starting material for the purification of SMA, SMC, IGF-I, and IGF-II. The first isolation was achieved by Rinderknecht and Humbel, who characterized two peptides termed IGF-I and IGF-II (Rinderknecht and Humbel, 1976a,b, 1978a,b; Humbel and Rinderknecht, 1978). IGF-I consists of 70 amino acid residues with a MW of 7649 and IGF-II consists of 67 amino acid residues with a MW of 7471. Their sequences share identical amino acids in 45 positions. These two homologs unequivocally show a close structural relationship to proinsulin. Like proinsulin, both are single-chain peptides with intrachain disulfide bridges. The homologous region to proinsulin corresponds to the a and b chains of insulin (Fig. 1). The connecting peptides of IGF-I and IGF-II are shorter (12 and 8 amino acids, respectively) and show no homology with the C-peptide of proinsulin (35 amino acids). In addition, IGF-I and IGF-II contain an extension at the carboxy terminal of 8 and 6 amino acid residues, respectively. Sequence similarities between IGF and proinsulin and the known three-dimensional structure of insulin, allow construction of three-dimensional models for IGF-I and IGF-II. These models indicate identical three-dimensional conformation of the parts corresponding to the a and b chains of insulin, while the connecting peptides cover less of the molecular surface than the C-peptide in proinsulin (Blundell *et al.*, 1978).

The sequence and structural similarity between IGF and proinsulin led to the suggestion that these molecules diverged from a common ancestor hormone during evolution (Blundell and Humbel, 1980). Based on the differences in the amino acid sequences between insulins from different classes of vertebrates and IGF-I, this divergence was proposed to occur before the appearance of the vertebrates. The time of divergence of IGF-I and IGF-II was suggested to occur with the appearance of the first mammals on earth (Zapf *et al.*, 1981a).

The isolated SMC is a basic peptide with a molecular size of 8567 as calculated from its amino acid composition (Svoboda *et al.*, 1980). Partial sequence data on SMC already shows 22 of 25 amino acid positions identical to those of IGF-I. The nine N-terminal amino acid residues are identical to IGF-I, but two fragments of SMC containing eight and nine amino acids are not present in IGF-I. It is suggested that SMC contains an extension at the carboxy terminus, thus explaining the higher molecular size and content of histidine not found in IGF I

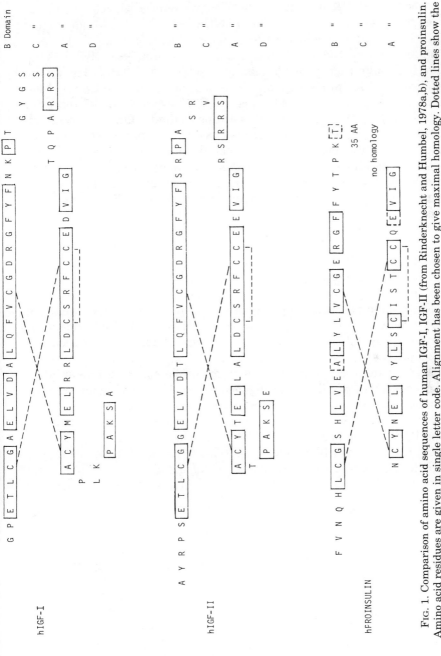

Fig. 1. Comparison of amino acid sequences of human IGF-I, IGF-II (from Rinderknecht and Humbel, 1978a,b), and proinsulin. Amino acid residues are given in single letter code. Alignment has been chosen to give maximal homology. Dotted lines show the conserved disulfide bridges. Homologous areas of IGF-I and IGF-II are marked with solid boxes. Residues of proinsulin homologous with either IGF-I or IGF-II are marked with dotted boxes.

(Svoboda *et al.*, 1980). The similarities in chemical structure and immunoreactivity between IGF-I and SMC have led to the introduction of the term SMC/IGF-I in referring to these peptides (van Wyk *et al.*, 1980). The basic SM, purified by Bala and Bhaumick (1979a), has the five N-terminal amino acids identical to SMC and IGF-I. The amino acid composition of the neutral SMA, previously purified by Fryklund *et al.* (1974, 1978) from Cohn fraction IV, shows several differences to IGF-I, notably the cysteine and histidine content (Hall and Fryklund, 1979). Recently, when whole plasma instead of Cohn fraction IV was used as starting material, immunoreactive SMA was recovered both in a neutral fraction designated SMA and in a more basic fraction, which probably represents IGF-I. The neutral fraction, although homogeneous according to HPLC, consisted of two peptides. Sequence determinations of 30 amino acids at the N-terminus disclosed that the major peptide differed from IGF-I in only two positions, whereas the other was identical with IGF-II (Enberg *et al.*, 1983). The peptide with 90% homology to IGF-I in the b chain is designated SMA. Although we cannot prove identity between this SMA peptide and the neutral peptide previously termed SMA, it has to be concluded that SMA is an IGF-I-related peptide and presumably similar to the immunoreactive IGF-I found in the neutral fraction (Zumstein *et al.*, 1983). Identity, however, can only be proved when the complete amino acid sequence is elucidated.

The existence of additional somatomedin homologs in human plasma is suspected by all groups engaged in purification of somatomedins. By use of different assays for identification and different purification schemes, peptides differing in charge and molecular size from IGF-I and IGF-II have been observed. Whether some of these peptides are identical to naturally occurring peptides or are products of the harsh purification procedures remains to be elucidated.

B. Nonprimate Somatomedins

Recently a somatomedin has been isolated from the plasma of rats bearing GH-producing tumors. This rat somatomedin shows striking sequence homology with IGF-I in the N-terminal region (Rubin *et al.*, 1982). Of the first 29 residues in the 2 molecules, there are 26 identities (Fig. 2). An IGF-II-like peptide has not yet been purified from the adult rat but one of the MSA peptides, purified from the conditioned medium from BRL-3A cells, shows 93% homology to IGF-II (Marquardt *et al.*, 1981). Based on the electrophoretic pattern and the elution volume after gel chromatography, the MSA peptides are grouped

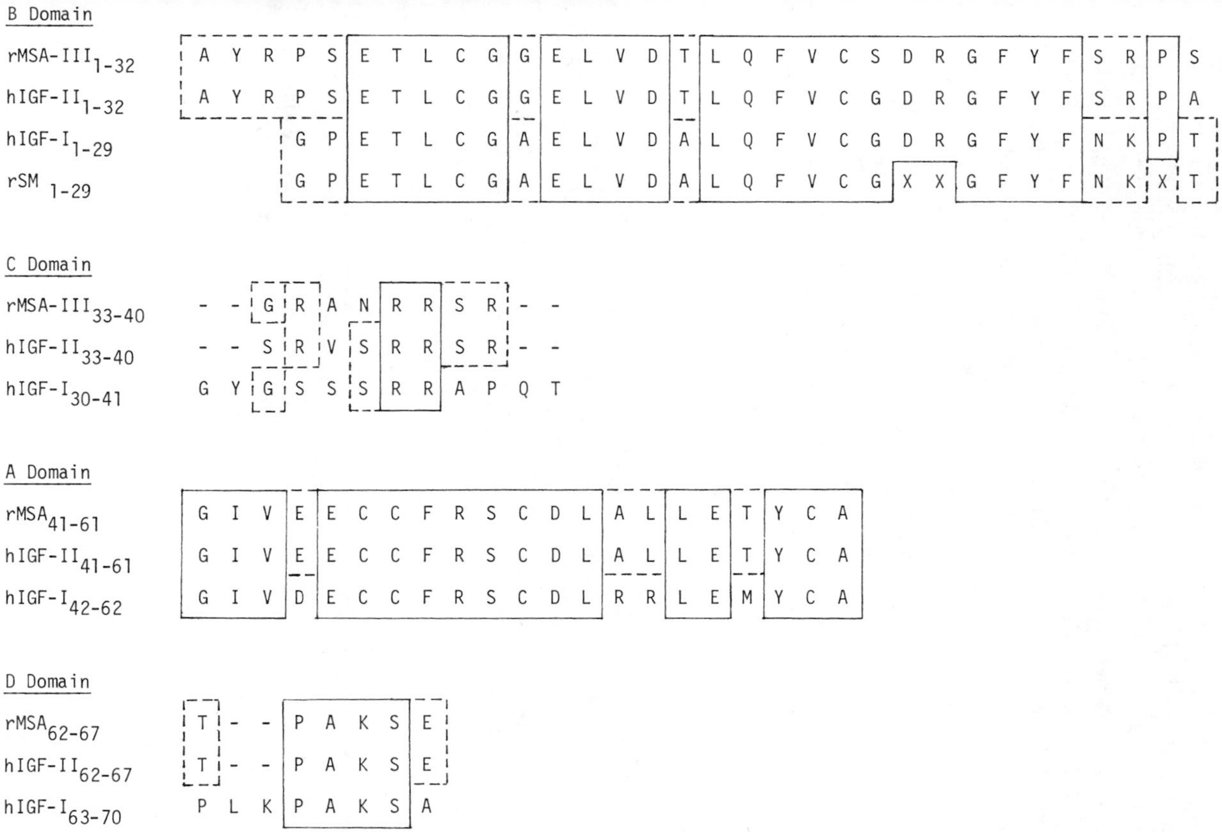

B Domain

$rMSA\text{-}III_{1-32}$	A	Y	R	P	S	E	T	L	C	G	G	E	L	V	D	T	L	Q	F	V	C	S	D	R	G	F	Y	F	S	R	P	S
$hIGF\text{-}II_{1-32}$	A	Y	R	P	S	E	T	L	C	G	G	E	L	V	D	T	L	Q	F	V	C	G	D	R	G	F	Y	F	S	R	P	A
$hIGF\text{-}I_{1-29}$				G	P	E	T	L	C	G	A	E	L	V	D	A	L	Q	F	V	C	G	D	R	G	F	Y	F	N	K	P	T
rSM_{1-29}				G	P	E	T	L	C	G	A	E	L	V	D	A	L	Q	F	V	C	G	X	X	G	F	Y	F	N	K	X	T

C Domain

$rMSA\text{-}III_{33-40}$	-	-	G	R	A	N	R	R	S	R	-	-
$hIGF\text{-}II_{33-40}$	-	-	S	R	V	S	R	R	S	R	-	-
$hIGF\text{-}I_{30-41}$	G	Y	G	S	S	R	R	A	P	Q	T

A Domain

$rMSA_{41-61}$	G	I	V	E	E	C	C	F	R	S	C	D	L	A	L	L	E	T	Y	C	A
$hIGF\text{-}II_{41-61}$	G	I	V	E	E	C	C	F	R	S	C	D	L	A	L	L	E	T	Y	C	A
$hIGF\text{-}I_{42-62}$	G	I	V	D	E	C	C	F	R	S	C	D	L	R	R	L	E	M	Y	C	A

D Domain

$rMSA_{62-67}$	T	-	-	P	A	K	S	E
$hIGF\text{-}II_{62-67}$	T	-	-	P	A	K	S	E
$hIGF\text{-}I_{63-70}$	P	L	K	P	A	K	S	A

FIG. 2. Primary structures of rat MSA-III, human IGF-I and IGF-II, and rat somatomedin (rSM). Alignment has been chosen to give maximal homology and the hyphen (-) indicates introduced gaps. Boxes in solid lines indicate residues identical in three or four of the peptides, whereas boxes in broken lines indicate identity between two of the peptides. X = unidentified. Data from Rinderknecht and Humbel (1978a,b), Rubin et al. (1982), and Marquardt et al. (1981).

into 3 regions, peak I with a molecular size of 16,300 daltons, peak II containing 4 closely migrating peptides with a molecular size of 8700 daltons, and peak III containing 2 closely migrating peptides with a molecular size of 7100 daltons (Rechler *et al.*, 1981). One of the MSA-III peptides has been isolated and sequenced (Marquardt *et al.*, 1981). This MSA peptide differs from IGF-II by only 5 conservative amino acid substitutions of which 3 are in the C-peptide region (Fig. 2).

The term insulin-related growth factor has been used by Bradshaw and Niall (1978) to refer to structural similarities between insulin and IGF, and also the polypeptides NGF and relaxin. The homology between insulin and the two growth factors, porcine relaxin and mouse NGF, is less pronounced than that between insulin and IGF (Bradshaw, 1980). These two factors show greater target tissue specificity than the somatomedins, with relaxin acting on the pubic symphysis and uterus and NGF being a maintenance factor for sensory and sympathetic neurons. Although relaxin stimulates thymidine uptake into human fibroblasts, it has no effect on embryonic chicken fibroblasts and does not cross-react with the receptors for insulin and IGF. Although chemical and possibly evolutionary relationships may exist between insulin and the more target tissue-specific factors NGF and relaxin, the functional relationship is much less than that between insulin and the somatomedins, which are more diverse in cellular effects. Interrelationship between the several somatomedin-type peptides are outlined in Table I.

TABLE I

SOMATOMEDIN STRUCTURES PARTIALLY OR FULLY CHARACTERIZED:
RELATED TO EITHER IGF-I OR IGF-II

	IGF-I related peptide	IGF-II related peptide
Human somatomedins		
Insulin-like growth factor I (IGF-I)	+	
Insulin-like growth factor II (IGF-II)		+
Somatomedin A (SMA)	+	
Somatomedin C (SMC)	+	
Basic somatomedin	+	
Nonprimate somatomedins		
Rat somatomedin	+	
Multiplication stimulating activity (MSA) family of peptides MSA-III-2		+

IV. Biological Effects of the Somatomedins

A. In Vitro

All the purified somatomedins act as anabolic hormones *in vitro*, as indicated in organ explants, primary cell cultures, and established cell lines (van Wyk *et al.*, 1978, 1981; Rechler *et al.*, 1981; Rothstein, 1982). In cells capable of proliferation, the somatomedins have been reported to stimulate thymidine uptake into DNA, DNA synthesis, and mitosis. Daughaday and Reeder (1966) first showed that GH-dependent factors in serum stimulate thymidine incorporation into the DNA of rat costal cartilage. Later this effect was shown to be due to the somatomedins (van Wyk *et al.*, 1975). Thymidine incorporation into the DNA of embryonic chicken fibroblasts was used in the bioassay for the purification of MSA (Dulak and Temin, 1973a,b; Nissley and Rechler, 1978).

Eventually somatomedins were shown to stimulate DNA synthesis and cell proliferation *in vitro* in a variety of cells, including human skin fibroblasts, embryonic chicken fibroblasts, embryonic chicken cartilage, rat myoblasts, rat and human fetal brain cells, and frog and rabbit lens epithelium (Table II). Rechler *et al.* (1976, 1978, 1980, 1981) have shown that not only MSA, but also SMA, SMC, IGF-I, and IGF-II stimulated both DNA synthesis and cell multiplication in embryonic chicken fibroblasts as well as human skin fibroblasts. Established and transformed cell lines have also been reported to respond to somatomedins. In contrast to primary cell systems, this effect is not universal. The explanation for this became apparent from findings that the BRL-3A and chondrosarcoma cells produce their own somatomedins. It is now clear that those cells capable of growing in serum-free medium and failing to respond to exogenous somatomedins produce them endogenously.

Detailed analyses of cell cycle influences exerted by SMC have been performed by Stiles, Pledger, and associates, using mouse BALB/c 3T3 cells (Stiles *et al.*, 1979a,b). They showed that SMC alone cannot completely replace the growth stimulatory effect of serum. Different growth factors are proposed to act at different stages of the cell cycle and are classified as either competence or progression factors. The cell cycle is initiated by competence factors such as platelet-derived growth factor (PDGF) or fibroblast growth factor (FGF), but progression factors are essential if the cell is to undergo DNA synthesis (Pledger *et al.*, 1977; Stiles *et al.*, 1979a,b; Leof *et al.*, 1980; Clemmons and van Wyk, 1981; Wharton *et al.*, 1981). The somatomedins act as progression fac-

TABLE II

Stimulatory Effects of Somatomedins *in Vitro* Demonstrated on Different Cells and Organs

Effect	Reference
Cell proliferation and/or DNA synthesis	
Amphibian lens epithelium	Rothstein (1982)
Human embryonic neuroblasts	Sara *et al.* (1980b)
Rat embryonic neuroblasts	Sara *et al.* (1980b)
Chick embryonic cartilage	Froesch *et al.* (1976)
Rat cartilage	van Wyk *et al.* (1978)
Rat myoblasts	Ewton and Florini (1980)
Chick embryonic fibroblasts	Rechler *et al.* (1978, 1980)
Rat fibroblasts	Zapf *et al.* (1981a)
Human embryonic lung fibroblasts	Weidman and Bala (1980)
Human skin fibroblasts	Rechler *et al.* (1978, 1980); Zapf *et al.* (1981a)
Mouse BALB/c 3T3 cells	Pledger *et al.* (1977); van Wyk *et al.* (1981)
HeLa cells	Hutchings and Sato (1978)
Protein synthesis	
Embryonic chick cartilage	Hall (1972); Froesch *et al.* (1976)
Rat cartilage	van Wyk *et al.* (1978); Zapf *et al.* (1978, 1981a)
Human skin fibroblasts	Rechler *et al.* (1981)
Glucose uptake and metabolism	
Rat adipose tissue	Zapf *et al.* (1981a)
Rat myoblasts	Ewton and Florini (1980)
Rat diaphragms	Zapf *et al.* (1981a)
Rat heart	Meuli and Froesch (1977)
Mouse soleus muscle	Poggi *et al.* (1979)

tors in the cell cycle. At high concentrations, the structural homolog insulin also acts as a progression factor.

The somatomedins stimulate not only mitotic division but also meiotic division as shown in *Xenopus laevis* oocytes (El-Etr *et al.*, 1979). The effects of somatomedins on cell differentiation have been relatively unexplored. Using rat myoblasts, Ewton and Florini (1981) observed that the somatomedins, while acting as mitogenic factors, also induce differentiation into myotubules, thus possibly acting as differentiation factors as well.

A prerequisite for DNA synthesis is an increase in protein synthesis. The somatomedins have been shown to stimulate both glucose uptake and the uptake of the nonmetabolizable amino acid (AIB) and the incorporation of amino acids into proteins in fibroblasts. Such an action still occurs in differentiated cells no longer capable of division where the somatomedins have an anabolic action and act as maintenance factors. These effects have been most thoroughly investigated in the target organs for insulin such as adipose tissue and muscle (Table II). In rat adipose tissue the somatomedins show complete insulin-like action (Froesch *et al.*, 1967; Werner *et al.*, 1974). They stimulate glucose transport, glucose incorporation into lipids, and conversion into CO_2, and inhibit the release of glycerol (Zapf *et al.*, 1978, 1981a). The order of potency for the different somatomedins in adipose tissues is IGF-II > IGF-I > SMA. Insulin, however, is more potent than any of the somatomedins and it has been suspected that the somatomedins act through the insulin receptor in adipose tissue. In rat diaphragm and heart muscle where the IGFs stimulate glucose incorporation into glycogen, glucose and amino acid transport, and lactate production, the somatomedins are more potent and appear to act via their own receptors.

The somatomedins, like insulin, increase the activity and the synthesis of enzymes involved in anabolism of cells. The induction of mRNA for specific enzymes and proteins is not yet explored. Only in the oviduct has it been shown that somatomedins, in combination with estrogens, induce the mRNA for ovalbumin (Evans *et al.*, 1981). The similarities between the somatomedins and insulin probably extend to the mechanism of action. The somatomedins inhibit the stimulated cyclic AMP production in rat hepatocytes and adipocytes (Hepp, 1972; Hall *et al.*, 1979b; Zederman *et al.*, 1980) (Fig. 3). This finding is in accordance with the observed decrease in cyclic AMP level in cells during rapid proliferation. Several hypotheses proposed for the mechanism of action of insulin have also been applied to the somatomedins. SMA has also been shown to inhibit the membrane-bound NADH dehydrogenase in isolated membranes from liver and adipose tissue (Löw *et al.*, 1978, 1979). Whether somatomedins act through a second messenger was not explored.

B. *In Vivo*

For a long period of time the demonstration of a growth-promoting effect of somatomedins *in vivo* has been hampered by the shortage of pure peptides. Partially purified preparations of somatomedins have been used to demonstrate an increase in body length and weight of the Snell dwarf mouse (van Buul and van den Brande, 1978; van Buul-Offers and van den Brande, 1981, 1982). In hypophysectomized rats,

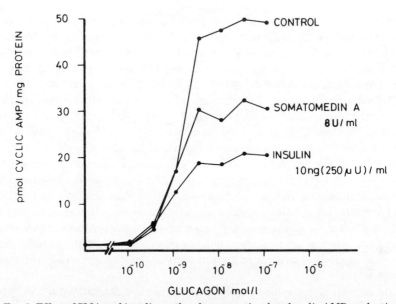

FIG. 3. Effect of SMA and insulin on the glucagon-stimulated cyclic AMP production in rat hepatocytes. The hepatocytes (4 × 10⁶ cells/ml) were preincubated without or with insulin or SMA for 15 minutes at 37°C. Glucagon in different concentrations was then added for 2 minutes incubation.

low doses of partially purified SMA stimulate sulfate uptake into cartilage, as well as leucine uptake into tissue protein (Fryklund *et al.*, 1974). However, in this study no effect was found on the growth of the epiphyseal plates, presumably due to the low dose used. In none of these studies, however, could interference by contaminating factors in the partially purified preparation be excluded.

The first study in which a pure peptide was used was performed in the frog (Rothstein *et al.*, 1980). Administration of SMC, via the dorsal lymph sac, to hypophysectomized frogs reinitiates DNA synthesis and mitosis in frog lens epithelium (Rothstein, 1982). Recently the growth-promoting effect of IGF-I and IGF-II has been clearly shown in the hypophysectomized rat, the classical experimental animal in GH studies (Schoenle *et al.*, 1982). IGF-I and IGF-II administered by continuous infusion (6 days) via implanted minipumps significantly increase the tibial epiphyseal width and body weight. In addition, the incorporation of tritiated thymidine into DNA thymidine is enhanced. IGF-I in daily doses of 103 μg is approximately equipotent to daily doses of 12.5 μg GH, but IGF-II is less potent per microgram. The potency difference between IGF-I and IGF-II is similar to that observed *in vitro* in the rat cartilage sulfation assay. The insulin-like action of somatomedins causing hypoglycemia has only been observed after intravenous or intraperitoneal administration to hypophysectomized or adrenalectomized rats, respectively (Froesch et al., 1967; Oelz et al., 1970; Skottner et al., 1980). The induced hypoglycemia is more long-lasting than that caused by insulin. It is not observed in intact rats, presumably due to binding of the administered somatomedins to endogenous carrier proteins.

Thus, convincing evidence has been provided for somatomedins as a growth factor in vivo. The somatomedin hypothesis which states that the somatomedins act as mediators of the growth-promoting action of GH is supported by these studies. The recent finding by Isaksson et al. (1982) that local injection of GH into the cartilage plate of hypophysectomized rats increases cartilage proliferation does not contradict this hypothesis. There may well be local production of somatomedins stimulated by GH. Several tissues appear to produce somatomedins locally and GH in vitro stimulates SMC release from fibroblasts (Clemmons et al., 1981b). However, it is surprising that Isaksson et al. (1982) found that 10 μg GH locally has such a small effect compared to the same dose given subcutaneously. It remains to be determined whether GH or somatomedins in the circulation are the endocrine hormone regulating cartilage anabolism.

V. RECEPTORS FOR THE SOMATOMEDINS

The binding of somatomedins to receptors on the cell surface is the first in a series of events leading to biological action. Somatomedin receptor sites have been detected and found to have a wide cellular and tissue distribution in man, monkey, pig, rat, mouse, and chicken (Hintz et al., 1972; Marshall et al., 1974; Megyesi et al., 1974b; Zapf et al., 1975a, 1978, 1981a; Takano et al., 1976a; Rechler et al., 1976, 1977, 1978, 1981; D'Ercole et al., 1976; Thorsson and Hintz, 1977; Daughaday et al., 1981a; Sara et al., 1980b, 1982d, 1983b).

The existence of more than one type of somatomedin binding site is recognized. Human placenta, for example, contains separate receptors for IGF-I- and IGF-II-related peptides. In the rat only IGF-II receptors are found in the placenta (Daughaday et al., 1981a). Three different patterns of cross reactivity have been described by Rechler et al. (1978, 1980, 1981). First, in embryonic chicken fibroblasts IGF-I and IGF-II were equipotent in competing with all the bound labeled somatomedins indicating a common receptor for the somatomedins. Insulin can also interact with this receptor. Second, in rat liver cells and rat liver membranes, labeled IGF-II was preferentially bound and IGF-I was 10–20 times less potent than IGF-II, but insulin does not interact. In addition, when IGF-I is used as a label, IGF-I and IGF-II were equipotent. This finding was interpreted as showing that two receptors exist: one specific for IGF-II and the other common to all somatomedins. Third, human fibroblasts preferentially bind IGF-I; IGF-II is one-third and insulin one-tenth as potent as IGF-I. Identical orders of cross-reactivity are seen with labeled IGF-II except that only 50% of the binding is inhibitable by IGF-I. This latter finding suggests that IGF-II binds to two receptors, an IGF-I receptor and an IGF-II receptor.

Direct evidence for the existence of more than one somatomedin receptor has been provided by the identification of two types of receptor structures. A structure similar to that for the insulin receptor is found for the IGF-I receptor in human placenta, human fibroblasts, embryonic chicken fibroblasts, and IM 9 cells (Bhaumick et al., 1981; Chernausek et al., 1981; Kasuga et al., 1981, 1982; Massaque et al., 1981). By photoaffinity coupling of SMC/IGF-I to placenta membrane, Bhaumick et al. (1981) identified a high-molecular-weight somatomedin receptor that was converted, under reducing conditions, to a smaller component with a molecular weight of about 140,000. The IGF-I receptor in human placenta has been further characterized by Massaque and Czech (1982), who suggested that the IGF-I receptor possessed a tetrameric structure composed of two α-units with a molecular weight of 130,000 and two β-units of 98,000 joined by interchain disulfide bridges. They proposed that the IGF-I receptor and the insulin receptor had evolved from a common ancestral molecule.

Evidence of a second somatomedin receptor was first described by Kasuga et al. (1981). They crosslinked labeled MSA to cultured rat liver cells (BRL) and found a complex of 260,000 MW, which was not dissociated by reducing agents. This type of receptor, identified by the binding of either MSA or IGF-II, has been found in rat liver membrane, rat adipocytes, rat embryonic fibroblasts, and chondrocytes from a rat chondrosarcoma. Both receptor types exist in human placenta but the IGF-I receptor predominates (Massaque and Czech, 1982).

The patterns of cross-reactivity cannot be explained by only two structural types of somatomedin receptors and additional types are thought to exist. In the human brain, which is rich in binding sites for both IGF-I and IGF-II, the pattern of cross-reactivity is different in early versus later life (Sara et al., 1983b,c). In the adult brain as well as in the human fetus after 25 weeks of gestation, IGF-I is three times more potent than IGF-II in inhibiting binding of labeled IGF-I, whereas the two peptides are equipotent against labeled IGF-II. In contrast before 17 weeks of gestational age, IGF-II is the most potent inhibitor of either labeled IGF-I or IGF-II from binding sites. Differences between the fetal and adult brain tissue led to the proposal of a fetal form of somatomedin receptor (Sara and Hall, 1980, 1983; Sara et al., 1981a).

Somatomedins induce down-regulation of their own binding sites. In children with GH deficiency GH treatment, which increases somatomedin levels in the circulation, also reduces the number of binding sites on circulating monocytes (Rosenfeld et al., 1981). The amount of SMA binding to plasma membranes from rat kidney and lung increases concomitantly with a decline in serum SMA levels during starvation (Takano et al., 1981). In vitro studies using IM 9 cells and human skin fibroblasts also indicate down-regulation by somatomedins of their own receptor (Rosenfeld and Dollar, 1982).

Insulin and proinsulin can interact with somatomedin receptors in some tissues such as embryonic chicken fibroblasts and human skin fibroblasts. The order of potency between somatomedins, insulin, and proinsulin is in accordance with their actions in stimulating thymidine incorporation into DNA. The growth-promoting effect of insulin in fibroblasts is thought to be mediated through the somatomedin receptors (Rechler et al., 1981). The Fab fragment, prepared from serum containing autoantibodies toward insulin, blocks the binding of insulin to insulin receptors but does not alter the insulin effect on thymidine incorporation (King et al., 1980; Rechler et al., 1981).

A pathogenetic role for the somatomedin receptors has also been suggested in some patients with leprechaunism. Leprechaunism is a rare, probably genetic disorder, characterized by low birth weight and length, poorly developed muscles, hyperinsulinemia, and insulin resistance. Two different types of leprechaunism have been observed, one lacking insulin and somatomedin receptors; the other has normal receptors but a postreceptor defect in the biological action of somatomedin and insulin on glucose and amino acid uptake in fibroblasts (D'Ercole et al., 1979; Knight et al., 1981; van Obberghen-Schilling et al., 1981; Kaplowitz and D'Ercole, 1982). A localized defect of brain somatomedin receptors has been proposed to occur in patients with senile dementia of the Alzheimer type (Sara et al., 1982b).

VI. Circulating Forms of the Somatomedins

The somatomedins are present in the circulation in heterogeneous forms. The majority of the somatomedins in human serum are found in the high-molecular-weight range with less than 1% being found in the molecular weight range of the isolated somatomedins (Koumans and Daughaday, 1963; van Wyk *et al.*, 1975; Zapf *et al.*, 1975b; Hall *et al.*, 1979a). After acid dissociation the serum somatomedins are recovered in the low-molecular-weight form. When added to serum, somatomedins reappear in the high-molecular-weight forms. These findings indicate that the somatomedins in serum are bound to carrier proteins. At least two forms of carrier proteins have been identified with molecular weights of 150,000 and 40–60,000 respectively. Neither of these carrier proteins has yet been purified to homogeneity. Acidification of the larger weight form of carrier protein reduces its apparent molecular size to that of the smaller form of carrier protein (Morris and Schalch, 1982). Some authors have proposed that the smaller carrier protein is a subunit of the larger form (Hintz *et al.*, 1978; Hintz and Liu, 1980; Furlanetto, 1980). However these forms differ in charge as well as binding characteristics and attempts to reconstitute the larger form from acidified binding proteins and other serum fractions have failed.

In serum from healthy subjects and patients with acromegaly most of the somatomedin, after gel chromatography at neutral pH, is recovered in the molecular range of 150,000 daltons, whereas in patients with GH deficiency, somatomedin is only found in the molecular range of 40–60,000 daltons (Fig. 4) (Hall *et al.*, 1979a). After GH administration to patients with GH deficiency, the somatomedins are again found in the 150,000-dalton range (Hintz *et al.*, 1981). After labeled somatomedin is added to serum from healthy subjects or patients with acromegaly, radioactivity is found both in the 150K and 60K regions (Zapf *et al.*, 1975b). In contrast, when added to the serum from patients with GH deficiency, the radioactivity is found only in the 60K complex which indicates the absence of the high molecular form of carrier protein. It is therefore generally agreed that the larger form of carrier protein is GH regulated.

The time of appearance of the GH-regulated carrier protein during development is debatable (Borsi *et al.*, 1982). In cord blood from premature infants of less than 27 weeks gestation only the smaller form of the carrier protein is observed. During development the appearance of the larger form of carrier protein was observed during the last 3 months (D'Ercole *et al.*, 1980b). In accordance with GH regulation of this later developing binding protein, this form was absent in a full term anencephalic child at birth. Similarily, in the rat, the appearance of the GH-regulated carrier protein in serum occurs first postnatally at the time when both growth and somatomedin production become GH regulated (Moses *et al.*, 1976; White *et al.*, 1982).

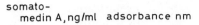

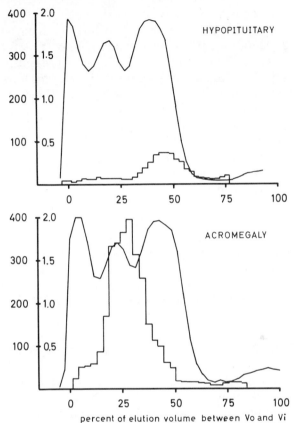

Fig. 4. Gel chromatography of sera from patients with GH deficiency and acromegaly, respectively, on Sephadex G-200 (42 × 2.6 cm) equilibrated with Tris–HCl, pH 7.4 (0.05 mol/liter) and NaCl (0.1 mol/liter). Histograms show immunoreactive SMA expressed in ng equivalents SMA (= mU SMA) per ml eluate; 5 ml of serum was applied to the column. From Hall *et al.* (1979a).

The presence of carrier proteins explains the long biological half-life of somatomedins in the circulation. After successful hypophysectomy of patients with acromegaly or withdrawal of GH treatment, the calculated half-life of the somatomedins is approximately 20 hours (Blethen *et al.*, 1982). In intact rats a half-life, about 4 hours, is reported after hypophysectomy (Takano *et al.*, 1977a). The half-lives, however, of administered MSA, IGF-I and IGF-II in hypophysectomized rats lacking the GH-regulated carrier protein are very much shorter.

The forms of somatomedins present in cerebrospinal fluid (CSF) appear to differ from those found in serum. After acidification of CSF, two IGF-II-like peptides have been found; one is similar to IGF-II purified from serum while the other is slightly larger having a molecular size of about 9000 daltons (Haselbacher and Humbel, 1982).

Although the somatomedins appear to be present in exocrine fluids, such as gastric fluid and breast milk, their forms have not been determined. In amniotic fluid the presence of somatomedins as well as their carrier proteins has been demonstrated (Bala *et al.*, 1978). The amniotic fluid carrier protein has a high affinity for the somatomedins (Chochinov *et al.*, 1976, 1977). The acidified carrier protein has been purified by Drop *et al.* (1979) and shown to have a molecular size of approximately 35,000.

The biological role of the somatomedin carrier proteins presumably is to assure a continuous supply to target cells. The anabolic effect of the somatomedins on the target tissues depends on the equilibrium between binding to the carrier proteins and to cell receptors. Only tissues with high affinity receptors can compete for the somatomedins. In low affinity tissues like the target organs of insulin, the somatomedins have scarcely any effect *in vivo*, thus explaining why somatomedins cannot replace insulin in patients with diabetes mellitus.

VII. ASSAYS FOR THE MEASUREMENT OF SOMATOMEDINS

Diverse assay techniques, such as bioassays, protein binding assays (PBA), radioreceptor assays (RRA), and radioimmunoassays (RIA) are currently used for the measurement of somatomedins. With the availability of pure peptides, radioligand assays have been developed with greater sensitivity and precision than the original bioassays and a higher specificity for the radioimmunoassays. Each assay system displays a characteristic order of cross-reactivity, which must be taken into consideration in the interpretation of results.

The lack of a common international standard causes difficulties in comparing results among laboratories. Pure peptides are only used as standards in the RIA-IGF-I and RIA-IGF-II assays where serum levels are expressed as nanogram equivalents of the respective peptide (Zapf *et al.*, 1981b). Because of the scarcity of pure peptides some groups choose an arbitrary serum standard assigned a value of 1 U/ml. Since age and other factors influence the somatomedin content of plasma, there is discordance between different serum standards, making interlaboratory comparisons difficult.

A. BIOASSAY

A variety of tissues and cells have been used as target organs in bioassay systems for the determination of somatomedin activity. Three classical bioassays have been employed. First, Salmon and Daughaday (1957) used the incorporation of [^{35}S]sulfate into hypophysectomized rat cartilage. Assays were developed using chicken embryo, weanling or fasted rats or porcine cartilage (Yde, 1968; Hall, 1970; van den Brande and Du Caju, 1974). These bioassays measure both IGF-I and IGF-II related peptides. IGF-I is slightly more potent than IGF-II in the chicken embryonic cartilage bioassay (Gibson et al., 1978; Zapf et al., 1978). Second, the epididymal fat pad bioassay measuring the conversion of [^{14}C]glucose to CO_2 was used to detect insulin-like activity (Froesch et al., 1963). In the fat pad bioassay IGF-II is more potent than IGF-I and SMA (Zapf et al., 1978). Third, the incorporation of tritiated thymidine into DNA of embryonic chicken fibroblasts was used to detect MSA. Although advantageous in biological relevance, bioassays show certain failings including lack of sensitivity, precision, and specificity. Inhibitory substances in serum influence the obtained results. The presence of other hormones in the sample must also be taken into account when interpreting the results. For example, thyroid hormones stimulate sulfate uptake into chicken embryo cartilage whereas cortisol inhibits this effect in porcine cartilage (Gibson et al., 1978; van den Brande, 1973).

When testing whole serum samples in the bioassay (and with certain other assays as well) the influence of carrier proteins must be considered. The results depend upon the equilibrium between the binding of somatomedins to the carrier protein and binding to the tissue receptor. With low affinity tissue such as fat cells it is impossible to measure quantitatively somatomedin in whole serum (Schlumpf et al., 1976). In contrast, high affinity tissues such as cartilage allow direct determinations with whole serum. These bioassays however do not detect the total amount of somatomedins present in serum, but rather reflect the biological significance of particular somatomedins for that target tissue.

B. RADIORECEPTOR ASSAY

The development of radioreceptor assay techniques provided opportunities to increase assay precision. The influence of nonspecific substances could be removed. As with bioassays, receptors on the target tissue determine the type of somatomedins detected. Human placenta membrane was first used as a matrix in a radioreceptor assay for SMC (Marshall *et al.,* 1974). In this assay, IGF-I and SMC are equipotent and all other somatomedins cross-react (van Wyk *et al.,* 1981). Regardless of whether IGF-I, SMA, SMC, or basic SM is used as ligand in the assay, similar results are obtained (Hall *et al.,* 1974; Takano *et al.,* 1976b; Baxter *et al.,* 1982). Human fetal brain tissue, in addition to measuring SMA, SMC, IGF-I and IGF-II, also detects an additional hormone in the human fetal circulation (Sara *et al.,* 1981a). This assay is therefore used to identify human fetal somatomedin (Sara *et al.,* 1981a).

Radioreceptor assays with animal tissues as the matrix have also been developed. Both rat placenta and liver have been used (Megyesi *et al.,* 1974a,b; Daughaday *et al.,* 1981a,b). Rat placenta RRA displays a different pattern of cross-reactivity than found with human placenta RRA and like rat liver shows preferential binding of IGF-II related peptides.

C. Protein Binding Assay

The acidified binding proteins of human serum have been used to establish a protein binding assay with IGF-II as ligand (Zapf *et al.,* 1972; Schalch *et al.,* 1978). In this assay IGF-II is preferentially detected and serum samples can only be measured after dissociation from the carrier proteins. Surprisingly the protein binding assay, using the acidified carrier protein from rat liver media, seems to measure IGF-I related peptides (Binoux *et al.,* 1982).

D. Radioimmunoassay

The highest specificity as well as precision is obtained with radioimmunoassays (RIA). The radioimmunoassays developed for somatomedins can be divided into those preferentially measuring IGF-I-related peptides and those measuring IGF-II-related peptides. The currently used radioimmunoassays for IGF-I-related peptides are RIA–IGF-I by Zapf *et al.* (1981b), RIA-IGF-I with antisera raised against its C-peptide by Hintz *et al.* (1980a, 1982), RIA–SMC by Furlanetto *et al.* (1977), RIA-SMA by Hall *et al.* (1979a), and RIA-basic SM by Bala and Bhaumick (1979b) and Baxter *et al.* (1982). IGF-II-related peptides are measured by the RIA-IGF-II developed by Zapf *et al.* (1981b) and RIA developed by Hintz and Liu (1982) with antisera raised against the connecting peptide of IGF-II. In addition an RIA for

MSA (rat IGF-II) has been developed by Moses *et al.* (1980a). Other than the antisera raised against the C- and D-peptides of IGF-I and C-peptide of IGF-II, antibodies have yet to be classified by specificity for particular sequences with somatomedin molecules. Only partial information concerning cross-reactivity is available for different radioimmunoassays.

Early attempts to immunize animals against somatomedins met with little success, probably due to the close homology of somatomedins between the species utilized. This was overcome either by coupling the somatomedins to larger proteins (Furlanetto *et al.*, 1977) or by immunizing hens, whose serum somatomedin does not interact with the receptor of human placenta (Hall *et al.*, 1979a). Furlanetto *et al.* (1977) were the first to develop an RIA allowing determination in whole serum samples. In this assay SMC and IGF-I are equally potent in competing with labeled SMC for binding to the antibodies. SMA, IGF-II, MSA-III, and MSA-II are, respectively, 5, 2, 1 and 0.1% as potent as IGF-I (van Wyk *et al.*, 1980). Equipotency between IGF-I and SMC also exists in the RIA, with antibodies raised against the C-peptide and D-peptide of IGF-I (Hintz *et al.*, 1980a,b, 1982). In the former, SMA and IGF-II do not cross-react, while in the latter, IGF-II and MSA show 10% cross-reactivity. No report is available concerning the potency of SMC in the RIA for IGF-I (Zapf *et al.*, 1981b). In this RIA, IGF-I is 10 times more potent than SMA and 100 times more potent than its close homolog IGF-II. An identical order of potency between IGF-I, SMA, and IGF-II is seen in the RIA for SMA, in spite of the fact that SMA is used as ligand and antibodies were raised against SMA (Hall *et al.*, 1979a) (Fig. 5). The order of potency in RIA-SMA is difficult to explain. Either the antisera raised contain antibodies directed at an immunoreactive sequence more exposed in IGF-I than SMA or the SMA was not pure.

The RIA-IGF-II mainly measures IGF-II. SMA and IGF-I are, respectively, 10 and 100 times less potent than IGF-II (Zapf *et al.*, 1981b). The cross-reactivity of SMC and MSA in the RIA-IGF-II has not been reported. With antisera raised against the C-peptide of IGF-II no cross-reaction occurs with SMC or IGF-I; the interaction of the MSA peptides has not been described (Hintz and Liu, 1982). In the RIA with antisera raised against rat MSA-II-1 by Moses *et al.* (1980a) a different pattern of cross-reactivity is obtained depending on the MSA peptide used as ligand (Rechler *et al.*, 1981). When labeled MSA-III is used, all MSA peptides cross-react in parallel, suggesting a common antigenic determinant. Human somatomedins also cross-react in this RIA, but their dose−response curves are not superimposable on that for MSA and the

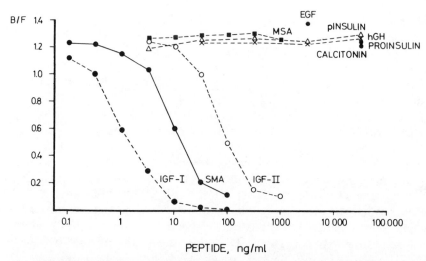

PEPTIDE, ng/ml

Fig. 5. Dose–response curves for the peptides SMA, IGF-I, IGF-II in the RIA for SMA with ^{125}I-SMA as ligand and antisera raised in hens against SMA. Antibody dilution 1:1200, free and antibody-bound radioactivity are separated with charcoal. From Hall *et al* (1979a).

potency is approximately 100-fold less than MSA. With labeled MSA-II used as a ligand human somatomedins do not cross-react.

Some of the radioimmunoassays developed for human somatomedins can be used for somatomedin determination in serum from other species. Both RIA-SMA and RIA-SMC but not RIA-IGF-I and RIA-IGF-I C-peptide measure GH-regulated somatomedins in the rat (Sara *et al.*, 1980a). The purified rat somatomedins also cross-react in a RIA with IGF-I as ligand and antibodies directed at human SMC (Daughaday *et al.*, 1982). Since IGF-I and rat somatomedin are homologous in the N-terminal but not in the C-peptide the different polyclonal antisera seem to be directed against different sequences of IGF-I. Surprisingly the RIA for rat MSA is reported not to detect IGF-II in human serum in spite of the close homology between MSA-III and IGF-II.

In order to measure the total amounts of somatomedins present in serum it has generally been necessary to separate the somatomedins from the carrier proteins by acidification and gel chromatography at low pH or by acid–ethanol precipitation before assay (Hintz, 1981; Daughaday *et al.*, 1980; Zapf *et al.*, 1981b; Bala *et al.*, 1981). In both the RIA-SMA and the RIA-SMC, determinations are performed directly in serum samples and total amounts are claimed to be measured (Furlanetto *et al.*, 1977; Hall *et al.*, 1979a). In these assays, the dose–response curve of serum is superimposable on that for the pure peptide. However parallelism does not ensure that total amounts in serum are quantitatively measured. The assay conditions were adjusted until equal amounts were obtained in whole serum and after acid dissociation. This was achieved in the RIA-SMC by the use of disequilibrium conditions and in the RIA-SMA by coupling the antibodies to Sepharose and elongation of the incubation period (Hall *et al.*, 1979a). Later changes in assay procedures for RIA-SMC, however, resulted in failure to measure total serum content and caused discrepancies in determinations in serum or plasma samples (Furlanetto, 1982). Such discrepancies have not yet been observed in the RIA-SMA.

VIII. CONTENT OF SOMATOMEDINS IN THE CIRCULATION

A. CONCENTRATION IN BLOOD

1. *Normal Concentrations Throughout Life*

Somatomedin concentrations change throughout life. This age-dependent variation differs according to the specificity of the assay used. Such knowledge is essential for the interpretation of serum levels in various disorders. No obvious diurnal rhythm has been observed although a slight temporal relationship to the nocturnal GH-peak has been reported (Minuto *et al.*, 1981). No differences in somatomedin concentrations before or after meals have been found, but fasting more than 24 hours causes a decrease (Clemmons *et al.*, 1981a; Merimee *et al.*, 1982b).

Mean results for immunoreactive SMA throughout life in healthy subjects are shown in Fig. 6. RIA-SMA is scarcely detectable in the human fetus and low amounts are found at birth (Hall *et al.*, 1980, 1981). During childhood there is a gradual rise toward adult concentrations, which are reached at about 10 years of age (Hall *et al.*, 1980). After a temporary peak during puberty (2.4 U/ml) the values remain at about 1 U/ml until approximately 40 years of age when they start to decline (Hall *et al.*, 1981) until old age when concentrations approach those of the newborn. A sex difference is observed with girls who show a somewhat higher concentration during childhood and an earlier onset of the pubertal peak (Fig. 7). In girls, the amount of RIA-SMA starts to rise between ages 10 and 12 and the peak (2.41 U/ml) is reached at 12.9 years. In boys, RIA-SMA increases by 12–14 years with the peak value (2.45 U/ml) being reached 2 years later than in girls. The pubertal peak is related in time to the growth spurt. In boys with delayed puberty the prepubertal values persist until the testes

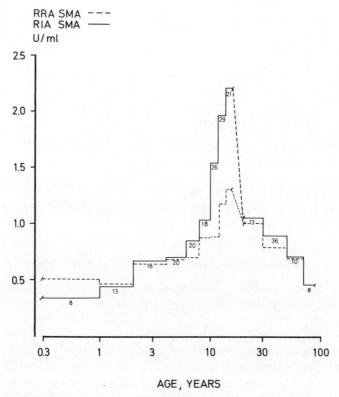

FIG. 6. Serum levels of immunoreactive SMA (RIA-SMA) and placental RRA-SMA in relation to age (logarithmic scale) for healthy Swedish children (n = 168) aged 0.3–16 years and healthy adults (n = 67) aged 20–80 years. Mean for each age group is given without regard to sex. From Hall *et al.* (1981).

reach a size of 5 to 8 ml (Hall *et al.*, 1981). During puberty the results correlate better to pubertal stage and skeletal age than to chronological age.

The age-related pattern for RIA-SMA is similar to that found with all assays preferentially measuring IGF-I-related peptides (Underwood *et al.*, 1980a; Bala *et al.*, 1981; Zapf *et al.*, 1981b). An identical pattern during childhood and puberty is obtained by determination of either RIA-SMA in whole serum or RIA-IGF-I in acid-dissociated serum. Although a pubertal peak was not reported in the first publication on RIA-SMC in children, later data have confirmed the presence of a pubertal peak as well as a sex difference in time of onset (Furlanetto *et al.*, 1977; Underwood *et al.*, 1980a). Similarily, low amounts of serum RIA-SMC are found in old age (Johansson and Blizzard, 1981).

The age-dependent pattern for RIA-IGF-II is different from that found for RIA-IGF-I (Zapf *et al.*, 1981b). Although low amounts are found at birth, they rise to adult values by the first year of life and there is no transient rise during puberty (Zapf *et al.*, 1981b). The differences between patterns for IGF-I and IGF-II peptides during life cause differences in radioreceptor and bioassay results. However, the observed discrepancies between the different assay results at different ages cannot be completely accounted for by the presently purified somatomedins. Rather these differences suggest the presence of other forms of somatomedins which predominate at different stages of life.

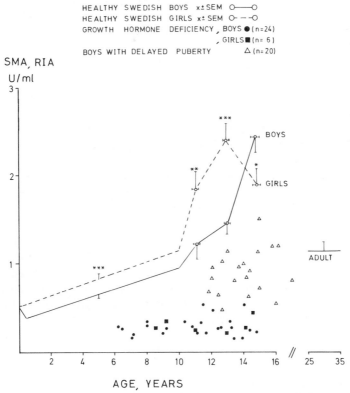

FIG. 7. Immunoreactive somatomedin A (RIA-SMA) in serum in relation to age from 188 healthy children (○), 30 children with GH deficiency (● boys, ■ girls), and 20 boys with delayed puberty (△). The regression lines for SMA on age are drawn for healthy girls and boys for the age group 2 months to 10 years. For the age groups 10–12, 12–14, and 14–16 years the means are shown separately. The bars indicate ± SEM. The significances of the differences between girls and boys are shown (* $p < 0.05$, ** $p < 0.01$, *** $p < 0.001$). From Hall *et al.* (1980).

The serum content of somatomedins throughout life determined by the three different assay systems used by us is shown in Fig. 6. Compared to IGF-I, the potency of IGF-II is as follows: RIA-SMA 1%, placenta RRA-SMA 30%, fetal brain RRA-SMA 100%. Discrepancies in the serum amounts determined by these assays are observed at three stages—old age, puberty, and fetal life. In old age, a pronounced decline is found only with RIA-SMA and fetal brain RRA–SMA methods. The pubertal peak is easily detected by both RIA-SMA and fetal brain RRA–SMA. However only a small increase is observed with the placenta RRA–SMA. This latter finding is in agreement with the results obtained using rat or porcine cartilage bioassays (Almqvist and Rune, 1961; van den Brande and Du Caju, 1973). Failure to detect the pubertal peak with some assays suggests either an interference by binding proteins or the existence of a pubertal form of somatomedin not detectable by those assays.

At birth, the content of somatomedin detected in cord serum by both RIA-SMA and placenta RRA-SMA is approximately half of that found in adults age 20–40. No such difference is observed with the fetal brain RRA–SMA. This assay difference is magnified in the fetus where extremely high amounts are measured by fetal brain RRA-SMA, yet values by RIA–SMA are below the level of detection (Sara et al., 1981a). Indeed, in all assays developed to measure the somatomedins purified from adult human plasma, low amounts are found at birth (Furlanetto et al., 1977; Sara and Hall, 1980; Zapf et al., 1981b). Initially it was thought that the elevated concentrations found with fetal brain RRA-SMA could be attributed to IGF-II but this was not supported by later studies which showed low RIA-IGF-II values in fetal serum. Since the elevated fetal brain RRA-SMA values could not be attributed to either immunoreactive IGF-I or IGF-II, we proposed the presence of an additional fetal form of somatomedin in man (Sara et al., 1980b, 1981a). The elevated amounts detected with fetal brain RRA-SMA decline with advancing gestational age to become concordant with RIA-SMA results within the first week after birth (Blom et al., 1983) (Fig. 8). This change in the serum pattern has led us to propose that there is a switch from the production of fetal to adult forms of somatomedins which is complete by approximately the first week of life. The trigger for this switching mechanism is still unknown in man. In the rat a similar pattern is observed (Moses et al., 1980c; Sara et al., 1980a, 1981a). Immunoreactive MSA is high in the fetal rat and declines with advancing age to become undetectable by the approximate postnatal age of 3 weeks (Moses et al., 1980c). Immunoreactive SMA, on the other hand, is low in the fetal and young rat until approx-

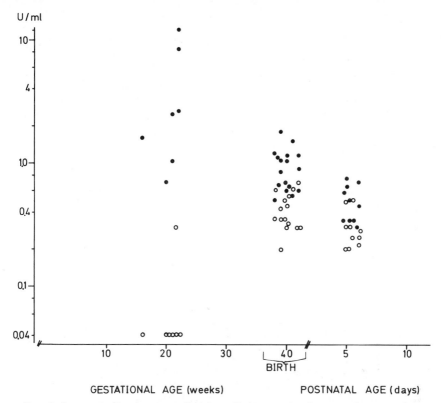

FIG. 8. Somatomedins in serum during early human development determined with fetal brain RRA-SMA (●) and RIA-SMA (○). Fetal samples were taken by fetoscopy.

imately 20 days of age when a large increase in RIA-SMA is seen. In the rat, therefore, the switch from fetal to adult somatomedin production probably occurs around the time of weaning when growth becomes GH regulated (Sara *et al.*, 1980a). The trigger in the rat may be related to nutrition or growth hormone.

Maternal serum values during pregnancy determined by our three different assay systems are illustrated for one healthy woman in Fig. 9. A rise during pregnancy is found with both RIA-SMA and fetal brain RRA-SMA while no change is observed with measurements by placenta RRA-SMA. The elevation in maternal immunoreactive SMA is similar to the increased immunoreactive SMC values found during a cross-sectional study of pregnant women (Furlanetto *et al.*, 1978). Recently these results have been confirmed by a determination performed in acid-dissociated plasma samples (Wilson *et al.*, 1982). The IGF-II-like

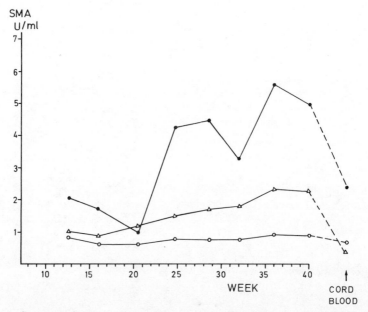

FIG. 9. Somatomedin A in serum determined by RIA-SMA (△—△), placenta RRA-SMA (○—○), and fetal brain RRA-SMA (●—●) in a healthy woman during pregnancy and in cord blood.

peptides also appear to rise during pregnancy. In a longitudinal study of pregnant women Franklin *et al.* (1979), using the adipocyte bioassay, demonstrated a steady rise in activity in acid–ethanol extracted serum. In cross-sectional studies a significant increase in these peptides in pregnant women is found when determined either by competitive protein binding assay or by RIA-IGF-II assay (C-peptide) (Heinrich *et al.*, 1979; Wilson *et al.*, 1982). In spite of the rise in both IGF-I- and IGF-II-like peptides during pregnancy, the placenta RRA-SMA does not detect increased amounts in whole serum. This is presumably due to an increase in the carrier protein which competes with the placental receptors for the peptides because an elevation is observed after dissociation from the carrier proteins (Wilson *et al.*, 1982). Since a marked elevation is observed with the fetal brain RRA-SMA method the equilibrium for somatomedin between the fetal brain receptor and the carrier-protein must differ from that for the placental receptor.

Preliminary studies suggest that maternal somatomedin values may provide a marker for fetal growth. In a longitudinal study, maternal fetal brain RRA-SMA values during the last trimester of pregnancy correlated with fetal growth, determined by ultrasound, and to birth weight and length (Sara *et al.*, 1982a). At caesarian delivery, maternal serum RIA-SMA values correlated significantly to the children's birth weight and length (Sara *et al.*, 1981a).

2. *Disease State*

The somatomedin concentrations during normal development reflect anabolism with peak values occurring during periods of rapid growth; similarly, the amounts associated with disease seem to be markers for the overall anabolic state. The earliest recognized diseases of somatomedin production were those secondary to changes in growth-hormone production. In patients with acromegaly, high concentrations of somatomedins are always detected by assays preferentially measuring IGF-I-related peptides (Furlanetto *et al.*, 1977; Clemmons *et al.*, 1979; Hall *et al.*, 1979a; Zapf *et al.*, 1981b; Bala *et al.*, 1981). The concentrations of immunoreactive SMA are 2- to 10-fold higher in patients with acromegaly than in age-matched controls (Fig. 10). A 10-fold elevation of immunoreactive SMC above normal is also found (Underwood *et al.*, 1980a,b). The "clinical activity" in acromegaly is better correlated with somatomedins than with GH concentrations (Clemmons *et al.*, 1979). These assays have proven to be valuable tools in the evaluation of therapy in patients with acromegaly.

In contrast to the results of assays for IGF-I-related peptides, no elevation in immunoreactive IGF-II is observed in acromegalic patients (Zapf *et al.*, 1980, 1981b). Other assays measuring IGF-II-related peptides such as the protein binding assay and the rat liver radioreceptor assays similarily show no increase in acromegaly (Megyesi *et al.*, 1974a,b; Zapf *et al.*, 1980).

Regardless of the assay used for somatomedin determination, decreased concentrations of somatomedins are always found in growth hormone deficiency (Underwood *et al.*, 1980b). No patient has yet been found with a complete lack of somatomedins. The low amounts in GH deficiency can be attributed to both decreased production of somatomedins and a decrease in the GH-regulated carrier protein. After GH administration there is a delay of up to 3 hours before any elevation is observed in serum. A peak response is observed within approximately 24 hours and returns to the starting value after 3 days (Takano *et al.*, 1977b).

In addition to GH deficiency low amounts of somatomedins are found in other conditions associated with growth retardation including malnutrition, malabsorption, liver disease, and Laron dwarfism. In addi-

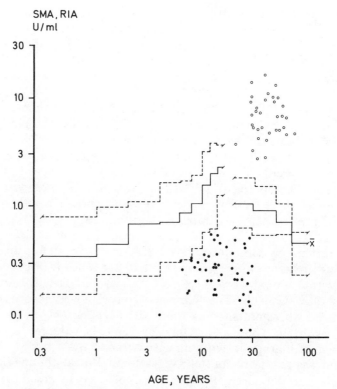

SMA, RIA
U/ml

AGE, YEARS

Fig. 10. Somatomedin A (RIA-SMA) in serum of patients with acromegaly (○, n = 34) and patients with growth hormone deficiency (●, n = 55) compared with healthy subjects (n = 255) (mean ± range in each age group). Both X and Y axis are logarithmic scales. From Hall et al. (1981).

tion, the easy availability of the somatomedin C screening assay for short children led to the detection of an additional group of somatomedin-deficient children. Rudman et al. (1981a,b) reported on some children with low immunoreactive SMC whom he found normal in immunoreactive GH but low in radioreceptor assayable GH. These children, who are 10 times more common than GH-deficient children, respond to GH treatment by an increase in immunoreactive SMC and in growth rate.

Starvation and malnutrition with concomitant catabolic status are associated with low concentrations of somatomedins. The importance of nutrition is emphasized by the dramatic decrease in somatomedins in patients with anorexia nervosa (Rappaport et al., 1978, 1980; Hall et *al.*, 1981; Hall and Sara, 1983). The levels of RIA-SMA decline concomitantly with growth retardation and rise again with improvement and increased growth. These low concentrations persist in spite of normal or high amounts of GH. The somatomedin activity is low in serum from children with protein caloric malnutrition (Grant *et al.*, 1973; van den Brande and Du Caju, 1973). Since these sera also contain substances with an inhibitory effect in the bioassay it has been difficult to evaluate their somatomedin content. However, low concentrations of RIA-SMC have been observed in children with kwashiorkor. In various malabsorption syndromes such as ulcerative colitis and Crohn's disease, low amounts of immunoreactive SMA have been found in association with growth retardation. Low somatomedin activity is also found in serum from growth-retarded children with celiac disease. A rapid normalization occurs on a glutamine-free diet (Lecornu and Francois, 1978).

Liver disorders often cause primary somatomedin deficiency. In the metabolic disorder morbus Gaucher, low amounts of somatomedins are found in children with growth retardation (Hall and Sara, unpublished results). In chronic liver disease like cirrhosis and in alcoholism, low amounts are found by bioassays, radioreceptor assays, and radioimmunoassays (Wu *et al.*, 1974; Schimpff *et al.*, 1978; Takano *et al.*, 1977c; Zapf *et al.*, 1981b). This is to be expected since the liver is one site for somatomedin production. In thalassemia, which also involves the liver, decreased amounts of somatomedins have been reported in childhood as well as in fetal life (Werther *et al.*, 1981; Sara *et al.*, 1981a; Herington *et al.*, 1981).

Patients with Laron dwarfism who are phenotypically similar to growth hormone-deficient children show low concentrations of both RIA-IGF-I and RIA-IGF-II in spite of an elevated concentration of GH (Laron *et al.*, 1971; Zapf *et al.*, 1981b). Further studies showed their endogenous GH to be normal as expected by their failure to respond to exogenous GH (Laron, 1982). Recently, it has been shown that patients with Laron dwarfism have a defect in the GH receptor in the liver (Laron, 1982). Normal GH production is also found in pygmies who display a deficiency in immunoreactive IGF-I with normal concentrations of immunoreactive IGF-II (Merimee *et al.*, 1981). The pygmy may represent the first example found of a selective deficiency in one of the somatomedins. A recent report suggests that patients with Down's syndrome may also display a selective deficiency in IGF-I-like peptides (Sara *et al.*, 1983a). In these growth-retarded patients, immunoreactive SMA fails to rise after birth and remains in the low infant range throughout life. In contrast, somatomedins determined with fetal brain RRA-SMA remain elevated, even in old age. These findings suggest a lack of GH-regulated IGF-I-related peptides and seem to represent failure to switch from the production of fetal to adult forms of somatomedins in Down's syndrome.

A disturbance of somatomedin production has been suggested in endocrine disorders characterized by catabolic status. Although a decrease was first suggested in Cushing's disease when serum levels were determined by porcine cartilage bioassay, later studies using radioreceptor and radioimmunoassay showed values within the normal range (van den Brande and Du Caju, 1973; Thorén *et al.*, 1981) (Fig. 11). Cortisol has a direct inhibitory effect on porcine cartilage. In children with inadequately controlled diabetes the decreased concentrations of immunoreactive IGF-I return toward normal after treatment

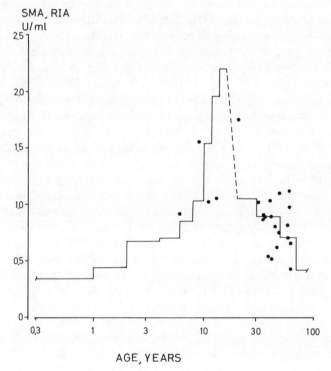

FIG. 11. Somatomedins in serum (RIA-SMA) in 23 patients with Cushing's disease (●). Results displayed on distribution of values for normal subjects. Data from Thorén *et al.* (1981).

to restore glucose homeostasis (Tamborlane *et al.*, 1981). The somatomedin status in thyroid hormone disorders has yet to be clarified.

A discrepancy between assay results is observed in chronic renal failure; somatomedin activity is low, but both radioreceptor assayable and immunoreactive SMA levels are elevated (Saenger *et al.*, 1974; Schwalbe *et al.*, 1977; Takano *et al.*, 1979). This difference is likely to be due to the presence of inhibitory substances which interfere with somatomedin activity in bioassays.

Somatomedin values above the normal range are unusual other than in acromegaly. Megyesi *et al.* (1974a) first reported elevated concentrations in patients with tumor hypoglycemia when using rat liver radioreceptor assay with NSILA or MSA as ligand. Similar results were reported by Daughaday *et al.* (1981b) using the rat placenta radioreceptor assay with IGF-II as ligand. However these high concentrations cannot be attributed to immunoreactive IGF-I or IGF-II because low or normal values are found in patients with tumor hypoglycemia (Zapf *et al.*, 1981a; Widmer *et al.*, 1982). The findings suggest tumor production of an IGF-II-related peptide. Todaro and De Larco (1978) have reported the production of such a peptide from human fibrosarcoma. There has not been extensive use of diverse RIAs in screening of patient material in malignancy. No elevation of RIA-SMA levels was found in patients with osteosarcoma (Adamson *et al.*, 1980).

B. Cerebrospinal Fluid (CSF)

Somatomedin activity in CSF was first demonstrated by Beaton *et al.* (1975). More recently a radioreceptor assay using adult human brain membrane as matrix and IGF-II as ligand was developed to detect neuroactive somatomedin-like peptides (Sara *et al.*, 1983a). In this assay IGF-I and IGF-II are equipotent. In 10 healthy volunteers the concentration determined with brain RRA-IGF-II in the CSF was 0.25 ± 0.05 U/ml and no gradient was observed in fractionated spinal fluid obtained from patients with subarachnoid hemorrhage (von Holtz and Sara, 1983). The amounts of IGF-I-related peptides are extremely low in cerebrospinal fluid. With the immunoreactive SMA method ranges between 0.01 and 0.03 U/ml were found in adults. Immunoreactive IGF-I was scarcely detectable in CSF whereas immunoreactive IGF-II and a further species, big IGF-II, were present at approximately 30 and 22 ng/ml, respectively (Haselbacher and Humbel, 1982).

Somatomedins in CSF appear to be independent of amounts of

somatomedins and growth hormone in serum. RIA-SMA and brain RRA-IGF-II methods show no differences between acromegaly and growth hormone deficiency in CSF content indicating that production is independent of growth hormone.

Somatomedins in the CSF have been determined in several patient groups using the brain RRA-IGF-II method. In subarachnoid hemorrhage, 12 out of 24 patients showed marked elevations in somatomedins in fractionated spinal fluid (von Holtz and Sara, 1983). Although no correlation with neurological condition or cerebral vasospasm was observed, the highest values were found in the only patient who later died. In two cases of head injury, the amounts of somatomedins in CSF were scarcely detectable even 10 days before death in spite of normal amounts in serum. This latter finding suggests endogenous CNS production of somatomedins.

Normal values were obtained in schizophrenic patients (Sara et al., 1983c). Elevated amounts of somatomedins in both CSF and serum have been found in dementia disorders of the Alzheimer type where a localized somatomedin receptor deficiency in the brain has been proposed (Sara et al., 1982b).

C. Exocrine Fluid

The somatomedins appear to be present in exocrine fluids, such as breast milk, intestinal fluids, and amniotic fluid. These fluids cross-react in RIA-SMA, fetal brain RRA-SMA, and placenta RRA-SMA. However the molecular forms present in exocrine fluids remain to be characterized. Additionally, synovial fluid has been demonstrated to contain both bioassayable somatomedin activity and immunoreactive SMA.

IX. Source of the Somatomedins

No endocrine cell has yet been found for the production of the somatomedins. The liver is considered to be the primary source of somatomedins in the circulation. This concept is supported by both direct and indirect evidence. In patients with severe liver disease somatomedin concentrations are low; arteriovenous gradients have been found for somatomedins across the liver (Wu et al., 1974; Takano et al., 1977c; Schimpff et al., 1978). Both immunoreactive IGF-I and IGF-II are reduced in liver disease (Zapf et al., 1981b). Rat liver explants and perfused rat liver release somatomedins together with their carrier proteins. This release is stimulated by GH and blocked by protein inhibitors like puromycin (McConaghey and Sledge, 1970; Phillips *et al.*, 1976; Schalch *et al.*, 1979; Binoux *et al.*, 1982). Hepatocytes from adult rats release somatomedins into the media as found both by radioreceptor and by protein binding assays (Spencer, 1979). Fetal rat liver cells in primary culture release peptides similar to the MSA peptides produced by the established rat liver cell line BRL 3A (Rechler *et al.*, 1979, 1981). The mRNA isolated from BRL 3A cells and translated in a cell-free system directs synthesis of proteins specifically precipitated by antisera against MSA (Acquaviva *et al.*, 1982). The precipitated protein, with a molecular size of 21,600, is proposed to represent prepro-MSA. The direct demonstration of mRNA for MSA in hepatocytes unequivocally shows the liver to be a site of production for somatomedins.

Production from fetal cells, however, does not seem to be simply restricted to the liver. Rather, all fetal cells may produce somatomedins. Explants of various tissues prepared from the human fetus release fetal brain somatomedins (detected by RRA-SMA) into the incubation medium (Sara *et al.*, 1983c). Primary culture of human fetal brain cells release similar material (fetal brain RRA-SMA) but scarcely detectable amounts of immunoreactive SMA (Sara *et al.*, 1983c). Somatomedin release has been found in the youngest fetus examined (10 weeks of gestational age). Acid extracts of human fetal tissue display similar values (fetal brain RRA-SMA) as found in conditioned media. An established cell line of human embryonic lung fibroblasts produces immunoreactive basic somatomedin (Atkinson and Bala, 1980, 1981). A somatomedin-like peptide has recently been purified from fetal bovine cartilage (Kato *et al.*, 1981). D'Ercole *et al.* (1980a) have shown that slices of fetal mouse organs release immunoreactive SMC into the incubation medium as early as day 11 of gestation. Higher concentrations are measured by placenta RRA-SMC than by RIA-SMC assay. Primary cell culture of rat fibroblasts produces different somatomedins according to the age of the donor. Fibroblasts derived from fetal and neonatal rats release immunoreactive MSA, whereas fibroblasts taken from more mature rats release only immunoreactive IGF-I into the incubation medium (Nissley *et al.*, 1983). This finding supports the concept of a switch from the production of fetal to adult forms of somatomedins during development.

As supported by the study with rat fibroblasts, cells other than hepatocytes can produce somatomedins in adults. Clemmons *et al.* (1981b) have shown that human skin fibroblasts release immunoreactive SMC into the conditioned medium. In early studies Hall and

Bozović (1969) reported that extracts from rat skeletal muscle, brain, and liver contained a low-molecular-weight fraction which stimulated sulfate uptake into embryonic chicken cartilage. Similarly, Salmon (1972) found that extracts from pancreas, kidney, heart, and pituitary stimulated sulfate uptake by rat cartilage. Utilizing placenta RRA-SMA, Kawai *et al.* (1979) demonstrated somatomedins in extracts from liver, kidney, lung, and pancreas. In these studies, when extraction was performed at neutral pH, no organ or tissue was found to contain more somatomedin activity than serum itself. However when extraction is performed at low pH, which inhibits degradation of somatomedins, significantly higher amounts of somatomedin activity are recorded. For example, somatomedin activity is found in acid extracts of rat liver at twice the concentration in rat serum (Vassilopoulou-Sellin and Phillips, 1982). Using acid extraction, immunoreactive SMA has been found widely distributed throughout the nervous system of the adult cat (Sara *et al.*, 1982c). The adult nervous system is believed to produce its own somatomedins since there is no correlation between amounts found in serum and CSF (von Holtz and Sara, 1983). Other adult tissues that appear to produce somatomedins include rat testis which in explants release considerable amounts of immunoreactive SMA. This production has been attributed to Sertoli cells (Hall *et al.*, 1983).

Thus, it is clear that the liver can no longer be considered the only site of somatomedin production. All fetal cells produce somatomedins and it would appear that this synthesis may be continued throughout life in certain cell types such as liver and neural tissue. In other cells the ability to produce somatomedins may be repressed except during certain stages of development or when derepressed in neoplastic growth. Both tumor tissue and transformed cell lines produce MSA-like peptides (De Larco and Todaro, 1978; Knauer *et al.*, 1980).

These studies have led to the concept of the somatomedins as both paracrine and endocrine hormones. In some organs such as the brain, the somatomedins may be secreted locally to act on neighboring cells. The somatomedins produced in the liver, however, are released into the circulation and thereby act on distant cells. Other cells or organs may also contribute to the circulating amounts of somatomedins.

X. REGULATION OF SOMATOMEDINS

Just as the somatomedin content of blood varies throughout life so does their regulation. Different regulatory factors influence so-

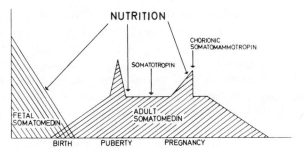

Fɪɢ. 12. Schematic diagram showing somatomedin concentrations throughout life and proposed regulation at different stages of development.

matomedin production at specific stages during life. Our present knowledge of this regulation is summarized in Fig. 12. The onset of the GH regulation of somatomedin production occurs during the first year of life and corresponds to the time when growth becomes growth hormone dependent. In the human fetus, neither growth nor somatomedins appear to be regulated by growth hormone, as evidenced by the normal growth hormone and somatomedin concentrations in the anencephalic fetus (Sara et al., 1981a). In general, the growth retardation in children with isolated GH deficiency is observed first at the age of 6–12 months, which corresponds to the period when RIA-SMA levels start to increase in healthy children. The onset of GH-regulated growth varies between species (Table III) and corresponds to the rise of IGF-I-related peptides. In the rat, RIA-SMA starts to increase at the time of weaning, when growth becomes GH dependent (Sara et al., 1980a). In the guinea pig, neither hypophysectomy nor GH administration influences growth. Moreover, neither of these treatments affects RIA-SMA concentrations (Hall and Sara, unpublished results).

TABLE III
Pɪᴛᴜɪᴛᴀʀʏ Dᴇᴘᴇɴᴅᴇɴᴛ Gʀᴏᴡᴛʜ

Species	Time of onset	Reference
Sheep	Prenatal	Robinson et al. (1978)
Rat	4 weeks	Walker et al. (1950)
Chick	14 weeks	Groussopoulos (1978)
Rabbit	15 weeks	Vezinhet (1968)
Man	First year	Root (1976)
Guinea pig	Never	Knobil and Greep (1959)

There is no indication that the rise in somatomedin concentration during childhood is due to an increase in GH production. The rise is more probably related to changing sensitivity to GH in the organs producing somatomedins. In children with GH deficiency the maximal concentration achieved as well as the percentage increase in somatomedins after GH administration increases toward puberty (Takano *et al.*, 1977b). Thus the temporary peak in somatomedin concentration during puberty cannot be explained by a change in growth hormone production (Hall *et al.*, 1980, 1981). The pubertal peak in somatomedins appears to be unique as no other hormone has yet been observed to display such a temporary rise. In children with primary hypogonadism, and high concentrations of gonadotropins, the pubertal somatomedin peak as well as the growth spurt is lacking.

Growth hormone is undoubtedly one of the major regulators of somatomedin production postnatally. A 10-fold elevation above normal is observed in patients with acromegaly by use of assays measuring IGF-I-related peptides, whereas low amounts are observed in GH-deficient patients (Furlanetto *et al.*, 1977; Hall *et al.*, 1979a; Clemmons *et al.*, 1979; Zapf *et al.*, 1980, 1981b; Bala *et al.*, 1981). Growth hormone directly stimulates somatomedin production from hepatocytes and fibroblasts *in vitro* (Clemmons *et al.*, 1981b). The fall in somatomedin with old age may be related to either a decline in growth hormone production or decreased sensitivity to growth hormone, secondary to either receptor or postreceptor defects. Johansson and Blizzard (1981) reported that the nocturnal peak in GH release is reduced in old age but the somatomedin response after high doses of GH is normal. In contrast, the findings of Thorén and Hall (1983) indicate a decline in GH sensitivity. These authors observed that GH administered in doses of 4 mg for 3 days, which causes a significant 40% increase in RIA-SMA in healthy subjects aged 25–50 years, has no effect in healthy subjects approximately 70 years of age.

During pregnancy somatomedin production is not primarily regulated by growth hormone. Rather the close GH homolog, chorionic somatomammotropin (CS), appears to regulate production. This lack of GH dependency is most elegantly demonstrated by the normal amounts of immunoreactive IGF-I and IGF-II in a GH-deficient woman before delivery (Merimee *et al.*, 1982a). Similarly, immunoreactive SMA rises during the last trimester of pregnancy in GH-deficient women (Hall *et al.*, 1983). In the rat, hypophysectomy does not influence the rise in somatomedin during pregnancy (Daughaday and Kapadia, 1978). Perfusion by hCS stimulates the release of somatomedins from the maternal rat liver (Skottner et al., 1980). Other GH homologs such as ovine prolactin also stimulate somatomedin production in the hypophysectomized rat (Hurley et al., 1977). It is unclear, however, whether human prolactin, which displays less homology with GH, could have a similar effect.

Several other hormones have been implicated in somatomedin regulation. Insulin may play a role in some animals such as the rat and the dog in which insulin deficiency is associated with a decreased serum somatomedin activity (Phillips and Orawski, 1977; Eigenmann et al., 1977). It is doubtful whether insulin has any direct influence in man as normal amounts of somatomedins are found in patients with insulinomas. Estrogens and androgens affect somatomedin production. In patients with acromegaly, high estrogen doses decrease RIA-SMC content and lead to clinical improvement without affecting GH values (Clemmons et al., 1980). In tall girls, high doses of estrogen suppress immunoreactive SMA as well as growth rate (Hall et al., 1981). Similarily, high doses of androgen cause a decrease in RIA-SMA in tall boys (Hall et al., 1981). The effect of substitution therapy of estrogens and androgens has yet to be elucidated. Cortisol has no effects on either immunoreactive SMA or SMC content as evidenced by the normal values obtained in patients with Cushing's syndrome (Thorén et al., 1981; Underwood et al., 1980a,b). Corticosteroid-induced growth retardation is believed to be due to its direct effect on the tissue.

Adequate nutrition is a prerequisite for the effect of GH on somatomedin production. During fasting the GH stimulated increase in RIA-IGF-I and RIA-IGF-II is inhibited (Merimee et al., 1982b). In starving girls with anorexia nervosa and high GH concentrations, the immunoreactive SMA is as reduced as in GH deficiency. With improvement of the disease the concentrations return to normal concomitantly with resumption of growth (Hall et al., 1981; Hall and Sara, 1983). Fasting in healthy subjects causes a slow decline in immunoreactive SMC to the hypopituitary range over approximately 5 days (Clemmons et al., 1981a). This decline is more dramatic in the rat where concentrations characteristic of hypophysectomy are found within 24 hours of fasting (Takano et al., 1977a, 1978, 1980a,b). Only refeeding and not GH administration allows return to normal values. Dietary studies in the rat indicate that protein in the diet is necessary to achieve restoration (Takano et al., 1978, 1980a,b; Phillips and Vassilopoulou-Sellin, 1980a,b; Prewitt et al., 1982). The contribution made by different amino acids has yet to be determined. Preliminary studies showing low amounts of immunoreactive SMA in patients on complete intravenous nutrition suggest that the gastrointestinal hormones may be involved. Nutrition during early development is especially important for growth. In rats, undernutrition induced by altered litter size results in decreased immunoreactive SMA in lactating mothers and their growth-retarded offspring (Sara *et al.*, 1979).

The regulation of somatomedin production from the nervous system appears to be independent of that in the periphery. This is well illustrated by the normal amounts in CSF observed in patients with acromegaly or hypopituitarism and the lack of CSF somatomedin in spite of normal amounts in serum after head injury. The normal CSF content found in patients with GH deficiency suggests that GH does not have a direct regulatory influence on somatomedin production within the nervous system. Other types of regulation must be considered. Electrical stimulation of the sciatic and brachial nerves in the perfused cat leg causes a rapid release of fetal brain RRA-SMA either from the nerve or muscle (Sara *et al.*, 1982c).

Little is known about the regulation of somatomedin production in the fetus; both somatomedin concentrations and growth are independent of GH. It is unlikely that the maternal somatomedin passes the placental barrier because immunoreactive SMA is undetectable in the fetus at the time it starts to rise in the mother (Sara *et al.*, 1981a). This is confirmed by experiments in dogs in which labeled SMC, injected during pregnancy, does not cross to the fetus. Rather the source of the embryonic somatomedin appears to be the fetus itself. Nutritional factors have been proposed to play a primary role in the regulation of production of somatomedins in the fetus. Figure 13 shows the hypothetical model previously proposed for the regulation of both maternal and fetal somatomedin production (Sara and Hall, 1980).

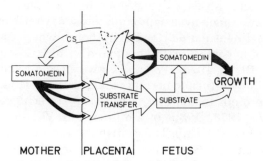

FIG. 13. Hypothetical somatomedin regulatory system for fetal growth. CS, Chorionic somatomammotropin. From Sara and Hall (1980).

XI. Conclusion: A Proposed Integrated Biological Role for the Somatomedins

It is now clear that the somatomedins are involved in a much broader range of biological functions than originally suspected. Their action is not restricted to the regulation of growth but applies also to the maintenance of mature cells. Similarly, these hormones now appear to be ubiquitous throughout the body, with target tissues ranging from cartilage to the nervous system. In view of such widespread action it is essential to consider the somatomedins as anabolic hormones rather than simply growth factors.

There is broader clinical significance as well. Earlier these hormones were believed of importance only in the regulation of skeletal growth throughout childhood. Now it is essential to consider their role in catabolism and anabolism in all tissues throughout life in health and disease. The somatomedins apparently act from the earliest embryonic and fetal stages where they regulate cellular growth, until maturity and old age where they have a maintenance function and may well prove to play a role in the aging process. Clinically their importance may range from intrauterine growth retardation to senile dementia.

Our concepts of the somatomedins must also involve fluidity and change during the life cycle. It is becoming obvious the somatomedins do not represent a single structure. Rather, different forms of somatomedins may predominate at different stages of life. Both sources and the regulation of production may also vary with period of life cycle. This cannot be a random process but possibly follows the principle that somatomedins are produced locally and act as paracrine hormones in rapidly dividing cells. The fetal form of somatomedin is produced by fetal cells. Production of this hormone may be repressed in most tissues only to be derepressed under certain conditions when there is intense local cellular growth such as in neoplastic tissue. In cells with a high metabolic rate, such as the nervous system, local production of this paracrine somatomedin may be maintained throughout life. Other mature cells, however, may rely on somatomedins supplied through the circulation. One source for the serum somatomedins is the liver, but other cells and organs may contribute to the circulating amounts of somatomedins. No cells are yet found for the storage of somatomedins. It has been suggested that the somatomedins are released continuously as befits their roles as anabolic hormones. The change in predominance of paracrine to endocrine action may follow the switch over from production of fetal to adult forms of somatomedins.

There is still controversy concerning the number of members that constitute the somatomedin family. This issue might be settled in the near future when the exciting techniques of molecular biology are applied to identify the several genomes for the somatomedins. This new technology should also provide sufficient amounts of pure somatomedins to allow us to fully examine their biological role.

REFERENCES

Acquaviva, A. M., Bruni, C. B., Nissley, S. P., and Rechler, M. M. (1982). Cell-free synthesis of rat insulin-like growth factor II. *Diabetes* **31**, 656–658.

Adamson, U., Broström, L. Å., Efendić, S., and Hall, K. (1980). Glucose tolerance, growth hormone and somatomedin levels in osteosarcoma patients. *Acta Endocrinol. (Copenhagen)* **94**, 517–522.

Almqvist, S., and Rune, I. (1961). Studies on sulfation factor (SF) activity of human serum: The variation of serum SF with age. *Acta Endocrinol. (Copenhagen)* **36**, 566–576.

Antoniades, H. N. (1961). Studies on the state of insulin in blood: The state and transport of insulin in blood. *Endocrinology* **68**, 7–16.

Atkinson, P. R., and Bala, R. M. (1980). Further studies of somatomedin-like activity produced by cultured human embryonic lung fibroblasts. *Clin. Res.* **28**, 669A.

Atkinson, P. R., and Bala, R. M. (1981). Partial characterization of a mitogenic factor with somatomedin-like activity produced by culture WI-38 human fibroblasts. *J. Cell. Physiol.* **107**, 317–327.

Bala, R. M., and Bhaumick, B. (1979a). Purification of a basic somatomedin, from human plasma Cohn fraction IV-1, with physiochemical and radioimmunoassay similarity to somatomedin-C and insulin-like growth factor. *Can. J. Biochem.* **57**, 1289–1298.

Bala, R. M., and Bhaumick, B. (1979b). Radioimmunoassay of a basic somatomedin: Comparison of various assay techniques and somatomedin levels in various sera. *J. Clin. Endocrinol. Metab.* **49**, 770–777.

Bala, R. M., Wright, C., Bardal, A., and Smith, G. R. (1978). Somatomedin bioactivity in serum and amniotic fluid during pregnancy. *J. Clin. Endocrinol. Metab.* **46**, 649–652.

Bala, R. M., Lopata, J., Leung, A., McCoy, E., and McArthur, R. G. (1981). Serum immunoreactive somatomedin levels in normal adults, pregnant women at term, children at various ages, and children with constitutionally delayed growth. *J. Clin. Endocrinol. Metab.* **52**, 508–512.

Baxter, R. C., Brown, A. S., and Turtle, J. R. (1982). Radioimmunoassay for somatomedin C: Comparison with radioreceptor assay in patients with growth-hormone disorders, hypothyroidism, and renal failure. *Clin. Chem.* **28**, 488–495.

Beaton, G. R., Sagel, J., and Distiller, L. A. (1975). Somatomedin activity in cerebrospinal fluid. *J. Clin. Endocrinol. Metab.* **40**, 736–737.

Bhaumick, B., Bala, R. M., and Hollenberg, M. D. (1981). Somatomedin receptor of human placenta: Solubilization, photolabeling, partial purification, and comparison with insulin receptor. *Proc. Natl. Acad. Sci. U.S.A.* **78**, 4279–4283.

Binoux, M., Lassarre, C., and Hardouin, N. (1982). Somatomedin production by rat liver in organ culture. III. Studies on the release of insulin-like growth factor and its carrier protein measured by radioligand assays. Effects of growth hormone, insulin and cortisol. *Acta Endocrinol. (Copenhagen)* **99**, 422–430.

Blethen, S. L., Daughaday, W. H., and Weldon, V. V. (1982). Kinetics of the somatome-din C/insulin-like growth factor I: Response to exogenous growth hormone (GH) in GH-deficient children. *J. Clin. Endocrinol. Metab.* **54**, 986–990.

Blom, L., Sara, V. R., Larsson, A., and Hall, K. (1983). Neonatal levels in healthy fullterm infants. *Acta Paediatr. Scand.*, submitted.

Blundell, T. L., and Humbel, R. E. (1980). Hormone families: Pancreatic hormones and homologous growth factors. *Nature (London)* **287**, 781–787.

Blundell, T. L., Bedarkar, S., Rinderknecht, E., and Humbel, R. E. (1978). Insulin-like growth factor: A model for tertiary structure accounting for immunoreactivity and receptor binding. *Proc. Natl. Acad. Sci. U.S.A.* **75**, 180–184.

Borsi, L., Rosenfeld, R. G., Liu, F., and Hintz, R. L. (1982). Somatomedin peptide dis-tribution and somatomedin-binding protein content in cord plasma: Comparison to normal and hypopituitary plasma. *J. Clin. Endocrinol. Metab.* **54**, 223–228.

Bradshaw, R. A. (1980). Nerve growth factor, relaxin and the somatomedins: The in-sulin-related growth factors. *Proc. Int. Congr. Endocrinol. 6th, 1980*, 532–535.

Bradshaw, R. A., and Niall, H. D. (1978). Insulin-related growth factors. *Trends Bio-chem. Sci.* **3**, 274–278.

Brasel, J. A., and Gruen, R. K. (1978). Postulated Growth. *In* "Human Growth" (F. Falkner and J. M. Tanner, eds.), pp. 3–19. Plenum, New York.

Bürgi, H., Müller, W. A., Humbel, R. E., Labhart, A., and Froesch, E. R. (1966). Non-suppressible insulin-like activity of human serum. I. Physiochemical properties, extraction and partial purification. *Biochim. Biophys. Acta* **121**, 349–359.

Carpenter, C., and Cohen, S. (1979). Human epidermal growth factor. *Annu. Rev. Bio-chem.* **48**, 193–216.

Chernausek, S. D., Jacobs, S., and van Wyk, J. J. (1981). Structural similarities between human receptors for somatomedin C and insulin: Analysis by affinity labeling. *Biochemistry* **20**, 7345–7350.

Chochinov, R. H., Ketupanya, A., Mariz, I. K., Underwood, L. E., and Daughaday, W. H. (1976). Amniotic fluid reactivity detected by somatomedin C radioreceptor assay: Correlation with growth hormone, prolactin and fetal renal maturation. *J. Clin. Endocrinol. Metab.* **42**, 983–986.

Chochinov, R. H., Mariz, I. K., Hajek, A. S., and Daughaday, W. H. (1977). Characteriza-tion of a protein in mid-term human amniotic fluid which reacts in the somatome-din-C radioreceptor assay. *J. Clin. Endocrinol. Metab.* **44**, 902–908.

Clemmons, D. R., and van Wyk, J. J. (1981). Somatomedin-C and platelet-derived growth factor stimulate human fibroblast replication. *J. Cell. Physiol.* **106**, 361–367.

Clemmons, D. R., van Wyk, J. J., Ridgway, E. C., Kliman, B., Kjellberg, R. N., and Underwood, L. E. (1979). Evaluation of acromegaly by radioimmunoassay of somatomedin-C *N. Engl. J. Med.* **301**, 1138–1142.

Clemmons, D. R., Underwood, L. E., Ridgway, E. C., Kliman, B., Kjellberg, R. N., and van Wyk, J. J. (1980). Estradiol treatment of acromegaly. Reduction of immunoreac-tive somatomedin-C and improvement in metabolic status. *Am. J. Med.* **69**, 571–575.

Clemmons, D. R., Klibanski, A., Underwood, L. E., McArthur, J. W., Ridgway, E. C., Beitins, I. Z., and van Wyk, J. J. (1981a). Reduction of plasma immunoreactive somatomedin C during fasting in humans. *J. Clin. Endocrinol. Metab.* **53**, 1247–1250.

Clemmons, D. R., Underwood, L. E., and van Wyk, J. J. (1981b). Hormonal control of immunoreactive somatomedin production by cultured human fibroblasts. *J. Clin. Invest.* **67**, 10–19.

Daughaday, W. H., and Kapadia, M. (1978). Maintenance of serum somatomedin activity in hypophysectomized pregnant rats. *Endocrinology* **102**, 1317–1320.

Daughaday, W. H., and Reeder, C. (1966). Synchronous activation of DNA synthesis in hypophysectomized rat cartilage by growth hormone. *J. Lab. Clin. Med.* **68**, 357–368.

Daughaday, W. H., Hall, K., Raben, M. S., Salmon, W. D., Jr., Van den Brande, J. L., and van Wyk, J. J. (1972). Somatomedin: Proposed designation for sulphation factor. *Nature (London)* **235**, 107.

Daughaday, W. H., Mariz, I. K., and Blethen, S. L. (1980). Inhibition of access of bound somatomedin to membrane receptor and immunobinding sites: A comparison of radioreceptor and radioimmunoassay of somatomedin in native and acid-ethanol-extracted serum. *J. Clin. Endocrinol. Metab.* **51**, 781–788.

Daughaday, W. H., Mariz, I. K., and Trivedi, B. (1981a). A preferential binding site for insulin-like growth factor II in human and rat placental membranes. *J. Clin. Endocrinol. Metab.* **53**, 282–288.

Daughaday, W. H., Trivedi, B., and Kapadia, M. (1981b). Measurement of insulin-like growth factor II by a specific radioreceptor assay in serum of normal individuals, patients with abnormal growth hormone secretion, and patients with tumour-associated hypolycemia. *J. Clin. Endocrinol. Metab.* **53**, 289–294.

Daughaday, W. H., Parker, K. A., Borowsky, S., Trivedi, B., and Kapadia, M. (1982). Measurement of somatomedin-related peptides in fetal, neonatal, and maternal rat serum by insulin-like growth factor (IGF)-I radioimmunoassay, IGF-II radioreceptor assay (RRA), and multiplication-stimulating activity RRA after acid-ethanol extraction. *Endocrinology* **110**, 575–581.

D'Ercole, A. J., Foushee, D. B., and Underwood, L. E. (1976). Somatomedin-C receptor ontogeny and levels in porcine fetal and human cord serum. *J. Clin. Endocrinol. Metab.* **43**, 1069–1077.

D'Ercole, A. J., Underwood, L. E., Groelke, J., and Plet, A. (1979). Leprechaunism: Studies of the relationship among hyperinsulinism, insulin resistance, and growth retardation. *J. Clin. Endocrinol. Metab.* **48**, 495–502.

D'Ercole, A. J., Applewhite, G. T., and Underwood, L. E. (1980a). Evidence that somatomedin is synthesized by multiple tissues in the fetus. *Dev. Biol.* **75**, 315–328.

D'Ercole, J., Willson, D. F., and Underwood, L. E. (1980b). Changes in the circulating form of serum somatomedin-C during fetal life. *J. Clin. Endocrinol. Metab.* **51**, 674–676.

De Larco, J. E., and Todaro, G. J. (1978). A human fibrosarcoma cell line producing multiplication stimulating activity (MSA) related peptides. *Nature (London)* **272**, 356–358.

Dobbing, J., and Sands, J. (1973). Quantitative growth and development of human brain. *Arch. Dis. Child.* **48**, 757–767.

Drop, S. L. S., Valiquette, G., Guyda, H. J., Corvol, M. T., and Posner, B. I. (1979). Partial purification and characterization of a binding protein for insulin-like activity (ILAs) in human amniotic fluid: A possible inhibitor of insulin-like activity. *Acta Endocrinol. (Copenhagen)* **90**, 505–518.

Dulak, N. C., and Temin, H. M. (1973a). A partially purified polypeptide fraction from rat liver cell conditioned medium with multiplication-stimulating activity for embryo fibroblast. *J. Cell. Physiol.* **81**, 153–160.

Dulak, N. C., and Temin, H. M. (1973b). Multiplication stimulating activity for chick embryo fibroblasts from rat liver cell conditioned medium: A family of small polypeptides. *J. Cell. Physiol.* **81**, 161–170.

Eigenmann, J. E., Becker, M., Kommermann, B., Leemann, W., Heiman, R., Zapf, J., and Froesch, E. R. (1977). Decrease of nonsuppressible insulin-like activity after pancreatectomy and normalization by insulintherapy. *Acta Endocrinol. (Copenhagen)* **85**, 818–822.

El-Etr, M., Shorderet-Slatkine, S., and Baulien, E. E. (1979). Meiotic maturation in *Xenopus laevis* oocytes initiated by insulin. *Science* **205**, 1397–1399.

Ellis, S., Hublé, J., and Simpson, M. E. (1953). Influence of hypophysectomy and growth hormone on cartilage sulfate metabolism. *Proc. Soc. Exp. Biol. Med.* **84**, 603–605.

Enberg, G., Jörnvall, H., Carlqvist, M., and Hall, K. (1983). Somatomedin A, purification and primary structure. In preparation.

Evans, H. M., and Long, J. A. (1921). The effect of feeding the anterior lobe of the hypophysis on the oestrous cycle of the rat. *Anat. Rec.* **21**, 42–64.

Evans, H. M., Simpson, M. E., Marx, W., and Kibrick, E. A. (1943). Bioassay of pituitary growth hormone. Width of proximate, epiphyseal cartilage of tibia in hypophysectomized rats. *Endocrinology* **32**, 13–16.

Evans, M. I., Hager, L. J., and McKnight, G. S. (1981). A somatomedin-like peptide hormone is required during the estrogen-mediated induction of ovalbumin gene transcription. *Cell* **25**, 187–193.

Ewton, D. Z., and Florini, J. R. (1980). Relative effects of the somatomedins, multiplication-stimulating activity, and growth hormone on myoblasts and myotubes in culture. *Endocrinology* **106**, 577–583.

Ewton, D. Z., and Florini, J. R. (1981). Effects of the somatomedins and insulin on myoblast differentiation in vitro. *Dev. Biol.* **86**, 31–39.

Franklin, R. C., Pepperell, R. J., Rennie, G. C., and Cameron, D. P. (1979). Acid ethanol-extractable nonsuppressible insulinlike activity (NSILA-s) during pregnancy and the puerperium and in cord serum at term. *J. Clin. Endocrinol. Metab.* **48**, 695–699.

Froesch, E. R., Bürgi, H., Müller, W. A., Humbel, R. E., Jacob, A., and Lambert, A. (1963). Antibody-suppressible and nonsuppressible insulin-like activity in human serum and their physiologic significance. An insulin assay with adipose tissue of increased precision and specificity. *J. Clin. Invest.* **42**, 1816–1834.

Froesch, E. R., Bürgi, H., Müller, W. A., Humbel, R. E., Jakob, A., and Labhart, A. (1967). Nonsuppressible insulinlike activity of human serum: Purification, physicochemical and biological properties and its relation to total serum ILA. *Rec. Prog. Horm. Res.* **23**, 565–616.

Froesch, E. R., Zapf, J., Audhya, J. K., Ben-Porath, E., Segen, B. J., and Gibson, K. D. (1976). Nonsuppressible insulin-like activity and thyroid hormones major pituitary-dependent sulfation factors for chick embryo cartilage. *Proc. Natl. Acad. Sci. U.S.A.* **73**, 2904–2908.

Fryklund, L., and Sievertsson, H. (1978). Primary structure of somatomedin B. A growth hormone dependent serum factor with protease inhibiting activity. *FEBS Lett.* **87**, 55–60.

Fryklund, L., Uthne, K., and Sievertsson, H. (1974). Identification of two somatomedin A active polypeptides and in vivo effects of a somatomedin A concentrate. *Biochem. Biophys. Res. Commun.* **61**, 957–962.

Fryklund, L., Skottner, A., and Hall, K. (1978). Chemistry and biology of the somatomedins. *Proc. FEBS Meet.* **48**, 65–73.

Furlanetto, R. W. (1980). The somatomedin-C binding protein: Evidence for a heterologous subunit structure. *J. Clin. Endocrinol. Metab.* **51**, 12–19.

Furlanetto , R. W. (1982). Pitfalls in the somatomedin-C radioimmunoassay. *J. Clin. Endocrinol. Metab.* **54**, 1084–1086.

Furlanetto, R. W., Underwood, L. E., van Wyk, J. J., and D'Ercole, A. J. (1977). Estimation of somatomedin-C levels in normals and patients with pituitary disease by radioimmunoassay. *J. Clin. Invest.* **60**, 648–657.

Furlanetto, R. W., Underwood, L. E., van Wyk, J. J., and Handwerger, S. (1978). Serum immunoreactive somatomedin-C is elevated late in pregnancy. *J. Clin. Endocrinol. Metab.* **47**, 695–698.

Gibson, K. D., Ben-Porath, E., Doller, H. J., and Segen, B. J. (1978). Influence of thyroid hormones on growth and growth related processes. *Proc. FEBS Meet.* **48**, 101–110.

Grant, D. B., Hambley, J., Becker, D., and Pimstone, B. L. (1973). Reduced sulphation factor in undernourished children. *Arch. Dis. Child.* **48**, 596–600.

Groussopoulos, J. (1978). Etude de la croissance relative postnatale chez le poulet. Principaux tissue et organes muscle et os individuels. Influence de l'hypophysectomi. Thesis, Univ. Montpellier.

Hall, K. (1970). Quantitative determination of sulphation factor activity in human serum. *Acta Endocrinol. (Copenhagen)* **63**, 338–350.

Hall, K. (1972). Human somatomedin: Determination, occurrences, biological activity and purification. *Acta Endocrinol. (Copenhagen)* **163**, 1–52.

Hall, K., and Bozović, M. (1969). Stimulation of ^{35}S incorporation into embryonic chick cartilage by extracts from rat muscle. *Horm. Metab. Res.* **1**, 235–240.

Hall, K., and Fryklund, L. (1979). Somatomedins. *In* "Hormones in Blood" (C. H. Gray and V. H. T. James, eds), 3rd Ed., Vol. 1, pp. 255–278. Academic Press, New York.

Hall, K., and Sara, V. R. (1983). Somatomedin levels throughout life. *Proc. Asia Oceania Congr. Endocrinol., Int. Congr. Ser. Excerpta Medica,* No. 598, 218–222.

Hall, K., and Uthne, K. (1971). Some biological properties of purified sulfation factor (SF) from human plasma. *Acta Med. Scand.* **190**, 137–143.

Hall, K., Takano, K., and Fryklund, L. (1974). Radioreceptor assay for Somatomedin A. *J. Clin. Endocrinol. Metab.* **39**, 973–976.

Hall, K., Brandt, J., Enberg, G., and Fryklund, L. (1979a). Immunoreactive somatomedin A in human serum. *J. Clin. Endocrinol. Metab.* **48**, 271–278.

Hall, K., Fryklund, L., Grebing, C., Löw, H., Sara, V. R., and Zederman, R. (1979b). Comparison between the action of somatomedin A and insulin. *Horm. Cell. Regul.* **3**, 139–148.

Hall, K., Enberg, G., Ritzén, M., Svan, H., Fryklund, L., and Takano, K. (1980). Somatomedin A levels in serum from healthy children and from children with growth hormone deficiency or delayed puberty. *Acta Endocrinol. (Copenhagen)* **94**, 155–165.

Hall, K., Sara, V. R., Enberg, G., and Ritzén, E. M. (1981). Somatomedins and postnatal growth. *In* "Biology of Normal Human Growth" (M. Ritzén, A. Aperia, K. Hall, A. Larsson, A. Zetterberg, and R. Zetterström, eds.), pp. 275–283. Raven, New York.

Hall, K., Ritzén, E. M., and Johnsonbaugh, R. E. (1983). Pubertal rise of immunoreactive somatomedin and its eventual source. *In* "Insulin-like Growth Factors/Somatomedins." Basic Chemistry, Biology and Clinical Importance (E. M. Spencer, ed.). de Gruyter, Berlin, in press.

Haselbacher, G., and Humbel, R. (1982). Evidence for two species of insuline-like growth factor II (IGF II and "big" IGF II) in human spinal fluid. *Endocrinology* **110**, 1822–1824.

Heinrich, U. E., Schalch, D. S., Jawede, M. H., and Johnson, C. J. (1979). NSILA and foetal growth. *Acta Endocrinol. (Copenhagen)* **90**, 534–543.

Heldin, C. H., Westermark, B., Mellström, K., Johnsson, A., Ek, B., Nister, M., Betsholtz, C., Rönnstrand, L., and Wasteson, Å. (1983). Platelet derived growth factor. In press.

Hepp, K. D. (1972). Adenylate cyclase and insulin action: Effect of insulin, nonsuppressible insulin-like material, and diabetes on adenylate cyclase activity in mouse liver. *Eur. J. Biochem.* **31**, 266–276.

Herington, A. C., Werther, G. A., Mattews, R. N., and Burger, H. G. (1981). Studies on the possible mechanism for deficiency of nonsuppressible insulin-like activity in thalassemia major. *J. Clin. Endocrinol. Metab.* **52**, 393–398.

Hintz, R. L. (1981). The somatomedins. *Adv. Pediatr.* **28**, 293–317.

Hintz, R. L., and Liu, F. (1980). Somatomedin plasma binding proteins. *Proc. Int. Symp. Growth Horm., 2nd, Int. Congr. Excerpta Med.* No. 244, 133–143.

Hintz, R. L., and Liu, F. (1982). A radioimmunoassay for insulin-like growth factor II specific for the C-peptide region. *J. Clin. Endocrinol. Metab.* **54**, 442–446.

Hintz, R. L., Clemmons, D. R., Underwood, L. E., and van Wyk, J. J. (1972). Competetive binding of somatomedin to the insulin receptors of adipocytes, chondrocytes, and liver membranes. *Proc. Natl. Acad. Sci. U.S.A.* **69**, 2351–2353.

Hintz, R. L., Liu, F., Horner, J. M., and Thorsson, A. (1978). Characterization of somatomedin binding to a specific plasma-binding protein. *Clin. Res.* **26**, 128A.

Hintz, R. L., Liu, F., Marshall, L. B., and Chang, D. (1980a). Interaction of somatomedin-C with an antibody directed against the synthetic C-peptide region of insulin-like growth factor-I. *J. Clin. Endocrinol. Metab.* **50**, 405–407.

Hintz, R. L., Liu, F., and Rinderknecht, E. (1980b). Somatomedin-C shared the carboxy-terminal antigenic determinants with insulin-like growth factor-I. *J. Clin. Endocrinol. Metab.* **51**, 672–673.

Hintz, R. L., Liu, F., Rosenfeld, R. G., and Kemp, S. F. (1981). Plasma somatomedin-binding proteins in hypopituitarism: Changes during growth hormone therapy. *J. Clin. Endocrinol. Metab.* **53**, 100–104.

Hintz, R. L., Liu, F., and Seegan, G. (1982). Characterization of an insulin-like growth factor-1/somatomedin C radioimmunoassay specific for the C-peptide region. *J. Clin. Endocrinol. Metab.* **55**, 927–930.

Humbel, R. E., and Rinderknecht, E. (1978). Chemistry of NSILA (= IGF): Structural homology to proinsulin. *Proc. FEBS Meet.* **48**, 55–58.

Hurley, T. W., D'Ercole, A. J., Handwerger, S., Underwood, L. E., Furlanetto, R. W., and Fellows, R. E. (1977). Ovine placental lactogen induces somatomedin: A possible role in fetal growth. *Endocrinology* **101**, 1635–1688.

Hutchings, S. E., and Sato, G. H. (1978). Growth and maintenance of HeLa cells in serum-free medium supplemented with hormones. *Proc. Natl. Acad. Sci. U.S.A.* **75**, 901–904.

Isaksson, O. G. P., Jansson, J. O., and Gause, I. A. M. (1982). Growth hormone stimulates longitudinal bone growth directly. *Science* **216**, 1237–1239.

Johansson, A. J., and Blizzard, R. M. (1981). Low somatomedin-C levels in older men rise in response to growth hormone administration. *Johns Hopkins Med. J.* **149**, 115–117.

Kaplowitz, P. B., and D'Ercole, A. J. (1982). Fibroblasts from a patient with leprechaunism are resistant to insulin, epidermal growth factor (EGF) and somatomedin-C. *J. Clin. Endocrinol. Metab.,* **55**, 741–748.

Kasuga, M., Van Obberghen, E., Nissley, S. P., and Rechler, M. M. (1981). Demonstration of two subtypes of insulin-like growth factor receptors by affinity cross-linking. *J. Biol. Chem.* **256**, 5305–5308.

Kasuga, M., Van Obberghen, E., Nissley, S. P., and Rechler, M. M. (1982). Structure of the insulin-like growth factor receptor in chicken embryo fibroblasts. *Proc. Natl. Acad. Sci. U.S.A.* **79,** 1864–1868.

Kato, Y., Nomura, Y., Tsuji, M., Kinoshita, M., Ohmae, H., and Suzuki, F. (1981). Somatomedin-like peptide(s) isolated from fetal bovine cartilage (cartilage-derived factor): Isolation and some properties. *Proc. Natl. Acad. Sci. U.S.A.* **78,** 6831–6835.

Kawai, K., Takano, K., Hizuka, N., and Shizume, K. (1979). Properties and concentrations of somatomedin A in various rat tissues. *Endocrinol. Jpn.* **26,** 559–565.

King, G. L., Kahn, C. R., Rechler, M. M., and Nissley, S. P. (1980). Direct demonstration of separate receptors for growth and metabolic activities of insulin and multiplication-stimulating activity (an insulinlike growth factor) using antibodies to the insulin receptor. *J. Clin. Invest.* **66,** 130–140.

Knauer, D. J., Iyer, A. P., Banerjee, M. R., and Smith, G. L. (1980). Identification of somatomedin-like polypeptides produced by mammary tumours of BALB/c mice. *Cancer Res.* **40,** 4368–4372.

Knight, A. B., Rechler, M. M., Romanus, J. A., Van Obberghen-Schilling, E. E., and Nissley, S. P. (1981). Stimulation of glucose incorporation and amino acid transport by insulin and an insulin-like growth factor in fibroblasts with defective insulin receptors cultured from a patient with leprechaunism. *Proc. Natl. Acad. Sci. U.S.A.* **78,** 2554–2558.

Knobil, E., and Greep, R. O. (1959). The physiology of growth hormone with particular references to its action in rhesus monkey and the "species specificity" problem. *Recent Prog. Horm. Res.* **3,** 3–44.

Koumans, J., and Daughaday, W. H. (1963). Amino acid requirements for activity of partial purified sulfation factor. *Trans. Assoc. Am. Physicians* **76,** 152–162.

Laron, Z. (1982). Somatomedin, insulin, growth hormone and growth: A review. *Isr. J. Med. Sci.* **18,** 823–829.

Laron, Z., Pertzelan, A., Karp, M., Kowadio-Silbergeld, A., and Daughaday, W. H. (1971). Administration of growth hormone to patients with familial dwarfism with high plasma immunoreactive growth hormone. Measurement of sulfation factor, metabolic and lineal growth response. *J. Clin. Endocrinol. Metab.* **33,** 332–342.

Lecornu, M., and Francois, D. R. (1978). Low serum somatomedin activity in celiac disease. *Helv. Paediatr. Acta* **33,** 509–516.

Leof, E. B., Wharton, W., van Wyk, J. J., and Pledger, W. J. (1980). Epidermal growth factor and somatomedin C control G_1 progression of competent BALB-c-3T3 cells: Somatomedin C regulates commitment to DNA synthesis. *J. Cell. Biol.* **87,** 5.

Levi-Montalcini, R., and Calissana, P. (1979). The nerve factor. *Sci. Am.* **240,** 44–53.

Löw, H., Crane, F. L., Grebing, C., Tally, M., and Hall, K. (1978). Hormone control of plasma membrane oxidation-reduction reactions. Effects of insulin. *FEBS Lett.* **91,** 166–168.

Löw, H., Crane, F. L., Grebing, C., Hall, K., and Tally, M. (1979). Metabolic milieu and insulin action. *Proc. 10th Congr. Int. Diabetes Fed. Int. Congr. Ser. Excerpta Med.,* No. 500, 209–213.

McConaghey, P., and Sledge, C. B. (1970). Production of "sulphation factor" by the perfused liver. *Nature (London)* **225,** 1249–1250.

Marie, P. (1889). Acromegali. *Brain* **13,** 59.

Marquardt, H., Todaro, G. J., Henderson, L. E., and Oroszlan, S. (1981). Purification and primary structure of a polypeptide with multiplication-stimulating activity from rat liver cell cultures. *J. Biol. Chem.* **256,** 6859–6865.

Marshall, R. N., Underwood, L. E., Voina, S. J., Foushee, D. B., and van Wyk, J. J.

(1974). Characterization of the insulin and somatomedin-C receptors in human placental cell membranes. *J. Clin. Endocrinol. Metab.* **39**, 283–292.

Massaque, J., and Czech, M. (1982). The subunit structures of two distinct receptors for insulin-like growth factors 1 and 2 and their relationship to the insulin receptor. *J. Biol. Chem.* **257**, 5038–5045.

Massaque, J., Guillette, B. J., and Czech, M. P. (1981). Affinity labeling of multiplication stimulating activity receptors in membranes from rat and human tissues. *J. Biol. Chem.* **256**, 2122–2125.

Megyesi, K., Kahn, C. R., Roth, J., and Gorden, P. (1974a). Hypoglycemia in association with extrapancreatic tumors: Demonstration of elevated plasma NSILA-s by a new radioreceptor assay. *J. Clin. Endocrinol. Metab.* **38**, 931–934.

Megyesi, K., Kahn, C. R., Roth, J., Neville, D. M., Jr., Nissley, S. P., Humbel, R. E., and Froesch, E. R. (1974b). The NSILA-s receptor in liver plasma membranes: Characterization and comparison with insulin receptor. *J. Biol. Chem.* **250**, 8990–8996.

Merimee, T. J., Zapf, J., and Froesch, E. R. (1981). Dwarfism in the pygmy. An isolated deficiency of insulin-like growth factor 1. *N. Engl. J. Med.* **305**, 965–968.

Merimee, T. J., Zapf, J., and Froesch, E. R. (1982a). Insulin-like growth factor in pregnancy: Studies in a growth hormone deficient dwarf. *J. Clin. Endocrinol. Metab.* **54**, 1101–1103.

Merimee, T. J., Zapf, J., and Froesch, E. R. (1982b). Insulin-like growth factors in the fed and fasted states. *J. Clin. Endocrinol. Metab.* **55**, 999–1002.

Meuli, C., and Froesch, E. R. (1977). Insulin and non suppressible insulin-like activity (NSILA-s) stimulated the same glucose transport system via two separate receptors in rat heart. *Biochem. Biophys. Res. Commun.* **75**, 689–695.

Minuto, F., Underwood, L. E., Grimaldi, P., Furlanetto, R. W., van Wyk, J. J., and Giordano, G. (1981). Decreased serum somatomedin C concentrations during sleep: Temporal relationship to the nocturnal surges of growth hormone and prolactin. *J. Clin. Endocrinol. Metab.* **52**, 399–403.

Morris, D. H., and Schalch, D. S. (1982). Structure of somatomedin-binding protein: Alkaline GH induced dissociation of an acid-stable, 60,000 molecular weight complex into smaller components. *Endocrinology* **111**, 801–805.

Moses, A. C., Nissley, S. P., Cohen, K. L., and Rechler, M. M. (1976). Specific binding of a somatomedin-like polypeptide in rat serum depends on growth hormone. *Nature (London)* **263**, 137–140.

Moses, A. C., Nissley, S. P., Short, P. A., and Rechler, M. M. (1980a). Immunological cross-reactivity of multiplication-stimulating activity polypeptides. *Eur. J. Biochem.* **103**, 401–408.

Moses, A. C., Nissley, S. P., Short, P. A., Rechler, M. M., and Podskalny, J. M. (1980b). Purification and characterization of multiplication-stimulating activity. Insulin-like growth factors purified from rat-liver-conditioned medium. *Eur. J. Biochem.* **103**, 387–400.

Moses, A. C., Nissley, S. P., Short, P. A., Rechler, M. M., White, R. M., Knight, A. B., and Higa, O. Z. (1980c). Increased levels of multiplication-stimulating activity an insulin-like growth factor, in fetal rat serum. *Proc. Natl. Acad. Sci. U.S.A.* **77**, 3649–3653.

Nissley, S. P., and Rechler, M. M. (1978). Multiplication-stimulating activity (MSA): A somatomedin-like polypeptide from cultured rat liver cells. *Natl. Cancer Inst. Monogr.* **48**, 167–177.

Nissley, S. P., Adams, S. O., Acquaviva, A. M., Yang, Y. W-H., Bruni, C. B., August, G. P., White, R. M., Foley, T. P., Jr., Moses, A. C., Cohen, K. L., and Rechler, M. M.

(1983). Multiplication activity for cells in culture. *In* "Insulinlike Growth Factors/Somatomedins. Basic Chemistry, Biology and Clinical Importance" (E. M. Spencer, ed). de Gruyters, Berlin, in press.

Oelz, O., Jakob, A., and Froesch, E. R. (1970). Nonsuppressible insulin-like activity (NSILA) of human serum. V. Hypoglycemia and preferential metabolic stimulation of muscle by NSILA-s. *Eur. J. Clin. Invest.* **1**, 48–53.

Phillips, L. S., and Orawski, A. T. (1977). Nutrition and somatomedin. III. Diabetic control, somatomedin and growth in rats. *Diabetes* **26**, 864–869.

Phillips, L. S., and Vassilopoulou-Sellin, R. (1980a). Somatomedins. *N. Engl. J. Med.* **302**, 371–380.

Phillips, L. S., and Vassilopoulou-Sellin, R. (1980b). Somatomedins. *N. Engl. J. Med.* **302**, 438–446.

Phillips, L. S., Herington, A. C., Korl, J. E., and Daughaday, W. H. (1976). Comparison of somatomedin activity in perfusates of normal and hypophysectomized rat liver with and without added growth hormone. *Endocrinology* **98**, 606–614.

Pledger, W. J., Stiles, C. D., Antoniades, H. N., and Scher, C. D. (1977). Induction of DNA synthesis in BALB/c 3T3 cells by serum components: Reevaluation of the commitment process. *Proc. Natl. Acad. Sci. U.S.A.* **74**, 4481–4485.

Poffenbarger, P. L. (1975). The purification and partial characterization of an insulin-like protein from human serum. *J. Clin. Invest.* **56**, 1455–1463.

Poggi, C., Le Marchand-Brustedl, Y., Zapf, J., and Froesch, E. R. (1979). Effects and binding of insulin-like growth factor I in the isolated soleus muscle of lean and obese mice: Comparison with insulin. *Endocrinology* **105**, 723–730.

Preece, M. A., and Holder, A. T. (1982). The somatomedins: A family of serum growth factors. *In* "Recent Advances in Endocrinology and Metabolism 2" (J. L. H. O'Riorelou, ed.), pp. 37–72. Churchill, London.

Prewitt, T. E., D'Ercole, A. J., Switzer, B. R., and van Wyk, J. J. (1982). Relationship of serum immunoreactive somatomedin-C to dietary protein and energy in growing rats. *J. Nutr.* **112**, 144–150.

Raben, M. (1958). Treatment of pituitary dwarf with human growth hormone. *J. Clin. Endocrinol. Metab.* **18**, 901–903.

Rappaport, R., Czernichow, P., and Prevot, C. (1978). Plasma GH and somatomedin activity (SMA) in relation to growth retardation and weight changes in anorexia nervosa (AN). *Pediatr. Res.* **12**, 153.

Rappaport, R., Prevot, C., and Czernichow, P. (1980). Somatomedin activity and growth hormone secretion. 1. Changes related to body weight in anorexia nervosa. *Acta Paediatr. Scand.* **69**, 37–41.

Rechler, M. M., Podskalny, J. M., and Nissley, S. P. (1976). Interaction of multiplication stimulating activity with chick embryo fibroblasts demonstrates a growth receptor. *Nature (London)* **259**, 134–136.

Rechler, M. M., Nissley, S. P., Podskalny, J. M., Moses, A. C., and Fryklund, L. (1977). Identification of a receptor for somatomedin-like polypeptides in human fibroblasts. *J. Clin. Endocrinol. Metab.* **44**, 820–831.

Rechler, M. M., Fryklund, L., Nissley, S. P., Hall, K., Podskalny, J. M., Skottner, A., and Moses, A. C. (1978). Purified human somatomedin A and rat multiplication stimulating activity. Mitogens for cultured fibroblasts that crossreact with the same growth peptide receptors. *Eur. J. Biochem.* **82**, 5–12.

Rechler, M. M., Eisen, H. J., Higa, O. Z., Nissley, S. P., Moses, A. C., Schilling, E. E., Fennoy, I., Bruni, C. B., Phillips, L. S., and Baird, K. L. (1979). Characterization of a somatomedin (insulin-like growth factor) synthetized by fetal rat liver organ cultures. *J. Biol. Chem.* **254**, 7942–7950.

Rechler, M. M., Zapf, J., Nissley, S. P., Froesch, E. R., Moses, A. C., Podskalny, J. M., Schilling, E. E., and Humbel, R. E. (1980). Interactions of insulin-like growth factors I and II and multiplication-stimulating activity with receptors and serum carrier proteins. *Endocrinology* **107**, 1451–1459.

Rechler, M. M., Nissley, S. P., King, G. L., Moses, A. C., Van Obberghen-Schilling, E. E., Romanus, J. A., Knight, A. B., Short, P. A., and White, R. M. (1981). Multiplication stimulating activity (MSA) from the BRL 3A rat liver cell line: Relation to human somatomedins and insulin. *J. Supramol. Struc. Cell. Biochem.* **15**, 253–286.

Rinderknecht, E., and Humbel, R. E. (1976a). Polypeptides with nonsuppressible insulin-like and cell-growth promoting activities in human serum: Isolation, chemical characterization, and some biological properties of forms I and II. *Proc. Natl. Acad. Sci. U.S.A.* **73**, 2365–2369.

Rinderknecht, E., and Humbel, R. E. (1976b). Amino-terminal sequences of two polypeptides from human serum with nonsuppressible insulin-like and cell-growth-promoting activities. Evidence for structural homology with insulin B chain. *Proc. Natl. Acad. Sci. U.S.A.* **73**, 4379–4381.

Rinderknecht, E., and Humbel, R. E. (1978a). The amino acid sequence of human insulin-like growth factor I and its structural homology with proinsulin. *J. Biol. Chem.* **253**, 2769–2776.

Rinderknecht, E., and Humbel, R. E. (1978b). Primary structure of human insulin-like growth factor II. *FEBS Lett.* **89**, 283–286.

Robinson, I. S., Hart, J., Jones, C. T., and Thorburn, G. F. (1978). Observation of experimental growth retardation in sheep. *Br. J. Obstet. Gynaecol.* **84**, 555.

Root, A. W. (1976). Growth hormone and prolactin in the fetus. *In* "Diabetes and other Endocrine Disorders during Pregnancy and in the Newborn" (M. I. New and R. H. Fisher, Jr., eds.). Liss, New York.

Rosenfeld, R. G., and Dollar, L. A. (1982). Characterization of the somatomedin-C/insulin-like growth factor 1 (SM-C/IGF-1) receptor on cultured human fibroblast monolayers: Regulation of receptor concentrations by SM-C/IGF-1 and insulin. *J. Clin. Endocrinol. Metab.* **55**, 434–440.

Rosenfeld, R. G., Kemp, S. F., Gaspich, S., and Hintz, R. L. (1981). In vivo modulation of somatomedin receptor sites: Effects of growth hormone treatment of hypopituitary children. *J. Clin. Endocrinol. Metab.* **52**, 759–764.

Ross, R., and Glomset, J. A. (1976). The pathogenesis of arthero sclerosis. *N. Engl. J. Med.* **295**, 369–377.

Rothstein, H. (1982). Regulation of the cell cycle by somatomedins. *Int. Rev. Cytol.* **78**, 127–232.

Rothstein, H., van Wyk, J. J., Hayden, J. H., Gordon, S. R., and Weinsieder, A. (1980). Somatomedin C: Restoration in vivo of cycle traverse in G_0/G_1 blocket cells of hypophysectomized animals. *Science* **208**, 410–412.

Rubin, J. S., Mariz, I., Jacobs, J. W., Daughaday, W. H., and Bradshaw, R. A. (1982). Isolation and partial sequence analysis of rat basic somatomedin. *Endocrinology* **110**, 734–740.

Rudman, D., Kutner, M. H., Blackstone, D. R., Cushman, R. A., Bain, R. P., and Patterson, J. H. (1981a). Children with normal-variant short stature: Treatment with human growth hormone for six months. *N. Engl. J. Med.* **305**, 123–131.

Rudman, D., Moffitt, S. D., Fernhoff, P. M., McKenzie, W. J., Kenny, J. M., and Bain, R.

P. (1981b). The relation between growth velocity and serum somatomedin C concentration. *J. Clin. Endocrinol. Metab.* **52**, 622–627.

Saenger, P., Wiedmann, E., Schwartz, E., Korth-Schutz, S., Lewy, J. E., Riggio, R. R., Rubin, A. L., Stenzel, K. H., and New, M. I. (1974). Somatomedin and growth after renal transplantation. *Pediatr. Res.* **8**, 163–169.

Salmon, W. D., Jr. (1972). Investigation with a partially purified preparation of serum sulfation factor. Lack of speciality for cartilage sulfation. *In* "Growth and Growth Hormone," *Proc. Int. Symp. Growth Horm., 2nd, Int. Congr. Excerpta Med.* No. 244, 180–191.

Salmon, W. D., Jr., and Daughaday, W. H. (1957). A hormonally controlled serum factor which stimulates sulfate incorporation by cartilage in vitro. *J. Lab. Clin. Med.* **49**, 825–836.

Samaan, N. A., Dempster, W. J., Fraser, R., Please, M. W., and Stillman, D. (1962). Further immunological studies on the form of circulating insulin. *J. Endocrinol.* **24**, 263–277.

Sara, V. R., and Hall, K. (1980). Somatomedins and the fetus. *In* "Clinical Obstetrics and Gynecology" (R. Chez, ed), Vol. 23, pp. 765–778. Harper, New York.

Sara, V. R., and Hall, K. (1983). Somatomedin receptors in the human brain throughout life. *In* "Insulin-like Growth Factors/Somatomedins. Basic Chemistry, Biology and Clinical Importance" (E. M. Spencer, ed). de Gruyter, Berlin, in press.

Sara, V. R., Hall, K., Sjögren, B., Finnson, K., and Wetterberg, L. (1979). The influence of early nutrition on growth and the circulating levels of immunoreactive somatomedin A. *J. Dev. Physiol.* **1**, 343–350.

Sara, V. R., Hall, K., Lins, P. E., and Fryklund, L. (1980a). Serum levels of immunoreactive somatomedin A in the rat. Some developmental aspects. *Endocrinology* **107**, 622–625.

Sara, V. R., Hall, K., Ottosson-Seeberger, A., and Wetterberg, L. (1980b). The role of the somatomedins in fetal growth. *Proc. Int. Congr. Endocrinol., 6th, 1980*, pp. 453–456.

Sara, V. R., Hall, K., Rodeck, C. H., and Wetterberg, L. (1981a). Human embryonic somatomedin. *Proc. Natl. Acad. Sci. U.S.A.* **78**, 3175–3179.

Sara, V. R., Hall, K., Rutter, M., Wetterberg, L., and Yuwiter, A. (1981b). Hormonal regulation of brain growth: Implications for mental retardation. *Proc. World Congr. Biol. Psychiatry, 3rd, 1981*, pp. 1316–1319.

Sara, V. R., Gennser, G., and Persson, P. H. (1982a). Somatomedins during pregnancy and their relationship to fetal growth. *J. Dev. Physiol.* **4**, 187–193.

Sara, V. R., Hall, K., Enzell, K., Gardner, A., Morowski, R., and Wetterberg, L. (1982b). Somatomedins in aging and dementia disorders of Alzheimer type. *Neurobiol. Aging* **3**, 117–120.

Sara, V. R., Uvnäs-Moberg, K., Uvnäs, B., Hall, K., Wetterberg, L., Posloncec, B., and Goiny, M. (1982c). The distribution of somatomedin in the nervous system of the cat and their release following neural stimulation. *Acta Physiol. Scand.* **115**, 466–470.

Sara, V., Hall, K., von Holtz, H., Humbel, R., Sjögren, B., and Wetterberg, L. (1982d). Evidence for the presence of insulin-like growth factors I and II and insulin receptors throughout the adult human brain. *Neurosci. Lett.*, **34**, 39–44.

Sara, V. R., Gustavsson, K.-H., Anneren, G., Hall, K., and Wetterberg, L. (1983a). Somatomedins in Downs syndrome. *Biol. Psychiat.*, **18**, 803–811.

Sara, V. R., Hall, K., Mizaki, M., Fryklund, L., and Wetterberg, L. (1983b). The ontogenesis of somatomedin and insulin receptors in the human fetus. *J. Clin. Invest.*, in press.

Sara, V. R., Hall, K., and Wetterberg, L. (1983c). The role of somatomedins in psychiatric disorders. *In* "Insulinlike Growth Factors/Somatomedins. Basic Chemistry, Biology and Clinical Importance" (E. M. Spencer, ed). de Gruyter, Berlin, in press.

Schalch, D. S., Heinrich, U. E., Koch, J. G., Johnson, C. J., and Schlueter, R. J. (1978). Nonsuppressible insulin-like activity (NSILA). I. Development of a new sensitive competitive proteinbinding assay for determination of serum levels. *J. Clin. Endocrinol. Metab.* **46**, 664–671.

Schalch, D. S., Heinrich, U. E., Draznin, B., Johnson, C. J., and Miller, L. L. (1979). Role of the liver in regulating somatomedin activity: Hormonal effects of the synthesis and release of insulin-like growth factor and its carrier protein by the isolated perfused rat liver. *Endocrinology* **104**, 1143–1151.

Schimpff, R. M., Lebrec, D., and Donnadieu, M. (1978). Serum somatomedin activity measured as sulphation factor in peripheral hepatic and renal veins of patients with alcoholic cirrhosis. *Acta Endocrinol. (Copenhagen)* **88**, 729–736.

Schlumpf, U., Heimann, R., Zapf, J., and Froesch, E. R. (1976). Nonsuppressible insulin-like activity and sulphation activity in serum extracts of normal subjects, acromegalic and pituitary dwarfs. *Acta Endocrinol. (Copenhagen)* **81**, 28–42.

Schoenle, E., Zapf, J., Humbel, R. E., and Froesch, E. R. (1982). Insulin-like growth factor 1 stimulates growth in hypophysectomized rats. *Nature (London)* **296**, 252–253.

Schwalbe, S. L., Betts, P. R., Rayner, P. H. W., and Rudd, B. T. (1977). Somatomedin in growth disorders and chronic renal insufficiency in children. *Br. Med. J.* **6062**, 679–682.

Skottner, A., Fryklund, L., Forsman, A., and Castensson, S. (1980). Somatomedin A and B: Biological studies. *In Proc. Int. Symp. Growth Horm., 2nd, Int. Congr. Excerpta Med.* No. 244, pp. 65–72.

Smith, P. E. (1927). The disabilities caused by hypophysectomy and their repair. *J. Am. Med. Assoc.* **88**, 158–161.

Spencer, E. M. (1979). Synthesis by cultured hepatocytes of somatomedin and its binding protein. *FEBS Lett.* **99**, 157–161.

Stiles, C. D., Capone, G. I., Scher, C. D., Antoniades, H. N., van Wyk, J. J., and Pledger, W. J. (1979a). Dual control of cell growth by somatomedin and platelet-derived growth factor. *Proc. Natl. Acad. Sci. U.S.A.* **76**, 1279–1283.

Stiles, C. D., Pledger, W. J., van Wyk, J. J., Antoniades, H., and Scher, C. D. (1979b). Hormonal control of early events in the BALB/c-3T3 cell cycle. Commitment to DNA synthesis. *Horm. Cell Cult.* **6**, 425–439.

Svoboda, M. E., van Wyk, J. J., Klapper, D. G., Fellows, R. E., Grissom, F. E., and Schlueter, R. J. (1980). Purification of somatomedin-C from human plasma: Chemical and biological properties, partial sequence analysis and relationship to other somatomedins. *Biochemistry* **19**, 790–797.

Takano, K., Hall, K., Fryklund, L., and Sievertsson, H. (1976a). Binding of somatomedins and insulin to plasma membranes prepared from rat and monkey tissue. *Horm. Metab. Res.* **8**, 16–24.

Takano, K., Hall, K., Ritzén, M., Iselius, L., and Sievertsson, H. (1976b). Somatomedin A in human serum, determined by radioreceptor assay. *Acta Endocrinol. (Copenhagen)* **82**, 449–459.

Takano, K., Hizuka, N., and Shizume, K. (1977a). The effects of GH and fasting on the serum levels of somatomedin in rats and men determined by radioreceptor assay. *Acta Endocrinol. (Copenhagen)* **85**, 189.

Takano, K., Hizuka, N., Shizume, K., and Hall, K. (1977b). Effect of human growth hormone on serum somatomedin A in patients with growth hormone deficiency. *Endocrinol. Jpn.* **24**, 359–365.

Takano, K., Hizuka, N., Shizume, K., Hayashi, N., Motoike, Y., and Obata, H. (1977c). Serum somatomedin peptides measured by somatomedin A radioreceptor assay in chronic liver disease. *J. Clin. Endocrinol. Metab.* **45**, 828–832.

Takano, K., Hizuka, N., Kawai, K., and Shizume, K. (1978). Effect of growth hormone and nutrition on the level of somatomedin A in the rat. *Acta Endocrinol. (Copenhagen)* **87**, 458–494.

Takano, K., Hall, K., Kastrup, K. W., Hizuka, N., Shizume, K., Kawai, K., Akimoto, M., Takuma, T., and Sugino, N. (1979). Serum somatomedin A in chronic renal failure. *J. Clin. Endocrinol. Metab.* **48**, 371–376.

Takano, K., Hizuka, N., Shizume, K., Hasumi, Y., Kogawa, M., and Tsushima, T. (1980a). Effect of insulin and nutrition on serum levels of somatomedin A in the rat. *Endocrinology* **107**, 1614–1619.

Takano, K., Hizuka, N., Shizume, K., Hasumi, Y., and Tsushima, T. (1980b). Effect of nutrition on growth and somatomedin A levels in the rat. *Acta Endocrinol. (Copenhagen)* **94**, 321–326.

Takano, K., Kogawa, M., Asakawa, K., Hasumi, Y., and Shizume, K. (1981). Effect of food and GH on the binding of ^{125}I-somatomedin A to the membranes of rat lung and kidney. *Endocrinol. Jpn.* **28**, 669–675.

Tamborlane, W. V., Hintz, R. L., Bergman, M., Genel, M., Felig, P., and Sherwin, R. S. (1981). Insulin-infusion-pump treatment of diabetes. Influence of improved metabolic control on plasma somatomedin levels. *N. Engl. J. Med.* **305**, 303–307.

Temin, H. M. (1971). Stimulation by serum of multiplication of stationary chicken cells. *J. Cell. Physiol.* **78**, 161–170.

Temin, H. M., Pierson, R. W., Jr., and Dulak, N. K. (1972). The role of serum in the control of avian and mammalian cells in culture. *In* "Growth Nutrition and Metabolism of Cells in Culture" (S. H. Rothblat and V. J. Cristofalo, eds.), pp. 50–81. Academic Press, New York.

Thorén, M., and Hall, K. (1983). Somatomedin response to GH in healthy subjects. In preparation.

Thorén, M., Hall, K., and Rähn, T. (1981). Serum levels of somatomedin A in patients with Cushing's disease. *Acta Endocrinol. (Copenhagen)* **97**, 12–17.

Thorsson, A. V., and Hintz, R. L. (1977). Specific ^{125}I-somatomedin response on circulating human mononuclear cells. *Biochem. Biophys. Res. Commun.* **74**, 1566–1573.

Todaro, G. J., and De Larco, J. E. (1978). Growth factors produced by sarcoma virus-transformed cells. *Cancer Res.* **38**, 4147–4153.

Underwood, L. E., Copeland, K. C., Clemmons, D. R., Chatelain, P. G., Blethen, S. L., and van Wyk, J. J. (1980a). Radioimmunoassay of somatomedin-C: Clinical applications. *Proc. 10th Cong. Int. Diabetes Fed. Int. Congr. Ser. Excerpta Med.*, No. 500, 278–282.

Underwood, L. E., D'Ercole, A. J., and van Wyk, J. J. (1980b). Somatomedin-C and the assessment of growth. *Pediatr. Clin. North Am.* **27**, 771–782.

Uthne, K. (1973). Human somatomedins: Purification and some studies on their biological actions. *Acta Endocrinol. (Copenhagen)* **175**, 1–35.

van den Brande, J. L. (1973). Plasma somatomedin studies on some of its characteristics and on its relationship with growth hormone. Gemeentedrukkerij, 1–74. Rotterdam.

van den Brande, J. L., and Du Caju, M. V. L. (1973). Plasma somatomedin activity in children with growth disturbances. *In* "Advances in Human Growth Hormone Research" (S. Raiti, ed), pp. 98–115. DHEW(NIH) 74–612, Washington, D.C.

van den Brande, J. L., and Du Caju, M. V. L. (1974). An improved technique for measuring somatomedin activity in vitro. *Acta Endocrinol. (Copenhagen)* **75**, 233–242.

van Buul, S., and van den Brande, J. L. (1978). The Snell-dwarfmouse II. Sulphate and thymidine incorporation in costal cartilage and somatomedin levels before and during growth hormone and thyroxine therapy. *Acta Endocrinol. (Copenhagen)* **89**, 646–658.

van Buul-Offers, S., and van den Brande, J. L. (1981). The growth of different organs of normal and dwarfed Snell mice, before and during growth hormone therapy. *Acta Endocrinol. (Copenhagen)* **96**, 46–58.

van Buul-Offers, S., and van den Brande, J. L. (1982). Cellular growth in organs of dwarf mice during treatment with growth hormone, thyroxine and plasma fractions containing somatomedin activity. *Acta Endocrinol. (Copenhagen)* **99**, 150–160.

van Obberghen-Schilling, E. E., Rechler, M. M., Romanus, J. A., Knight, A. B., Nissley, S. P., and Humbel, R. E. (1981). Receptors for insulinlike growth factor I are defective in fibroblasts cultured from a patient with leprechaunism. *J. Clin. Invest.* **68**, 1356–1365.

van Wyk, J. J., and Underwood, L. E. (1978). The somatomedins and their actions. *Biochem. Actions Horm.* **5**, 101–148.

van Wyk, J. J., Underwood, L. E., Baseman, J. B., Hintz, R. L., Clemmons, D. R., and Marshall, R. N. (1975). Exploration of the insulin-like and growth-promoting properties of somatomedin by membrane receptor assay. *Adv. Metab. Disord.* **8**, 127–150.

van Wyk, J. J., Furlanetto, R. W., Plet, A. S., D'Ercole, A. J., and Underwood, L. E. (1978). The somatomedin group of peptide growth factors. *Natl. Cancer Inst. Monogr.* **48**, 141–147.

van Wyk, J. J., Svoboda, M. E., and Underwood, L. E. (1980). Evidence from radioligand assays that somatomedin-C and insulin-like growth factor-I are similar to each other and different from other somatomedins. *J. Clin. Endocrinol. Metab.* **50**, 206–208.

van Wyk, J. J., Underwood, L. E., D'Ercole, A. J., Clemmons, D. R., Pledger, W. J., Wharton, W. R., and Leof, E. B. (1981). Role of somatomedins in cellular proliferation. *In* "The Biology of Normal Human Growth" (M. Ritzén, A. Aperia, K. Hall, A. Larsson, A. Zetterberg, and R. Zetterstrom, eds.), pp. 223–240. Raven, New York.

Vassilopoulou-Sellin, R., and Phillips, L. S. (1982). Extraction of somatomedin activity from rat liver. *Endocrinology* **110**, 582–589.

Vezinhet, A. (1968). Effect de l'hypophysectomie sur la croissance ponderal du lapin. *C. R. Hebd. Sceances Acad. Sci. Ser. D* **266**, 2348–2351.

von Holtz, H., and Sara, V. R. (1983). The presence of somatomedin in fractionated cerebrospinal fluid following subarachnoid hemorrhage. *Acta Neurol. Scand,* submitted.

Walker, D. G., Simpson, M. E., Asling, C. N., and Evans, H. M. (1950). Growth and differentiation in the rat following hypophysectomy at 6 days of age. *Anat. Rec.* **106**, 539–554.

Weidman, E. R., and Bala, R. M. (1980). Direct mitogenic effects of human somatomedin on human embryonic lung fibroblasts. *Biochem. Biophys. Res. Commun.* **92**, 577–585.

Werner, S., Hall, K., and Löw, H. (1974). Similar effects of calcitonin, insulin and somatomedin A on lipolysis and uptake of calcium and glucose in rat adipose tissue in vitro. *Horm. Metab. Res.* **6**, 319–325.

Werther, G. A., Matthews, R. N., Burger, H. G., and Herington, A. C. (1981). Lack of response of nonsuppressible insulin-like activity to short term administration of human growth hormone in thalassemia major. *J. Clin. Endocrinol. Metab.* **53**, 806–809.

Wharton, W., van Wyk, J. J., and Pledger, W. J. (1981). Inhibition of BALB/c-3T3 cells in late G_1: Commitment to DNA synthesis controlled by somatomedin C. *J. Cell. Physiol.* **107**, 31–39.

White, R. M., Nissley, S. P., Short, A., Rechler, M. M., and Fennoy, I. (1982). Development pattern of a serum binding protein for multiplication stimulating activity in the rat. *J. Clin. Invest.* **69**, 1239–1252.

Widmer, U., Zapf, J., and Froesch, E. R. (1982). Is extrapancreatic tumor hypoglycemia associated with elevated levels of insulin-like growth factor II? *J. Clin. Endocrinol. Metab.* **55**, 833–839.

Widdowson, E. M. (1981). Growth of the body and its components and the influence of nutrition. *In* "The Biology of Human Growth" (M. Ritzén, A. Aperia, K. Hall, A. Larsson, A. Zetterberg, and R. Zetterstrom, eds.), pp. 253–263. Raven, New York.

Wilson, D. M., Bennett, A., Adamson, G. D., Nagashima, R. J., Liu, F., DeNatale, M. L., Hintz, R. L., and Rosenfeld, R. G. (1982). Somatomedins in pregnancy: A cross-sectional study of insulin-like growth factors I and II and somatomedin peptide content in normal human pregnancies. *J. Clin. Endocrinol. Metab.* **55**, 858–861.

Winick, M. (1968). Changes in nucleic acid and protein content of the human brain during growth. *Pediatr. Res.* **2**, 352–355.

Wu, A., Grant, D. B., Hambley, J., and Levi, A. J. (1974). Reduced serum somatomedin activity in patient with chronic liver disease. *Clin. Sci. Mol. Med.* **47**, 359–366.

Yde, H. (1968). A simplified technique for the determination of growth hormone dependent sulfation factor, using intact animals. *Acta Endocrinol. (Copenhagen)* **57**, 557–564.

Young, F. G. (1945). Growth and diabetes in normal animal treated with pituitary (anterior lobe) diabetogenic extract. *Biochem. J.* **39**, 515–536.

Zapf, J., Kaufmann, U., Eigenmann, E., and Froesch, E. R. (1972). Determination of nonsuppressible insulin-like activity in human serum by a sensitive proteinbinding assay. *Clin. Chem.* **23**, 677–682.

Zapf, J., Mäder, M., Waldvogel, M., Schalch, S., and Froesch, E. R. (1975a). Specific binding on nonsuppressible insulinlike activity to chicken embryo fibroblasts and to a solubilized fibroblast receptor. *Arch. Biochem. Biophys.* **168**, 630–637.

Zapf, J., Waldvogel, M., and Froesch, E. R. (1975b). Binding of nonsuppressible insulinlike activity to human serum: Evidence for a carrier protein. *Arch. Biochem. Biophys.* **168**, 638–645.

Zapf, J., Rinderknecht, E., Humbel, R. E., and Froesch, E. R. (1978). Nonsuppressible insulin-like activity (NSILA) from human serum: Recent accomplishments and their physiologic implications. *Metabolism* **27**, 1803–1828.

Zapf, J., Morell, B., Walter, H., Laron, Z., and Froesch, E. R. (1980). Serum levels of insulin-like growth factor (IGF) and its carrier-protein in various metabolic disorders. *Acta Endocrinol. (Copenhagen)* **95**, 505–517.

Zapf, J., Froesch, E. R., and Humbel, R. E. (1981a). The insulin-like growth factors (IGF) of human serum: Chemical and biological characterization and aspects of their possible physiological role. *Curr. Top. Cell. Regul.* **19**, 257–309.

Zapf, J., Walter, H., and Froesch, E. R. (1981b). Radioimmunological determination of insulinlike growth factors I and II in normal subjects and in patients with growth disorders and extrapancreatic tumor hypoglycemia. *J. Clin. Invest.* **68**, 1321–1330.

Zederman, R., Grebing, C., Hall, K., and Löw, H. (1980). Effect of somatomedin A and insulin on cyclic AMP generation in isolated rat hepatocytes. *Horm. Metab. Res.* **12,** 251–256.

Zumstein, P. P., Laubli, U. K., and Humbel, R. E. (1983). A simplified purification procedure for IGF-1 and IGF-2 and a preliminary characterization of two additional forms of IGF from human serum. *In* "Insulin-like Growth Factors/Somatomedins Basic Chemistry, Biology and Clinical Importance" (E. M. Spencer, ed). de Gruyter, Berlin, in press.

VITAMINS AND HORMONES, VOL. 40

Calciferols: Actions and Deficiencies in Action

STEPHEN J. MARX

*Metabolic Diseases Branch, National Institute of Arthritis,
Diabetes, Digestive, and Kidney Diseases, National Institutes of Health,
Bethesda, Maryland*

URI A. LIBERMAN

*Metabolic Diseases Branch, National Institute of Arthritis,
Diabetes, Digestive, and Kidney Diseases, National Institutes of Health,
Bethesda, Maryland
and Beilinson Medical Center, Tel Aviv University Medical School,
Tel Aviv, Israel*

CHARLES EIL

*Endocrinology Branch, Department of Medicine, National Naval
Medical Center and Uniformed Services University of the Health
Sciences, Bethesda, Maryland*

I. INTRODUCTION

The calciferols are a group of compounds also known as the D vitamins (D refers to vitamin D_2 and/or vitamin D_3); they are secosteroids, implying that they contain a steroidal configuration with one ring open (i.e., the B-ring at its 9–10 bond). Vitamin D is generally considered to be an inactive precursor form with several properties appropriate for classification as a vitamin; 1,25(OH)$_2$D is highly bioactive, adhering to the general model of action that characterizes the true steroidal hormones. We shall retain the traditional vitamin terminology for the calciferols while emphasizing their basically hormonal mechanism of action. This article will focus upon activation and

235

ISBN 0-12-709840-2

target interactions of calciferols, particularly aspects of these processes (1) that have been clarified since related topics were last covered in "Vitamins and Hormones" in 1974, and (2) that are relevant to states of deficiency in calciferol action.

II. NORMAL CALCIFEROL ACTION

A. PRODUCTION OF BIOACTIVE CALCIFEROLS

1. 25-Hydroxylation of Calciferols

The initial step in the activation of circulating vitamin D is enzymatic conversion to 25(OH) vitamin D. Reconstitution experiments have identified one essential component of the 25-hydroxylation system as a cytochrome, P-450, found in hepatic mitochondria (Bjorkhem and Holmberg, 1978; Bjorkhem et al., 1980) and in hepatic microsomes (Bjorkhem et al., 1979; Yoon and DeLuca, 1981). Incubation of a series of substrates with mitochondria gave the following relative rates of 25-hydroxylation: vitamin D_3, 1; 1α-(OH)D_3, 11; cholesterol, 1; and 7-dehydrocholesterol, 0.2 (Bjorkhem and Holmberg, 1979). Comparable studies with hepatic microsomes showed a relative rate of 0.12 with dihydrotachysterol$_3$ (Madhok and DeLuca, 1979). With perfused rat liver Fukushima et al. (1978) found that, at nanomolar concentrations of substrate, 25-hydroxylation of D_3 or of 1α(OH)D_3 proceeded at similar rates, but, at higher concentrations, 25-hydroxylation of D_3 was far less efficient. It is uncertain whether hepatic microsomes or mitochondria possess distinguishable enzymes or whether the enzyme is even distinct from that which catalyzes the 25- or 26-hydroxylation of cholesterol.

   a. Tissue Distribution of 25-Hydroxylase. The liver is the only organ where physiologically important amounts of this conversion are known to occur. Within the liver, this process is not uniformly distributed. Dueland et al. (1981) found that perfusion of rat liver with tritiated vitamin D_3 led to accumulation of the isotope by both hepatocytes and by nonparenchymal cells; with dispersed separated rat liver cells, however, the 25-hydroxylation was shown to occur in hepatocytes and not in nonparenchymal cells.

   b. Regulation of 25-Hydroxylation. The 25-hydroxylase exhibits regulation appropriate for a cytochrome P-450 dependent enzyme (i.e., phenobarbital treatment increases it and metapyrone inhibits it), but there is little or only modest regulation associated with perturbations in calcium homeostasis. In vitamin D deficiency there is little (Madhok and DeLuca, 1979) or no (Dueland *et al.*, 1981) stimulation; administration of 25(OH)D$_3$, the enzyme's product either *in vivo* (Rojanasathit and Haddad, 1976) or *in vitro* (Bjorkhem and Holmberg, 1979), causes no significant feedback inhibition of the D$_3$ 25-hydroxylase. Norman *et al.* (1979) have reported that one synthetic analog of the reaction product with a shortened side chain, 24-*nor*-25(OH)D$_3$, lacks intrinsic bioactivity in chicks but inhibits the conversion of D$_3$ to 25(OH)D$_3$ in this species, even when administered *in vivo* with D$_3$ at an equimolar dose. Onisko *et al.* (1979) tested 25-aza-vitamin D$_3$ for similar activity; this compound was a blocker of conversion of D$_3$ to 25(OH)D$_3$ but exhibited blockage of D$_3$ action only when administered *in vivo* at a very high dose ratio (3000:1).

2. 1α-Hydroxylation of Calciferols

The conversion of 25(OH)D to 1α,25(OH)$_2$D (the 1-hydroxyl is in alpha orientation on the vitamin D A-ring; we refer to the hydroxyl group interchangeably with the terms 1-alpha, 1α-, or 1-) is the focal point in regulation of calciferol metabolism. This conversion occurs principally in the kidney, mediated by a mitochondrial enzyme system of which one major component is a cytochrome *P*-450. Because of instability, low activity, and lack of purified preparations, detailed studies of substrate specificity have not been done on the 1-hydroxylase enzyme. However, a hydroxyl residue at carbon-25 appears to be one important requirement since 24(*R*)(OH)D$_3$ is a poor substrate (Tanaka *et al.*, 1977).

a. Tissue Distribution of 1α-Hydroxylase. Microdissection studies have localized this enzyme system to proximal portions of the nephron in birds (Brunette *et al.*, 1978) and mammals (Akiba *et al.*, 1980). While early studies suggested cessation of this hydroxylation following nephrectomy, small amounts of 1,25(OH)$_2$D are produced even by anephric humans (Lambert *et al.*, 1982) and pigs (Littledike and Horst, 1982). The site(s) of this extrarenal production are not known. Calvarial bone cells from chick fetus (Turner *et al.*, 1980), as well as cultured bone cells from adult man (Howard *et al.*, 1981), can mediate this conversion. In cultured bone cells the level of activity is similar to that in cultured kidney cells. The placenta (probably fetal components) exhibits similar activity (Weisman *et al.*, 1978; Whitsett *et al.*, 1981) as do cells from embryonic intestine (Puzas et al., 1983). Granuloma tissue may also have this capability (Barbour et al., 1981).

b. Regulation of 1α-Hydroxylation. In the renal proximal convoluted tubule, the enzyme is activated by parathyroid hormone (PTH) *in vivo* (Kawashima et al., 1981a). In similar experiments, 1α-hydroxylase activity was not present in the proximal straight tubule of the rat unless animals received calcitonin *in vivo* (Kawashima *et al.*, 1981b). Kawashima and associates have found with rat kidney that PTH and calcitonin activate the tubular 1-hydroxylase system through distinct mechanisms based on the following three observations. First, PTH activates the adenylate cyclase enzyme in proximal convoluted and proximal straight tubules, while calcitonin activates adenylate cyclase in neither. Second, cAMP given *in vivo* activated the 1-hydroxylase system of the proximal convoluted tubule but not that of the proximal straight tubule (Kawashima *et al.*, 1982). Third, systemic acidosis impairs activation of 1-hydroxylase by PTH but not by cAMP in the proximal convoluted tubule; however, identical acidosis did not impair calcitonin activation of 1-hydroxylase in the proximal straight tubule (Kawashima *et al.*, 1982). These findings have raised the interesting possibility that PTH activation of the 1-hydroxylase is mediated by intracellular cAMP, while calcitonin activation may occur through other mediators.

Under normal conditions, PTH is the major activator of vitamin D-1-hydroxylase; parathyroidectomy leads to a rapid and striking drop in circulating levels of $1,25(OH)_2D$. With kidney slices, activation of 1-hydroxylase has been detected as soon as 5 minutes after exposure to PTH (Kremer and Goltzman, 1982). Infusion of dibutyryl cAMP into thyroparathyroidectomized rats provoked elevations of circulating $1,25(OH)_2D$ levels similar to those provoked by PTH (Noriuchi *et al.*, 1977). Studies with cultured cells have thus far obtained only 50–100% stimulation of the enzyme by maximal doses of PTH. To demonstrate an effect of PTH on 1-hydroxylation, stringent culture conditions have been necessary including the use of insulin (Henry, 1981) and/or inhibitors of "basal" activity such as $1,25(OH)_2D$ and low calcium (Trechsel *et al.*, 1979).

A second class of regulators of the renal 1-hydroxylase is the calciferols themselves. $1,25(OH)_2D$ is a potent inhibitor of this enzyme system *in vivo* or *in vitro*. Omdahl *et al.* (1980) examined the specificity of this inhibition by exposing renal tubules from the chick to calciferol analogs for 10 hours. The seco-steroid configuration was essential, the following steroids were without effect: estradiol, testosterone, progesterone, corticosterone, cholesterol, and 25-hydroxycholesterol. In cultured kidney cells, $1,25(OH)_2D_3$ has been the most potent inhibitor of this enzyme (Henry, 1979; Trechsel *et al.*, 1979). Inhibition of the 1-hydroxylase by calciferol congeners may be mediated through the receptor for $1,25(OH)_2D$ although in one study (Omdahl *et al.*, 1980) $25(OH)D_3$ was more potent as an inhibitor than $1,25(OH)_2D_3$. This might be explained, however, by preferential uptake of 25(OH)D or preferential degradation of $1,25(OH)_2D_3$ in that system. The inhibition requires both RNA and protein synthesis (Omdahl et al., 1980).

Although sex steroids do not affect 1-hydroxylase directly in vitro, major regulatory effects have been noted in vivo. For example, 1-hydroxylase activity in castrated male chickens can be stimulated from a basal activity of 7 up to 190 fmol/mg/min by the synergistic effects of estradiol, testosterone, and progesterone (Tanaka et al., 1978). These striking effects may be mediated indirectly via changes in calcium turnover and in PTH levels.

The 1-hydroxylase regulation allows adaptation to variations in dietary supply of calcium and/or phosphate. Adaptation can occur slowly at the levels of enzyme synthesis and turnover (Henry et al., 1974) or rapidly as under the influence of cAMP (Larkins et al., 1975). While PTH seems to be the principal mediator of the adaptation to variation in calcium supplies, the 1-hydroxylase system can also be activated in vivo by calcium deficiency (Trechsel et al., 1980) or phosphate deficiency (Tanaka and DeLuca, 1973) in the total absence of PTH. Although cAMP probably accounts for the activation by PTH, the intracellular mediators of activation by calcitonin, calcium deficiency, and hypophosphatemia are unknown. Dispersed chick renal tubules exhibit activation of 1-hydroxylase when incubated in media deficient in calcium or phosphate (Bikle and Rasmussen, 1975); similar effects have not been reproduced with cultured chick kidney cells (Trechsel et al., 1979). Bikle and Rasmussen (1978) analyzed a series of ions and substrates interacting with renal mitochondria. They noted that all activators of the 1-hydroxylase were associated with enhancement of proton efflux from the mitochondria and speculated that proton fluxes could activate the 1-hydroxylase system at several distinct steps.

3. 24-Hydroxylation of Calciferols

The calciferol 1α-hydroxylase and 24-hydroxylase (the natural configuration of the hydroxyl at carbon 24 is R, but this designation will be used only where important) activities exhibit many similarities, suggesting that they share important components (Table I). Their apparent affinities for the 25(OH)D substrate differ; with primary cultures of chick kidney cells the apparent K_m for 25(OH)D was 2.1 μM for the 24(R)-hydroxylase but only 0.125 μM for the 1-hydroxylase activity (Trechsel et al., 1979). With a solubilized, partially purified renal enzyme, the affinities of 1-hydroxylase and 24-hydroxylase for substrates were close to identity (Warner, 1982). Hiwatashi et al. (1982) claim to have purified to homogeneity a renal mitochondrial

TABLE I

SIMILARITIES IN THE SYSTEMS THAT HYDROXYLATE CALCIFEROLS
AT POSITION 1α OR 24(R)[a]

1. Present in kidney, bone, intestine, and placenta
2. Renal location limited to proximal tubule
3. Preference for substrate with hydroxyl on carbon-25
4. Direct regulation by parathyroid hormone
5. Direct regulation by 1,25(OH)$_2$D
6. Regulation by 1,25(OH)$_2$D via nuclear action

[a]Documentation for each of these similarities is presented in the text.

cytochrome P-450 that is specific for the 1-hydroxylation reaction and does not mediate the 24-hydroxylation reaction in a reconstituted enzyme system.

  a. *Tissue Distribution of 24-Hydroxylase.* The majority of 24-hydroxylation is mediated by the kidney, and 24,25(OH)$_2$D is generally not detectable (less than one-twentieth the normal level) in the circulation of anephric humans (Taylor *et al.,* 1978). Microdissection experiments with rat kidney showed 24-hydroxylase activity to be present in the proximal convoluted tubule and proximal straight tubule (Kawashima *et al.,* 1981b). In related experiments, 1-hydroxylase activity was identified in the same segments (see Section II,A,2,a). Like the 1-hydroxylase, 24-hydroxylase activity has been identified in placenta (Weisman *et al.,* 1979), in bone cells (Turner *et al.,* 1980; Howard *et al.,* 1981), and in fetal intestine (Puzas *et al.,* 1983). However, 24-hydroxylation has been found in tissues (Garabedian *et al.,* 1978; Kumar *et al.,* 1978; Acker *et al.,* 1982) and in cell lines (Colston and Feldman, 1982; Haussler *et al.,* 1982; Feldman *et al.,* 1982) apparently lacking ability to express 1-hydroxylase activity. The 24-hydroxylation has exhibited similar stimulation by 1,25(OH)$_2$D$_3$ in kidney, bone, and cultured fibroblasts although the possibility of several distinct 24-hydroxylase systems is real.

  b. *Regulation of 24-Hydroxylation.* Like the 1-hydroxylase, the calciferol 24-hydroxylase is found principally in mitochondria and contains cytochrome P-450 (Kulkowski *et al.,* 1979). The 24-hydroxyl residue is inserted in the R configuration. The enzyme from renal mitochondria shows similar activity with 25(OH)D$_3$ or 1,25(OH)$_2$D$_3$ as substrate, but analogs [such as 1α(OH)D$_3$] that lack an hydroxyl group on carbon-25 are poor substrates (Tanaka *et al.,* 1977).

  Both *in vivo* and *in vitro,* the 24-hydroxylase responds to most of the factors regulating the 1-hydroxylase but in an opposite direction. However, the solubilized enzyme from renal mitochondria of vitamin D-deficient (versus replete) rats was associated not with contrasting changes but with parallel rises in both 1- and 24-hydroxylases, suggesting dissociation of the enzyme from regulatory factor(s) (Warner, 1982). In avian species, sex steroids exert opposing effects on the renal 24- and 1-hydroxylase systems (Tanaka *et al.*, 1976). Sex steroids and hormonal status modulate 24-hydroxylase activity in rat endometrial cells (Acker *et al.*, 1982). Serum phosphate in the rat causes opposing effects on the 24- and 1-hydroxylases (Tanaka and DeLuca, 1973). Administration of $1,25(OH)_2D_3$ to chicks causes approximately 10-fold stimulation of 24-hydroxylation within 24 hours, while PTH administration leads to suppression down to 50% of initial levels within 2 hours (Tanaka *et al.*, 1975). In this regard, it was surprising that aminophylline administration to chicks led to a 10-fold rise in renal 24-hydroxylating ability within 4 hours (Kulkowski *et al.*, 1979); however, it was not proven that this effect was mediated by the known capacity of aminophylline to raise intracellular cAMP. In separate studies cultured chick kidney cells responded to dibutyryl cAMP with increased 1-hydroxylation but no change in 24-hydroxylation of $25(OH)D_3$ (Henry, 1981).

The regulatory effects of $1,25(OH)_2D$ on the 24-hydroxylase, like those on the 1-hydroxylase, may be mediated by the receptor for $1,25(OH)_2D$. Omdahl *et al.* (1980) observed that with chick kidney tubules the stimulation of 24-hydroxylase and the inhibition of 1-hydroxylase activities occurred with similar doses of a series of calciferol analogs, and both hydroxylase activities were blocked by inhibitors of RNA or protein synthesis. With a cell line derived from porcine kidney Colston and Feldman (1982) observed that half-maximal stimulation of 24-hydroxylase was achieved at the same ambient concentration of $1,25(OH)_2D_3$ causing half-maximal occupancy of the receptor for $1,25(OH)_2D$ in that cell line. Cultured skin fibroblasts from a patient with hereditary deficiency in activity of receptors for $1,25(OH)_2D$ failed to show the usual stimulation of 24-hydroxylase activity by $1,25(OH)_2D_3$ (Feldman *et al.*, 1982).

4. *Other Calciferol Modifications Potentially Important in Activation*

Kumar *et al.* (1981b) administered D_3 orally to vitamin D-deficient rats and identified a plasma metabolite as 5,6-*trans*-$25(OH)D_3$. Of the total circulating $25(OH)D_3$, approximately 10% showed this 5,6-trans configuration. It is not known whether this metabolite is produced enzymatically; it was clearly not an artifact of the calciferol purification procedure. Cis–trans isomerization of the 5–6 diene bond could potentially activate a large series of metabolities possessing one or more side chain hydroxyl residues (see Section II,C,3,c).

Metabolites of calciferols are being identified at a rapidly increasing rate. Many contain side-chain oxidations at carbons 23 and/or 26 (Wichman et al., 1981b; Tanaka et al., 1981). At present there is no evidence that these oxidations are significant physiologically for calciferol activation (Esvelt and DeLuca, 1981). Perhaps the greatest importance of these further metabolites is as interfering substances in certain assays for biologically active metabolites. For example, $25(OH)D_3$-26,23-lactone, a major metabolite with little known bioactivity, competes for binding to the rat calciferol-transport globulin [used in radioligand assays for $25(OH)D$ or $24,25(OH)_2D$] with an affinity fivefold higher than that of $25(OH)D_3$ (Horst, 1979). Extrarenal production of $24,25(OH)_2D_3$, $25,26(OH)_2D_3$, and $1,25(OH)_2D_3$ but not of $25(OH)D_3$-26,23-lactone was documented in anephric pigs given high doses of vitamin D_3 (Littledike and Horst, 1982).

B. Actions of Bioactive Calciferols

1. $1,25(OH)_2D$

a. *Intestinal Transport of Ions.* The most important target tissue for $1,25(OH)_2D$ is the intestine. Administration of $1,25(OH)_2D_3$ to D-deficient animals causes an increase in intestinal lumen-to-plasma flux of calcium, phosphate, and magnesium. On a relative scale, the stimulation of calcium transport is far greater than that of phosphate or magnesium (Brickman et al., 1977; Hodgkinson et al., 1979); for this reason, most studies of the mechanism of action of vitamin D and $1,25(OH)_2D$ have focused upon intestinal transport of calcium. Pansu et al. (1981) showed that calcium transport by duodenal loops from the rat could be modeled as two processes, one saturable and one nonsaturable. At physiologic concentrations of intraluminal calcium, most flux would occur through the saturable mechanisms. The nonsaturable process was unaffected by dietary calcium while the saturable process was decreased by high dietary calcium. Since this regulation is thought to be through endogenous $1,25(OH)_2D$, this suggested that the hormone specifically affected saturable fluxes of calcium.

The principal intestinal cell rapidly responsive to $1,25(OH)_2D$ is the mucosal cell at the villus tip, but the details of its response are not completely understood. The time course of change in intestinal transport of calcium after intravenous $1,25(OH)_2D_3$ differs in chicks and rats. The chick intestine exhibits a monophasic response, whereas rat intestine shows a clearly biphasic response with a brief peak at 6 hours and a second, more lasting peak at 24 hours (Halloran and DeLuca, 1981). Such complex kinetics could reflect the lag required for villus crypt cells of the rat to differentiate or could reflect several fundamentally different mechanisms of action of the hormone within the same mature villus tip cell. $1,25(OH)_2D$ does not evoke major changes in the cytoskeletal protein structure of the intestinal mucosa. While minor degrees of stimulation of villus length have been noted (Bikle et al., 1977), a detailed analysis of composition of brush border microvilli from rachitic or D-replete chicks showed similar ultrastructure, protein composition, protein phosphorylation, and protein interaction with calmodulin (Howe et al., 1982).

The most striking molecular response to $1,25(OH)_2D_3$ is the increase in content of vitamin D-dependent calcium binding protein. The possible functions of this protein in calcium transport are discussed below (see Section II,C,5,a). Certain studies have suggested that $1,25(OH)_2D$ acts to facilitate carrier-mediated calcium entry at the mucosal face of the cell (Rasmussen et al., 1979). Others have suggested that $1,25(OH)_2D$ acts to facilitate energy-dependent calcium efflux at the serosal face (Lane and Lawson, 1978), or that the principal effects on calcium flux occur at intracellular locations (Freedman et al., 1977; Kretsinger et al., 1982). Administration of $1,25(OH)_2D$ leads to changes in activity of several plasma membrane-bound enzymes, potentially involved in ion flux. Ca-ATPase is one example at the basal–lateral face of the cell and has been suggested as a source of energy for calcium extrusion from the cell. While alkaline phosphatase activities, concentrated at the brush border, usually change simultaneously with the $1,25(OH)_2D$-induced change in calcium transport, blockade of protein synthesis and of alkaline phosphatase response need not result in blockade of response of brush border calcium transport to $1,25(OH)_2D_3$ (Rasmussen et al., 1979). An intravenous pulse of $1,25(OH)_2D_3$ given to chicks increases both the intestinal transport of calcium and Ca-ATPase activity in homogenates of intestinal mucosa with both peaking by 8 hours and then decaying to near baseline by 24 hours. Alkaline phosphatase activity reaches a peak at 24 hours and does not then decline (Lane and Lawson, 1978). Two laboratories have found that increasing membrane fluidity alone could increase calcium transport in a manner mimicking the actions of vitamin D. Adams et al. (1970) applied filipin to duodenal mucosa of vitamin D-deficient chicks and observed the induction of active transport of calcium; the mucosa from vitamin D-replete animals did not show this response to filipin. Fontaine et al. (1981) obtained analogous results by addition of *cis*-vaccinic acid to brush border membrane vesicles of D-deficient versus D-replete chicks. $1,25(OH)_2D_3$ administration is associated with rapid changes in phospholipid metabolism that might account for the suggested effects on membrane fluidity. O'Doherty (1979) showed that treatment of rat intestinal cells with $1,25(OH)_2D_3$ stimulated the phosphatidylcholine deacylation–reacylation cycle by two- to threefold within 3 hours. Matsumoto *et al.* (1981) have shown that treatment of the D-deficient chick with $1,25(OH)_2D_3$ leads to rapid and simultaneous changes at the level of the brush border membrane vesicle for calcium transport and phosphatidylcholine synthesis.

While $1,25(OH)_2D$-induced stimulation of transport for calcium and phosphate could result from the same cellular modifications, three interesting differences in the transport responses for these two ions have been noted: (1) $1,25(OH)_2D_3$ stimulates uptake of calcium and phosphate into explants of chick intestine; stimulation of phosphate uptake has been observed as early as 30 minutes after application of hormone while that for calcium begins only after 60 minutes (Birge and Miller, 1977). (2) In the rat duodenal mucosa, the active lumen-to-serosa flux is greater for calcium than phosphate, and $1,25(OH)_2D_3$ stimulates calcium flux more than phosphate flux; however, in the jejunum, basal flux is greater for phosphate than calcium, and $1,25$-$(OH)_2D_3$ results in greater stimulation of phosphate flux than calcium flux (Walling, 1977). (3) Administration of $1,25(OH)_2D_3$ *in vivo* leads to an increase in maximal uptake capacity for calcium and phosphate with brush border membrane vesicles from the chick; the saturable uptake of phosphate is sodium dependent (Matsumoto *et al.*, 1980) and that of calcium is not.

b. Bone Homeostasis. Efforts to detect direct anabolic effects of $1,25(OH)_2D_3$ on bone have been largely unsuccessful. For example, $1,25(OH)_2D_3$ inhibited the synthesis of collagen with cultured rat calvaria (Raisz *et al.*, 1978), and this effect is probably mediated through decreased levels of procollagen mRNA (Rowe and Kream, 1982). At the organ level, a major action of $1,25(OH)_2D$, proved beyond doubt, is the mobilization of skeletal mineral (Raisz *et al.*, 1972). $1,25(OH)_2D_3$, given intravenously to thyroparathyroidectomized vitamin D-deficient rats, causes striking changes in osteoclast morphology; within 6 hours their size, their ruffled border, and their clear zones enlarge (Holtrop *et al.*, 1981). Many aspects of bone response to $1,25(OH)_2D$ have been investigated including the issue of actions selective to osteoblasts or osteoclasts. By sequential release from calvaria, Wong *et al.* (1977) separated bone cells into a PTH-responsive (osteoblast-like) and a calcitonin-responsive (osteoclast-like) population. Culture of PTH-responsive cells with either PTH or $1,25(OH)_2D_3$ caused similar decreases of alkaline phosphatase, citrate decarboxylation, and collagen synthesis; culture of calcitonin-responsive cells with either hormone caused similar stimulation of acid phosphatase and hyaluronate synthesis. Thus, $1,25(OH)_2D_3$ and PTH evoked similar responses in separated bone cells; unlike PTH, however, $1,25(OH)_2D_3$ did not stimulate synthesis of cAMP. In fact, preincubation with $1,25(OH)_2D_3$ inhibited the cAMP response to PTH but not the cAMP response to calcitonin (Wong et al., 1977; Kent et al., 1980).

The subcellular mechanism of the bone cell response to $1,25(OH)_2D_3$ is not known and has been studied in less detail than that for the duodenal mucosa. $1,25(OH)_2D_3$ exerts complex effects on cultured rat osteosarcoma cells (osteoblast-like) (Majeska and Rodan, 1982). In early stages of culture when alkaline phosphatase activity is low, the hormone inhibits cell proliferation and stimulates alkaline phosphatase activity; in later stages when alkaline phosphatase activity is higher, the hormone at low concentrations reduces alkaline phosphatase and increases cell number. In the same cell line $1,25(OH)_2D_3$ stimulates intracellular and extracellular levels of a bone-specific protein containing γ-carboxy-glutamic acid (Price and Baukol, 1980). Although this protein (which binds calcium with an affinity in the millimolar range) is a major component of bone matrix, and its stimulation by $1,25(OH)_2D_3$ in tissue culture is dramatic, no function has yet been discovered for it. Vitamin D_3 also stimulates, in bone cells, the synthesis of another calcium-binding protein that is immunologically identical to that in intestinal cells (Christakos and Norman, 1978).

c. *Tissues Other Than Intestine and Bone.* The kidney is an important target organ for $1,25(OH)_2D$. This hormone regulates the renal metabolism of its own precursor, $25(OH)D$. In the proximal tubule, $1,25(OH)_2D$ inhibits 1α-hydroxylation and stimulates $24R$-hydroxylation; $1,25(OH)_2D$ similarly influences the metabolism of $25(OH)D$ in bone cells (see Sections II,A,2 and 3). Another location of feedback on calciferol metabolism is the skin where $1,25(OH)_2D$ stimulates accumulation of 7-dehydrocholesterol, the immediate precursor of cholecalciferol (Esvelt et al., 1980); it is not known if this reflects increased synthesis or decreased metabolism of 7-dehydrocholesterol. $1,25(OH)_2D$ effects little, if any, direct action on renal transport of calcium (Hugi et al., 1979), but significant actions on phosphate transport have been noted. Bonjour et al. (1977) observed a chronic phosphaturic action of $1,25(OH)_2D_3$ in thyroparathyroidectomized rats given a normal or high phosphate diet. It was not proved, however, that this action could be dissociated from changes in overall phosphate balance or in serum calcium levels. Moreover, it is difficult to reconcile these observations with others indicating that, in the thyroparathyroidectomized rat, acute administration of $1,25(OH)_2D_3$ could increase tubular resorption of calcium and phosphate; these latter actions could only be detected in the presence of an accompanying infusion of PTH or vasopressin (Puschett and Kuhrman, 1978; Nseir *et al.*, 1978). In this regard it is notable that $1,25(OH)_2D_3$, *in vitro,* directly inhibits PTH stimulation of adenylate cyclase activity in renal plasma membranes from D-deficient rats (Cloix *et al.*, 1980). With kidney cells isolated from D-deficient chicks, $1,25(OH)_2D_3$ stimulated sodium-dependent uptake of phosphate, reaching 130% of baseline by 2 hours of incubation (Liang *et al.*, 1982).

Receptors for $1,25(OH)_2D$ have been identified in the parathyroid gland, pancreatic beta cell, and pituitary (see Section II,C,3,a), and acute actions of $1,25(OH)_2D$ have been noted in preparations of all three tissues though these actions have sometimes been rather small in magnitude. In the rat parathyroid cell, $1,25(OH)_2D_3$ inhibits PTH release (Nko *et al.*, 1982); in the dog $1,25(OH)_2D_3$ can increase or decrease PTH concentrations depending upon the rate of administration (Oldham *et al.*, 1979). Insulin release, evoked by infusion of arginine plus glucose, is depressed in perfused pancreas from D-deficient rats but effects of chronic hypocalcemia were not controlled for (Norman *et al.*, 1980). Clark *et al.* (1981) showed that administration of $1,25(OH)_2D_3$ to D-deficient rats elevated insulin concentration by 100% at 48 hours, but this was also accompanied by small but significant elevations in serum calcium. In a rat pituitary cloned cell line, $1,25(OH)_2D_3$ inhibited basal prolactin production but enhanced maximal production rates under stimulation of TRH (Murdoch and Rosenfeld, 1981). With a similar cell line, cultured in a chemically defined medium, Wark and Tashjian (1982) observed potent stimulation of prolactin synthesis.

Direct actions observable by microscopy have been reported with cultured cells. Complex effects on proliferation of rat osteosarcoma cells have been cited above (see Section II,B,1,b). $1,25(OH)_2D_3$ inhibits proliferation in cultured malignant melanoma cells (Colston *et al.*, 1981) and stimulates (Freake *et al.*, 1981) or inhibits (Eisman *et al.*, 1982) proliferation in cultured human breast cancer cell lines. $1,25(OH)_2D_3$ restores normal phagocytic ability to macrophages from D-deficient mice (Bar-Shavit *et al.*, 1981). With a mouse myeloid leukemia cell line previously known to undergo differentiation into mature macrophages and granulocytes, $1,25(OH)_2D_3$ is the most potent known inducer of this differentiation (Abe *et al.*, 1981); whereas the minimal effective concentration of dexamethasone is 100 nM, that for $1,25(OH)_2D_3$ is 0.1 nM.

Analyses of dosage requirements have shown that $1,25(OH)_2D$ is the most potent calciferol metabolite to evoke the above effects on intestine, bone, and kidney. In general, $25(OH)D$ or $24,25(OH)_2D$ evokes a similar effect but at doses 10- to 100-fold higher than required for $1,25(OH)_2D_3$. Since these potencies correspond to the relative affinity of the $1,25(OH)_2D$ receptor for these analogs, it is likely that $25(OH)D$ or $24,25(OH)_2D$ exerts actions through direct low-affinity interaction with receptor.

2. 24,25(OH)$_2$D

$24,25(OH)_2D$ can express bioactivity by direct, weak interaction with receptors for $1,25(OH)_2D$ or interaction at a higher affinity after metabolism to $1,24,25(OH)_2D$. In contrast to these $1,25(OH)_2$ D-like actions, $24,25(OH)_2D$ exhibits several actions that may not be mimicked by $1,25(OH)_2D$, suggesting interaction with a different receptor–effector system.

a. *Bone Homeostasis.* Corvol *et al.* (1978) found that in rabbit growth plate chondrocytes grown in culture, calciferol analogs could stimulate sulfate incorporation into cellular proteoglycans by approximately 50%. The half-maximal dosages (molar) for this effect were as follows: $24,25(OH)_2D_3$, 7×10^{-12}; $25(OH)D_3$, 2×10^{-8}; the effect of $1,25(OH)_2D_3$ was smaller with half maximum at 2×10^{-12}. Endo *et al.* (1980) examined the effects of calciferol analogs on bone formation in cultured long bones of chick embryos. Calciferols or PTH alone were inadequate to promote development of mineralized bone. Mineralization required simultaneous presence of PTH, $1,25(OH)_2D_3$, and $24,25(OH)_2D_3$. Interactions of $24,25(OH)_2D$ with cAMP accumulation in bone tissue have been noted (Marcus *et al.*, 1980). Lieberherr *et al.* (1980) analyzed calvaria bones of 3-day-old rats. $1,25(OH)_2D_3$ inhibited cAMP content with half-maximal inhibition at $10^{-11}M$; $24,25(OH)_2D_3$ or $25(OH)D_3$ stimulated cAMP content with similar dosage for half-maximal effect, but the maximal stimulation by $25(OH)D$ was double that with $24,25(OH)_2D_3$. In an extension of those studies, Silve *et al.* (1981) examined regulation of calvarial cAMP by somatostatin at 1 mM calcium. Preincubation with $1,25(OH)_2D_3$ increased the sensitivity of the bones to the stimulatory effect of somatostatin on cAMP accumulation. Preincubation with the same dose of $24,25(OH)_2D_3$ elevated basal cAMP content and converted somatostatin to an inhibitor of cAMP accumulation. Marcus *et al.* (1980) evaluated effects of administration of calciferol analogs on the response of female rats to PTH *in vivo*. $24,25(OH)_2D_3$ increased the cAMP content in calvaria or renal cortex slices after PTH administration, while $1,25(OH)_2D_3$ in doses sufficient to evoke a calcemic response did not change the cAMP response to PTH. Administration of $24,25(OH)_2D_3$ had no effect on adenylate cyclase in membranes from kidney cortex but significantly inhibited phosphodiesterase activity.

Putative receptors specific for $24,25(OH)_2D$ have been identified in bone tissues. Corvol *et al.* (1980) observed high-affinity nuclear uptake of $[^3H]24,25(OH)_2D_3$ with cultured growth plate cartilage from the rabbit; neither $25(OH)D$ nor $1,25(OH)_2D_3$ competed for this process (but the tested doses of these metabolites were not specified). Somjen *et al.* have observed specific binding of $24,25(OH)_2D_3$ in extracts from developing long bones of newborn rats (1982b) and from chick limb bud mesenchyme (1982a). Although specificity for $24,25(OH)_2D_3$ has been demonstrated in these extracts, physicochemical separation of the putative receptor for $24,25(OH)_2D$ from the receptor for $1,25(OH)_2D_3$ has not been achieved.

b. Tissues Other Than Bone. Henry *et al.* (1977) observed that vitamin D_3 administration to D-deficient chicks caused a calcemic response and significant regression of parathyroid gland weight; doses of $1,25(OH)_2D_3$ causing a similar calcemic response did not lead to parathyroid gland regression. Addition of $24,25(OH)_2D_3$, in a dose that was ineffective alone, to $1,25(OH)_2D_3$, caused regression of parathyroid gland size. Analogous, mild suppressive effects of $24,25(OH)_2D$ on the parathyroid gland have been suggested in uremic dogs (Canterbury *et al.*, 1980), in uremic humans (Christiansen *et al.*, 1981), and in humans with D deficiency (Miravet *et al.*, 1981). A binding protein for $24,25(OH)_2D$ has been identified in soluble extracts from parathyroid gland (Merke and Norman, 1981), but competition studies with a series of calciferol analogs to distinguish it from the receptor for $1,25(OH)_2D$ have not been reported. $24,25(OH)_2D_3$ incubated at low concentrations with plasma membranes from human parathyroid adenoma inhibits the adenylate cyclase enzyme (Cloix *et al.*, 1981); similar inhibition could not be detected with 100-fold higher concentrations of $1,25(OH)_2D_3$.

Administration of $1,25(OH)_2D_3$ as the sole calciferol source to hens allows production of fertile eggs, but the majority fail to hatch (Henry and Norman, 1978). $24,25(OH)_2D_3$, at a dose insufficient to support production of normal numbers of eggs, permitted normal egg hatchability when combined with $1,25(OH)_2D_3$.

In order to evaluate the purported essentiality of $24,25(OH)_2D_3$ several studies have been done with $24,24$-difluoro-$25(OH)_2D_3$, a compound capable of hydroxylation at position 1-α but incapable of hydroxylation at carbon-24. (1) This compound was found to act similarly to

25(OH)D_3 in D-deficient rats with regard to intestinal transport of calcium, mobilization of calcium from bone, normalization of rachitic bone and cartilage, and normalization of serum phosphorus (Tanaka *et al.*, 1979). (2) It was similarly effective in treatment of pups born to D-deficient rats (Halloran *et al.*, 1981), and (3) in restoring normal egg hatchability after administration with 1,25(OH)$_2$$D_3$ to D-deficient hens (Ameenuddin *et al.*, 1982).

None of the above data is definitive evidence for or against a unique role for 24,25(OH)$_2$D. Full dose–response relationships between 1,25(OH)$_2$$D_3$ and 24,25(OH)$_2$$D_3$ have not been evaluated, and the role of metabolism of 24,25(OH)$_2$$D_3$ or of 1,25(OH)$_2$$D_3$ in target tissues has not been adequately explored. Similarly, work with 24-difluoro-25(OH)D is not conclusive since this compound could be a direct agonist at the putative receptor for 24,25(OH)$_2$$D_3$.

3. Other Metabolites

There is little evidence for specific effects of metabolites other than 1,25(OH)$_2$D or 24,25(OH)$_2$D. Birge and Haddad (1975) reported that 25(OH)D_3 at pharmacologic concentration acted *in vitro* on muscle of D-depleted rats to increase ATP content and protein synthesis; pharmacologic concentrations of 1,25(OH)$_2$$D_3$ or of D_3 did not reproduce these effects.

C. MOLECULAR ASPECTS OF 1,25(OH)$_2$D ACTION

1. Mechanism of Action

It is believed that vitamin D action is mediated largely through its dihydroxylated metabolite, 1,25(OH)$_2$D, in analogy to the actions of true steroid hormones (Fig. 1) whose structure the calciferols resemble. 1,25(OH)$_2$D circulates in blood mostly bound to a serum vitamin D binding protein (DBP). A small amount of the total circulating 1,25(OH)$_2$D, however, is free, and it is this unbound fraction that is presumably available to interact with the target tissues.

The first step probably involves diffusion of the free hormone across the plasma membrane of the cell which offers little resistance for entry into the cytoplasm since both the hormone and the membrane are lipophilic. Inside the cell, the hormone binds to a "receptor" protein which may be located either in the cytoplasm or in the nucleus. The binding of the hormone to the receptor protein (1) is highly specific for calciferols in general and 1,25(OH)$_2$$D_3$ in particular, (2) occurs with high affinity (at concentrations in the range of 10^{-10} to $10^{-9}M$), and

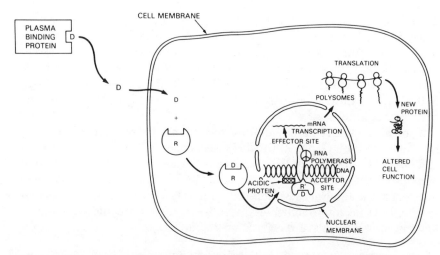

FIG. 1. Schematic representation of the nuclear mechanism of 1,25(OH)$_2$D action. Some aspects of this figure are controversial, such as the intracellular location of the receptor protein (R) and the change in the receptor state (R') prior to genomic action.

(3) is limited in capacity to approximately 10,000–20,000 high-affinity receptor sites/cell. A 3.2–3.6 S protein capable of specific, high-affinity, saturable binding of 1,25(OH)D can be extracted from the nuclei of vitamin D target tissues (Lawson and Wilson, 1974; Brumbaugh and Haussler, 1975a; Brumbaugh et al., 1975). Feldman et al. (1979) have shown that a 6.8 S binding protein from rat intestinal cytosol could be generated from the 3.2 S species merely by changing the ionic composition of sucrose density gradients from hypertonic to hypotonic. Regardless of where in the cell the hormone–receptor complex is formed, 1,25(OH)$_2$D$_3$ must be localized in the nucleus in order to induce all or many of its effects. Although there has been a report that 1,25(OH)$_2$D can influence calcium transport by directly altering the permeability of duodenal mucosal cell membranes via a "liponomic" (membrane interaction only) mechanism of action (Fontaine et al., 1981), this is a minority opinion and most investigators believe that 1,25(OH)$_2$D induces its effects via a nuclear mechanism. A direct effect of 1,25(OH)$_2$D at the membrane level is also suggested by the inhibition of adenylcyclase in rat kidney membranes in vitro (Cloix et al., 1980).

Once the hormone binds to the receptor protein, the hormone-receptor complex may require "activation," a poorly understood transformation of the receptor protein that allows it to bind to specific sites on the target cell genome. After proper nuclear-chromatin interaction of the hormone-receptor complex, a series of events is entrained in which

DNA-dependent RNA polymerase activity is initiated, RNA synthesis for specific messenger RNAs is activated and new proteins are ultimately synthesized. The fate of receptors after binding to the nuclear "acceptor" sites is unknown.

Details of this overall schema will be dealt with in separate sections below.

2. *Transport in Plasma*

Vitamin D metabolites are transported in blood bound to plasma proteins. These proteins have been characterized in man and other species (Haddad and Walgate, 1976a; Imawari *et al.*, 1976; Bouillon *et al.*, 1976). In comparison to that from man, monkey, or chick, serum (and presumably DBP) from the toad has 10-fold higher affinity and 100-fold lower capacity for 25(OH)D$_3$ (Bouillon *et al.* 1980b). DBP from man or rat has similar affinity for 25(OH)D$_2$ and 25(OH)D$_3$; but DBP from chicks has 10-fold lower affinity for 25(OH)D$_2$ (Belsey *et al.* 1974a). The purified human protein, vitamin D binding protein (DBP), is a major component of the α-globulin region and is known by immunologic cross-reactivity and electrophoretic mobility to be identical with human group specific component (Gc) protein (Daiger *et al.*, 1975; Bouillon *et al.*, 1976). It is characterized by a sedimentation coefficient of approximately 4 S, a molecular weight between 50,000 and 60,000, and preferential binding of 25(OH)D$_3$ with an affinity ($K_d \cong 1 \times 10^{-9}M$) greater than that of vitamin D$_3$ or 1,25(OH)$_2$D$_3$. 24,25(OH)$_2$D$_3$ and 25,26(OH)$_2$D$_3$ show affinities for DBP similar to that for 25(OH)D$_3$ (Horst, 1979). After immunoprecipitation, an antibody against the Gc protein inhibits all plasma binding of vitamin D$_3$, 25(OH)D$_3$, and 1,25(OH)$_2$D$_3$, indicating a common transport protein for all these steroids in human plasma (Haussler and McCain, 1977). The binding proteins from humans and rats are only 1–3% saturated with vitamin D sterol in blood *in vivo* (Haddad *et al.*, 1976; Rojanasathit and Haddad, 1977). Bouillon *et al.* (1981) showed a positive correlation between concentrations of DBP and 1,25(OH)$_2$D. A calculated index of free 1,25(OH)$_2$D concentration was normal in women using oral contraceptives and in early pregnancy, but during the last weeks of gestation the index of free 1,25(OH)$_2$D was elevated in maternal and cord blood.

The concentration of this protein is not altered in a number of calcium- and phosphorus-related pathologic states, but is moderately increased by estrogens (Haddad and Walgate, 1976a; Bouillon *et al.*, 1981). Although circulating DBP appears to be synthesized and secreted from the liver, Imawari *et al.* (1982) have shown that another protein, immunologically similar to DBP, but different physiochemically, is synthesized in but not secreted from the kidney. Together with a tissue component (presumably actin) this protein also forms a complex observed in almost all nucleated tissues (Van Baelen *et al.*, 1980; Haddad, 1982). Prior to the demonstration of a tissue DBP-binding component it was thought that "receptors" for 25(OH)D were universal in all tissues (Haddad and Birge, 1975). The issue of whether the DBP–actin complex forms because of serum contamination during cytosol preparation or because DBP was actively incorporated by cells *in vivo* has not been resolved (Cooke *et al.*, 1979).

Studies with isolated cells and an antibody against human sex-steroid binding protein suggest that this latter transport protein can cross the cell membrane, but does not enter the nucleus (Bordin and Petra, 1980). Despite its possible presence inside the cell, however, even slight amounts of DBP outside the cell are capable of preventing 25(OH)D extraction by tissues *in vivo* (Manolagas and Deftos, 1980a,b; Olgaard *et al.*, 1982); only $1,25(OH)_2D$ is taken up in important amounts by the cell under normal conditions *in vivo*.

DBP, which makes up approximately 6% of the α-globulin fraction, is heterogeneous due to genetic polymorphism (3 alleles Gc^{1F}, Gc^{1S}, Gc^2, and 26 known variants) (Cleve and Patutschnick, 1979). The Gc1F and Gc1S proteins each have two components probably due to posttranslational modification by differential sialylation (Svasti and Bowman, 1978). It appears that despite the heterogeneity of DBP the affinities of the proteins for $25(OH)D_3$ are not significantly different (Constans *et al.*, 1980; Kawakami *et al.*, 1979). DBP or the DBP–25(OH)D complex is removed from plasma by many tissues, the DBP moiety is degraded into small fragments which are excreted in the urine, and a significant recirculation of 25(OH)D probably occurs after renal clearance of the DBP–25(OH)D complex (Haddad *et al.*, 1981).

3. $1,25(OH)_2D$ Receptors

a. Tissue Distribution. With the availability of $[^3H]1,25(OH)_2D_3$ of higher and higher specific activity and the optimization of assay conditions, it is now apparent that receptors for $1,25(OH)_2D_3$ are present in many more tissues (Table II) and cell lines (Table III) than the classical targets (intestine and bone) in which they were first discovered (Tsai and Norman, 1973b; Brumbaugh and Haussler, 1973; Kream *et al.*, 1977a).

Putative receptors have been identified by virtue of their hormone binding properties. Two methods have been used: (1) injection of labeled $1,25(OH)_2D_3$ of high specific activity *in vitro* with autoradiography of tissue sections; or (2) homogenization of tissues and preparation

TABLE II
TISSUE DISTRIBUTION OF 1,25(OH)$_2$D RECEPTORS

Tissue	Species	References
Intestine	Chick	Brumbaugh and Haussler (1973); Tsai and Norman (1973a)
	Rat	Chen and DeLuca (1973)
	Human	Wecksler et al. (1979b)
	Eel	Marcocci et al. (1982)
Bone	Chick and rat	Kream et al. (1977a)
Kidney	Rat	Chandler et al. (1979); Stumpf et al. (1979)
	Chick	Christakos and Norman (1979)
Skin	Rat	Stumpf et al. (1979); Simpson and DeLuca (1980)
	Human	Feldman et al. (1980)
	Mouse	Colston et al. (1980)
Parathyroid	Chick	Brumbaugh et al. (1975)
	Rat	Stumpf et al. (1979)
	Human	Hughes and Haussler (1978)
Pancreas	Chick	Pike et al. (1980); Christakos and Norman (1979)
	Rat	Clark et al. (1980)
Pituitary	Rat	Stumpf et al. (1979); Haussler et al. (1980)
	Chick	Pike et al. (1980)
	Eel	Marcocci et al. (1982)
Mammary gland	Rat	Narbaitz et al. (1981)
	Mouse	Colston et al. (1980)
	Rabbit and human	Eisman et al. (1980)
Ovary	Chicken	Dokoh et al. (1983)
Uterus	Rat	Walters (1981)
Liver	Eel	Marcocci et al. (1982)
Thymus	Cow	Reinhardt et al. (1982)
Brain/spinal cord	Eel	Marcocci et al. (1982)
	Rat	Stumpf et al. (1982)
Placenta	Rat	Pike et al. (1980)
Yolk sac	Rat	Danan et al. (1981)

of extracts for incubation with [^{3}H]1,25(OH)$_2$D$_3$ *in vitro*. Using the former method, Stumpf and associates (Stumpf *et al.*, 1979, 1980, 1982; Clark *et al.*, 1980; Narbaitz *et al.*, 1981) have identified an impressive array of tissues that specifically concentrate the hormone. In the skin, for instance, the demonstration of [^{3}H]1,25(OH)$_2$D$_3$ in the hair follicle (Stumpf *et al.*, 1979) is particularly relevant to the observation that many patients with hereditary rickets (see Section III,B,2,b) show total

TABLE III

CELL LINES WITH RECEPTORS FOR $1,25(OH)_2D$

	Cell line	References
Transformed	Rat osteogenic sarcoma	Partridge et al. (1980)
	Rat osteogenic sarcoma	Manolagas et al. (1980)
	MCF-7 breast carcinoma	Eisman et al. (1979)
	T47-D breast carcinoma	Sher et al. (1981); Freake et al. (1981)
	HL-60 human myeloid leukemia	Tanaka et al. (1982)
	Hs 695T human melanoma	Colston et al. (1981)
	VX_2 rabbit skin carcinoma	Freake et al. (1980)
Nontransformed	Mouse bone	Chen et al. (1979); Walters et al. (1982)
	Chick kidney	Simpson et al. (1980)
	Porcine kidney (LLC PK)	Colston and Feldman (1982)
	GH_4 rat pituitary	Murdoch and Rosenfeld (1981)
	Human skin fibroblasts	Feldman et al. (1980); Eil and Marx (1981)
	Human skin keratinocytes	Feldman et al. (1980)
	Chinese hamster ovary	Dokoh et al. (1983)

alopecia. Thus, these observations have expanded the concept of what the target tissues for vitamin D are.

In a systematic investigation of mouse tissues Colston et al. (1980), using in vitro binding studies, showed that in addition to bone, intestine, and kidney, the $1,25(OH)_2D_3$ receptor is found in skin and mammary gland. The binder had an identical sedimentation constant (3.2 S) and affinity, suggesting that the receptor is the same in all tissues. The binder was not detectable in brain, lung, skeletal muscle, diaphragm, myocardium, or uterus, but varying amounts of a 6 S species were noted in all tissues, presumably representing the binding of $[^3H]1,25(OH)_2D_3$ to the complex generated from the association of DBP and actin (see Section II,C,2) (Van Baelen et al., 1980; Haddad, 1982). Recent studies have identified the receptor in bovine thymus gland (Reinhardt et al., 1982) and in rat uterus following estrogen priming (Walters, 1981). The physiological significance of the $1,25(OH)_2D_3$ receptors found in tissues not previously recognized as vitamin D targets, such as mammary gland and skin, is not known. In many tissues the presence of $1,25(OH)_2D_3$ receptors correlates with the presence of a vitamin D-dependent CaBP. Although some tissues, such as the parathyroid gland, clearly contain receptors and CaBP, CaBP synthesis in the parathyroid is not vitamin D dependent (Christakos *et al.*, 1979). Obviously, $1,25(OH)_2D$ regulates genes other than those for CaBP.

b. Properties. Receptors for $1,25(OH)_2D$ have been examined in greatest detail from chick duodenal mucosa. This receptor is a protein that sediments at $\cong 3.5$ S on sucrose gradients containing KCl and shows a Stokes molecular radius of 36–38 Å (Wecksler *et al.*, 1980). Molecular weight estimates for this receptor have varied from 47,000 to 68,000 suggesting that it had undergone proteolysis with varying degrees. Recently, Simpson and DeLuca (1982) reported that chick intestinal receptor, purified to apparent homogeneity by classical fractionation techniques and precipitation with polyethyleneimine, was a protein with a molecular weight of approximately 67,000 on SDS polyacrylamide gel electrophoresis and gel chromatography. The purified receptor had a p$I \cong 6.0$ and was highly pH labile, stability was optimal at pH 7.4. Bishop *et al.* (1982), using crude preparations, reported that the addition of phenylmethyl sulfonyl fluoride (PMSF), a protease inhibitor, with or without ligand, allowed recovery of the receptor with an apparent molecular weight of 99,700 by gel filtration. In the absence of PMSF, however, the unoccupied receptor showed an apparent molecular weight of 51,400. Interestingly, this smaller form of the receptor, upon incubation with $[^3H]1,25(OH)_2D_3$ and PMSF, migrated with an apparent molecular weight of 95,900, suggesting the presence of previously unappreciated multiple molecular forms of the receptor. Proteolysis, therefore, cannot completely account for the multiplicity of receptor sizes.

The $1,25(OH)_2D_3$ binding activity of the receptor can be destroyed by sulfhydryl alkylating agents such as N-ethylmaleimide and iodoacetamide (Mellon *et al.*, 1980; Wecksler *et al.*, 1980). The occupied receptor, however, is partially protected against the effects of these reagents, suggesting that there is a cysteine residue at or near the ligand binding site that is essential for maintenance of binding activity (Wecksler and Norman, 1980). Although the temperature of the assay affects the result obtained, the chick receptor, as for other tissues and species, shows a K_d of about $0.5–5.0 \times 10^{-10}$ M, clearly in the physiologic range of plasma $1,25(OH)_2D_3$ concentrations.

Although $1,25(OH)_2D_3$ receptors have been identified in avian tissues other than intestine (see Table II for distribution and references), the molecular properties of the receptor appear to be uniform, i.e., a protein which migrates at 3.5–3.7 S on 0.3 M KCl-containing sucrose gradients, possesses a K_d for $1,25(OH)_2D_3$ of 3×10^{-10} M at 4°C, and contains cysteine near the ligand binding site (Wecksler and Norman, 1980).

Physical and chemical properties such as sedimentation distribution on sucrose gradients, K_d, Stokes radius, ligand binding specificty, stabilization by salt, reducing agents, and low temperature are similar for the $1,25(OH)_2D_3$ receptors from mammalian and avian sources (Wecksler and Norman, 1980). The molecular weight estimates range from 60,000 for receptor from human intestine (Wecksler et al., 1980) to 80,000 for that from rat intestine (Wecksler et al., 1979a).

c. *Structure/Function Relationships.* The specificity of hormonal binding for the receptor has been extensively examined by competitive-binding studies with $[^3H]1,25(OH)_2D_3$ (Kream et al., 1977b; Procsal et al., 1975; Wecksler et al., 1980; Eisman and DeLuca, 1977). The results of these studies, using reconstituted chromatin–cytosol systems as well as competition binding assays with cytosol alone, have shown that the hydroxyl residues at 1α- and 25- are critical while that at 3β is less important.

The 23-keto metabolites of $25(OH)D_3$ and $1,25(OH)_2D_3$ show affinity for the receptor similar to that of the parent compound (Horst et al., 1982b). The D_2 form (characterized by the 24R-methyl group) of $1\alpha,25(OH)_2$ vitamin D seems to be equivalent to the D_3. However, the receptor will tolerate only small changes in the side chain. Shortening the side chain by one methylene group $[24\text{-}nor\text{-}1\alpha,25(OH)_2D_3]$ or by insertion of an —OH group at carbon 24 causes a 50–67% reduction in binding potency. The presence of an —OH group at either the 24 or 25 (but not both) position is equivalent since $1\alpha,24R(OH)_2D_3$ and $1,25(OH)_2D_3$, but not $1\alpha,24R,25(OH)_3D_3$, display similar receptor affinities and biopotencies. With 25-hydroxy analogs modification of the A-ring at C-1, C-3, C-4, C-10, or C-19 markedly reduces the affinity of binding while analogs modified in both the side chain and the A-ring show little binding activity (Procsal et al., 1975; Wecksler et al., 1978). A list of analog binding potencies for the $1,25(OH)_2D$ receptor and DBP is provided in Table IV.

Biologic potency, as judged by intestinal calcium transport and bone calcium mobilization, generally correlates well with binding affinity of calciferol metabolites (Holick et al., 1975; Stern et al., 1975; Mallon et al., 1981; Table IV). Receptor affinity does not predict whether the compound is an agonist or an antagonist. In fact, no receptor antagonist for the calciferols has yet been identified. *In vitro* testing with receptor preparations also does not take into consideration variable binding of the analogs to DBP or differences in metabolism by the kidney, liver, and other tissues which certainly can be expected to affect the activity of many calciferols *in vivo*. 25-Azavitamin D_3, for instance, is an antagonist of vitamin D action *in vivo* on the basis of its inhibition of 25-hydroxylation in the liver (Onisko et al., 1979).

TABLE IV

LIGAND SPECIFICITY OF THE CHICK INTESTINAL $1\alpha,25(OH)_2D_3$ RECEPTORS AND RAT PLASMA VITAMIN D BINDING PROTEIN (DBP): COMPETITIVE BINDING STUDIES OF ANALOGS OF VITAMIN D

	Relative competitive index	
Competitor	Receptor protein[a]	DBP[b]
Side chain analogs of 1α-hydroxyvitamin D_3		
$1\alpha,25$-Dihydroxyvitamin D_3, -D_2	100[c]	4.2
$1\alpha,24R$-Dihydroxyvitamin D_3	77	—
24-nor-$1\alpha,25$-Dihydroxyvitamin D_3	46	—
$1\alpha,24R,25$-Trihydroxyvitamin D_3	41	—
$1\alpha,24S,25$-Trihydroxyvitamin D_3	53	—
$1\alpha,24S$-Dihydroxyvitamin D_3	14	—
1α-Hydroxyvitamin D_3	0.4	—
1α-Hydroxy-$\Delta^{24,25}$-vitamin D_3	0.4	—
A-Ring analogs of 25-hydroxyvitamin D_3		
$1\alpha,25$-Dihydroxy-5,6-trans-vitamin D_3	12.8	—
3-deoxy-$1\alpha,25$-dihydroxyvitamin D_3	5.7	—
25-Hydroxyvitamin D_3	0.5	100
25-Hydroxydihydrotachysterol$_3$	0.64	29
25-Hydroxy-5,6-trans-vitamin D_3	0.51	—
19,25-Dihydroxydihydrovitamin-II	0.087	—
19,25-Dihydroxydihydrovitamin-III	0.087	—
Side chain analogs of 25-OH-D_3		
25-Hydroxyvitamin D_3	0.5	100
25-Hydroxyvitamin D2	—	87
$24R,25$-Dihydroxyvitamin D_3	0.03	100
$24S,25$-Dihydroxyvitamin D_3	0.03	—
25,26-Dihydroxyvitamin D_3	—	100
24-nor-25-Hydroxyvitamin D_3	0.012	41
24-homo-25-Hydroxyvitamin D_3	0.012	—
23,24-dinor-25-Hydroxyvitamin D_3	0	—
26,27-dinor-25-Hydroxyvitamin D_3	—	31
Analogs with both side chain and A-ring modifications		
24-nor-25-Hydroxy-5,6-trans-vitamin D_3	0.10	—
24-homo-25-Hydroxy-5,6-trans-vitamin D_3	0.06	—
3-deoxy-1α-hydroxyvitamin D_3	0.03	—
1α-Hydroxy-3-epi-vitamin D_3	0.01	—
3-deoxy-3α-methyl-1-hydroxyvitamin D_3	0	—
5,6-trans-Vitamin D_3	0	0.0014

(continued)

TABLE IV (*continued*)

Competitor	Relative competitive index	
	Receptor protein[a]	DBP[b]
Vitamin D_3	0	1.3
Vitamin D_2	0	1.2
Dihydroxytachysterol$_3$	0	0.13
Dihydrotachysterol$_2$	—	0
19-Hydroxydihydrovitamin D_3-II	0	—
19-Hydroxydihydrovitamin D_3-III	0	—

[a]Modified from Wecksler and Norman (1980). Binding with $1\alpha,25(OH)_2D_3$ is defined as 100 in a reconstituted chromatin cytosol system. Lower numbers indicate lower binding affinities.

[b]Adapted from Belsey *et al.* (1974a) and Horst (1979). Binding with $25(OH)D_3$ is defined as 100. Lower numbers indicate lower binding affinities.

[c]Jones *et al.* (1980a) found a receptor potency of 77 for $1\alpha,25(OH)_2D_2$.

d. Regulation. Cellular content of receptors is dependent on the rate of DNA synthesis; mouse bone cells at confluence contained mimimal concentrations of receptors (Chen and Feldman, 1981). Furthermore, Walters *et al.* (1982) found that the decrease in $1,25(OH)_2D$ receptor content in confluent osteoblast-like MMB-1 mouse bone cells was reflected in decreased hormonal responsiveness in that collagen synthesis by the cells was no longer inhibited by $1,25(OH)_2D_3$.

An extensive evaluation of total (occupied and unoccupied) receptor capacity of chick intestinal mucosa showed no evidence that this capacity was regulated by sex steroids (Hunziker *et al.*, 1982). Glucocorticoids do influence $1,25(OH)_2D$ receptors; some of the effects are species specific. Glucocorticoids prevent a decline in rat calvarial $1,25(OH)_2D$ receptors (Manolagas *et al.*, 1976), increase the number of receptors in rat osteosarcoma cells (Manolagas *et al.*, 1981), and increase receptor numbers in rat intestine (Massoro *et al.*, 1982). On the other hand, glucocorticoids inhibit $1,25(OH)_2D_3$ receptors in mouse bone cells (Chen *et al.*, 1982) and mouse intestine (Hirst and Feldman, 1981).

The refractoriness of rats in the early suckling period to stimulation of intestinal calcium uptake by $1,25(OH)_2D_3$ is explained by the relative paucity of receptors for $1,25(OH)_2D_3$ in intestinal mucosa (Halloran and DeLuca, 1981). Corticosteroids can participate in induction of these receptors with intestinal explants from suckling rats (Massoro *et al.,* 1982). Ontogeny, in addition to glucocorticoids, estrogens (Walters, 1981), and rate of cell division, can influence $1,25(OH)_2D$ receptor content.

4. *Nuclear Events*

In the current view of steroid hormone action, the steroid hormone receptor proteins do not bind to DNA or accumulate in nuclei until they undergo some structural alteration (Grody *et al.,* 1982). Receptor transformation or "activation" is presumed to be the critical event in mediating receptor translocation and occupation of chromatin acceptor sites because of free diffusion of proteins the size of receptors through nuclear pores. The changes have most often been elicited *in vitro* with temperature, salt concentration, dilution, or the addition of hormones. The transformation is associated with major changes in molecular weight, sedimentation properties, and other physical parameters (Grody *et al.,* 1982). In others, the attainment of nuclear and DNA binding ability is the only detectable alteration. The ability to bind to DNA-cellulose is used as a measure of "activation" for steroid hormone receptors that otherwise lack this ability without exposure to high salt concentrations or 37°C (Schmidt *et al.,* 1980). Interestingly, $1,25(OH)_2D$ receptors differ from other steroid hormone receptors in that "nonactivated" receptors appear capable of binding to DNA-cellulose (Pike, 1982; Radparvar and Mellon, 1982). This observation may explain why homogenization under low ionic strength conditions yields unoccupied $1,25(OH)_2D$ receptors apparently localized in the nucleus (Walters *et al.,* 1980); Pike (1982), however, claims that hormone binding is necessary for nuclear localization of receptors. An important observation to mention here is the demonstration by Liberman *et al.* (1983), in two families with a rare form of resistance to $1,25(OH)_2D$, that under physiologic conditions *in vitro* $1,25(OH)_2D$ does not accumulate in the nucleus of cultured skin fibroblasts despite the presence in the "cytosol" of adequate amounts of otherwise apparently normal receptors (see Section III,B,2,a). This has two implications: (1) receptors can be found in the cell without ultimate occupancy of nuclear binding sites, and (2) proper nuclear localization is required for normal $1,25(OH)_2D$ action. Pike (1982) has demonstrated that DNA itself is the critical nuclear binding component, and Radparvar and Mellon (1982) have shown that the $1,25(OH)_2D$–receptor complex is specific for AT-rich segments of double-stranded DNA. These latter authors claim that this interaction is not merely hydrostatic but involves hydrophobic interaction with the major and/or minor grooves of the DNA helix.

Based on the work of Pike (1982) and Radparvar and Mellon (1982) it seems clear that the ability of $1,25(OH)_2D$ receptors to bind to DNA *in vitro* is not dependent on temperature or high ionic strength. Pike (1982) also showed that the chick $1,25(OH)_2D$ receptor binds to RNA, albeit with a lower strength than to DNA. Receptor occupancy by hormone was not required for either interaction. Hormone binding, however, was critical for localization of the complex to nuclear chromatin. The nuclear binding of occupied receptors was temperature independent and was extremely sensitive to KCl concentration. Pike (1982) also found that the chick intestinal receptor–sterol complex bound to nuclei from chicken heart, chick liver, and rat liver nuclei with high affinity, albeit with lower affinity than to nuclei from chick intestine.

Observations several years ago (Hallick and Deluca, 1969; Tsai and Norman, 1973a; Zerwekh *et al.*, 1976) indicated that after nuclear localization, $1,25(OH)_2D_3$, like classical steroid hormones, stimulated *de novo* RNA and protein synthesis for $1,25(OH) D_3$-dependent calcium transport. However, *in vivo* studies with transcriptional and translational inhibitors have produced equivocal results regarding the requirement for RNA and protein synthesis for $1,25(OH)D$ mediated calcium transport (Tsai *et al.*, 1973; Tanaka *et al.*, 1971; Bikle *et al.*, 1978; Rasmussen *et al.*, 1979). *In vitro* studies using cultured embryonic chick duodenum have revealed more decisively that $1,25(OH)_2D_3$-dependent calcium uptake can be blocked by protein and RNA synthesis inhibitors (Corradino, 1973). More recently, Franceschi and DeLuca (1981), examining inhibitor effects at early times after the onset of the $1,25(OH)_2D_3$ response, showed that inhibition of RNA synthesis by greater than 50% caused a total blockade of calcium transport. Similar results were obtained with cycloheximide, anisomycin, and α-amanitin.

However, it should be noted that Lawson and co-workers have found some discrepancies in the *in vivo* chronology of $1,25(OH)_2D_3$-stimulated intestinal calcium absorption and appearance of CaBP (Spencer *et al*, 1976a,b, 1978). They have found that although calcium absorption was definitely stimulated within 1–2 hours in vitamin D-deficient chicks given $1,25(OH)_2D_3$, messenger RNA for CaBP was not detected until after 4 hours, and CaBP could not be detected until after 5–6 hours. Thus, although vitamin D mediates intestinal calcium transport and $1,25(OH)_2D_3$ specifically stimulates the synthesis of CaBP mRNA and not RNA in general (Charles *et al.*, 1981), it is unlikely that CaBP accounts for all of the hormone's effects on the intestine.

5. *Vitamin D-Induced Proteins*

a. Calcium Binding Protein (CaBP). The appearance of CaBP in the intestinal mucosa of the vitamin D-deficient chick or rat is totally dependent on the administration of vitamin D_3 or one of its active metabolites (Norman, 1979). Its *de novo* synthesis in response to vitamin D is abolished by prior administration of actinomycin D (Corradino and Wasserman, 1968). The amino acid sequence of vitamin D-induced CaBP classifies it as a member of the calmodulin family of calcium binding proteins, which includes myosin light chain, the S-100 protein, troponin C, and parvalbumin. It was first isolated from chick intestine by Wasserman and colleagues (1968) and subsequently from mammalian intestinal mucosa (Fullmer and Wasserman, 1973; Hitchman *et al.*, 1973; Bruns *et al.*, 1977). Vitamin D does not alter calmodulin concentration in intestine (Thomasset *et al.*, 1981) or in red blood cells (Halloran *et al.*, 1980).

There appear to be two types of CaBP: one, the avian type with MW of $\cong 27,000$, is immunologically similar in the kidney and cerebellum of many species; the other, with a MW of $\cong 7000$, found primarily in the gastrointestinal tract, is immunologically specific for mammals (Thomasset *et al.*, 1982). Material that cross-reacts immunologically with the avian type has been detected in mammalian tissues, such as rat and human kidney (Hermsdorf and Bronner, 1975; Piazolo *et al.*, 1971; Morrisey and Roth, 1974) and, more recently, in rat brain (Feldman and Christakos, 1983). As shown in Table V the tissue distribution of CaBP in chicks is widespread. However, vitamin D stimulated a significant rise in CaBP only in the GI tract, pancreas, kidney, bone, adrenal, and lungs. There were significant basal amounts of CaBP in hypothalamus, parathyroid, and cerebral cortex of D-deficient chicks; these levels did not rise with vitamin D treatment. In the study by Thomasset *et al.* (1982) vitamin D clearly stimulated rat intestinal CaBP (MW $\cong 7000$) and renal CaBP (MW $\cong 27,000$) but not cerebellar CaBP (MW $\cong 27,000$). A recent study by Thorens *et al.* (1982), using immunocytochemistry and both light and electron microscopy of chick duodenum, demonstrated convincingly that CaBP was localized in the cytosol and euchromatin of the absorptive cells of the villi, but not in the brush border or the goblet cells.

In addition to the studies of Lawson and co-workers cited above (see Section II,C,4), kinetic experiments by Morrisey *et al.* (1978), examining intestinal responses to $1,25(OH)_2D_3$ with changes in calcium and phosphorous uptake *in vitro* as well as *in vivo* calcium transport and accumlation, indicated the lack of correlation between the appearance of CaBP and the early rise in the transport rate of calcium across the brush border membrane from the gut lumen after treatment with $1,25(OH)_2D_3$. The biochemical evidence and immunocytochemical evidence are more consistent with the hypothesis that vitamin D-depen-

TABLE V
TISSUE DISTRIBUTION OF IMMUNOREACTIVE CaBP

Tissue	Species	Vitamin D dependence[a]	References
Small intestine	Chick	+	Wasserman and Taylor (1966)
	Cow	ND	Fullmer and Wasserman (1973)
	Pig	ND	Hitchman et al. (1973)
	Rat	ND	Bruns et al. (1977)
		+	Thomasset et al. (1982)
Caecum and stomach	Rat	ND	Thomasset et al. (1982)
Bone	Chick	+	Christakos et al. (1979)
	Rat	ND	Thomasset et al. (1982)
Kidney	Chick	+	Taylor and Wasserman (1967)
		+	Christakos et al. (1979)
	Rat	ND	Hermsdorf and Bronner (1975)
		+	Thomasset et al. (1982)
	Dog	ND	Sand and Kessler (1971)
	Human	ND	Piazolo et al. (1971)
Skin	Rat	+	Laouari et al. (1980)
Parathyroid	Chick	−	Christakos et al. (1979)
Pancreas	Chick	+	Christakos et al. (1979); Roth et al. (1982)
Lungs	Rat	ND	Thomasset et al. (1982)
Mammary gland	Rat and Cow	ND	Wasserman et al. (1978)
Adrenal	Chick	+	Christakos et al. (1979)
Cerebral cortex	Chick	−	Christakos et al. (1979)
	Rat	ND	Feldman and Christakos (1983)
Cerebellum	Rat	−	Thomasset et al. (1982)
Hypothalamus	Chick	−	Christakos et al. (1979)
Chorioallantoic membrane	Chick	ND	Tuan et al. (1978)

[a]The (+) indicates vitamin D dependence; (−) indicates lack of vitamin D dependence; ND indicates no data on D dependence reported.

dent intestinal CaBP plays a role in either regulation of intracellular calcium concentration or movement of calcium across the epithelial cell, rather than directly in the initial steps of calcium absorption across the brush border membrane.

Immunohistochemical studies with chick and mammalian kidney have localized the CaBP to the proximal and distal convoluted tubules, in all cases studied and some portions of the collecting system (Christakos *et al.*, 1981; Rhoten and Christakos, 1981; Roth *et al.*, 1981; Taylor *et al.*, 1982). Another function in the kidney induced by $1,25(OH)_2D$, $25(OH)D$-24-hydroxylase has been exclusively localized to the proximal nephron based on enzyme activity (Kawashima *et al.*, 1981a) (see Section II,A,3,b). Consistent with the intrarenal location of these vitamin D-sensitive processes is the demonstration by Kawashima and Kurokawa (1982) of $1,25(OH)_2D$ receptors in both the proximal and distal segments of the rat nephron.

As pointed out in the sections on the actions of $1,25(OH)_2D$ and $1,25(OH)_2D$ receptors the pancreas and the skin appear to be target organs. Immunocytochemical studies have also revealed the presence of vitamin D-dependent CaBP in these tissues. Roth *et al.* (1982) observed that CaBP in chick pancreatic islets was localized exclusively to the insulin-producing β-cells while Laouari *et al.* (1980) found a CaBP in rat skin with a molecular weight similar to intestinal CaBP (10,000) but immunologically different. The function of the skin CaBP is unknown, but recent purification of this protein has allowed it to be classified as a parvalbumin (Rinaldi *et al.*, 1982).

There have been no convincing studies with purified intestinal CaBP to show that the protein is directly responsible for mediating intestinal calcium transport. Only in one study (Corradino *et al.*, 1976) was it shown that highly purified chick intestinal CaBP added to embryonic chick intestine in organ culture caused an increase in calcium transport. Mathematical analysis by Kretsinger *et al.* (1982) using the calcium binding properties of CaBP showed that these properties were sufficient to account for calcium transport *in vivo*. Thus far, neither of these reports has been confirmed with additional experimental evidence.

b. Alkaline Phosphatase. Vitamin D increases intestinal mucosa alkaline phosphatase, calcium-stimulated ATPase, and phytase enzyme activites (Norman, 1979). Several groups of investigators (Norman *et al.*, 1970; Holdsworth, 1970; Haussler *et al.*, 1970) have documented a three- to fourfold rise in alkaline phosphatase, specifically associated with the brush border, after giving vitamin D_3 to rachitic chicks. Following administration of $1,25(OH)_2D_3$ to rachitic chicks the rise in intestinal alkaline phosphatase activity and in CaBP concentration occurs several hours after the rise in calcium transport (Morrisey *et al.*, 1978). The rise in enzyme activity precedes the intestinal calcium accumulation stimulated by $1,25(OH)_2D$, suggesting that the enzyme (or CaBP) is involved in the regulation of intracellular calcium content in the steady-state condition. Alkaline phosphatase has also been shown to be regulated in tissue culture by $1,25(OH)_2D_3$ with osteoblastic osteosarcoma cells (Majeska and Rodan, 1982).

c. *ATPase.* Brush border membranes from chick or rat intestinal mucosa *in vivo* respond to a vitamin D with an increase in calcium-stimulated ATPase (Martin *et al.,* 1969; Melancon and DeLuca, 1970). Based on inhibitor and temperature inactivation studies it appeared that intestinal alkaline phosphatase and calcium-ATPase were in fact the same protein (Haussler *et al.,* 1970; Holdsworth, 1970; Russell *et al.,* 1972). However, a subsequent study (Lane and Lawson, 1978) revealed differences in the activities after an intravenous pulse of $1,25(OH)_2D_3$, thereby questioning the identity of the two proteins.

d. *Peptide Hormones and Other Proteins.* As already stated in Section II,B, $1,25(OH)_2D$ can regulate the secretion of several protein hormones, including PTH (Nko *et al.,* 1982; Oldham *et al.,* 1979), insulin (Norman *et al.,* 1980; Clark *et al.,* 1981), and prolactin (Murdoch and Rosenfeld, 1981). The presence of $1,25(OH)_2D_3$ receptors in the parathyroid, pancreas, and pituitary (Table II) is consistent with the possibility of a regulatory role for $1,25(OH)_2D_3$ on the secretion of these and other hormones.

Another protein regulated by $1,25(OH)_2D_3$ is a major component of bone matrix and contains γ-carboxyglutamic acid (GLA-protein) (Price and Baukol, 1980). Its functional role is not known.

Finally, there are several other intestinal proteins that increase in response to $1,25(OH)_2D_3$ and may help elucidate the role of vitamin D in the regulation of intestinal calcium transport (Hobden *et al.,* 1980; Wilson and Lawson, 1981; Schachter and Kowarski, 1982; Mezzetti *et al.,* 1982). The $1,25(OH)_2D$-dependent spermine binding protein described by Mezzetti *et al.* (1982) appears within 1–2 hours after exposure of rachitic chicks to the hormone, making this one of the earliest protein responses induced in the duodenum by $1,25(OH)_2D_3$.

III. DEFICIENCIES IN CALCIFEROL ACTION

The clinical, biochemical, radiological, and histological manifestations of calciferol deficiency represent the combined end result of the deficiency itself and compensatory mechanisms. The main function of active calciferol metabolites is maintenance of calcium and possibly phosphorus homeostasis (see Section II,B). Disturbances in this function may lead, therefore, to hypocalcemia and secondary hyperparathyroidism. Hypophosphatemia can ensue from the primary defect in calciferol action on intestine and bone and from the consequence of secondary hyperparathyroidism to increase phosphate excretion by the kidney. Low concentrations of extracellular calcium and inorganic phosphate lead to defective mineralization of the protein matrix of bone and in the growing skeleton of the preosseous cartilage as well, causing morphological changes of bone, termed osteomalacia in adults and rickets in childhood. None of the signs, symptoms, or biochemical abnormalities is exclusively associated with calciferol deficiency; each can be an end result of different primary disturbances in mineral homeostasis or bone mineralization.

As mentioned above (Section I and II,A,B), 1,25-dihydroxycalciferol is produced in selected cells in a controlled manner, is secreted into the circulation, and acts on specific target tissues; it is recognized, therefore, as a true hormone. Vitamin D may be considered as a prohormone because its *de novo* production and availability are dependent on external factors—either ultraviolet light or dietary sources. Based on this schema and the availability of assays for serum levels of bioactive calciferol metabolites, we classify the calciferol deficiency states into (1) deficiency states with decreased or inappropriately low circulating levels of active calciferol metabolites, or (2) states with elevated plasma levels of $1,25(OH)_2D$.

Extensive reviews with detailed delineation of clinical features and differential diagnoses have been published recently (Stamp, 1982; Scriver *et al,* 1982; Dunnigan *et al,* 1982; Mawer, 1982; Coburn and Brautbar, 1980). The several etiologies for the calciferol deficiency states will be reviewed here, focusing on recent observations.

A. Decreased or Inappropriately Low Circulating Concentrations of Active Calciferol Metabolites

1. *Defective Production of Calciferol or Its Metabolites*

a. Inadequate Supply of Calciferol. i. Environmental effects. Vitamin D-deficient rickets or osteomalacia remains common in Asia, the Middle East, and Africa (Rizvi *et al.,* 1976; Salimpour, 1975; Pettifor *et al.,* 1978). The disease is rare in North America and Europe except among infants of impoverished background, eldery persons (Lawson *et al.,* 1979), and Asian immigrants (Dunningan, 1977; Ford *et al.,* 1976; Dunnigan *et al.,* 1982). In normal adults, even in northern latitudes, more than 90% of circulating serum 25(OH)D, as well as $1,25(OH)_2D$, is derived from synthesis in the skin (D_3 series), while dietary sources of vitamin D (usually as D_2) contribute little to the amount of calciferol in blood (Lawson 1979; Poskitt *et al.,* 1979; Preece *et al.,* 1975). The relative contribution of dietary cholecalciferol is unresolved, but it is believed that most animal food with the exception of liver and cod liver oil contains low amounts of vitamin D_3 (Dunnigan *et al.*, 1982). Ultraviolet radiation is therefore critical for normal supply of vitamin D (Stamp *et al.*, 1977; Lawson, 1979). The amount of UV radiation delivered to the skin will depend on the duration of exposure, latitude, and the filtering effect of environmental and intrinsic factors. Urbanization, atmospheric pollution, and habits of dress contribute toward the development of vitamin D deficiency as shown by several epidemiological studies (Loomis, 1970; Preece *et al.*, 1975; Dunnigan *et al.*, 1982). Both experimental and clinical studies demonstrate that pigmented skin does not transmit UV radiation as well as white skin. Holick and associates (1982) have shown that there is a need to increase exposure time to simulated solar radiation in order to maximize previtamin D_3 formation in pigmented human skin *in vitro*. The same investigators (Clemens *et al.*, 1982) observed that one minimal erythemal dose of UV radiation increased serum vitamin D concentration by up to 60-fold in 2 lightly pigmented caucasians, whereas this dose did not produce any significant change in serum vitamin D concentrations in 3 heavily pigmented volunteers. Reexposing one of the pigmented volunteers to a six times larger UV radiation dose increased circulating vitamin D to concentrations similar to those recorded after the lower exposure dose in the caucasian volunteers. Skin pigmentation may therefore contribute to the development of calciferol deficiency states, especially if additional risk factors are present.

Although it usually makes a marginal contribution, dietary supplementation with vitamin D may be essential under situations of limited exposure to UV light and/or increased demands for the hormone, such as in infancy, adolescence, pregnancy, and institutionalization. Moreover, there is some evidence that prolonged breast feeding associated with delayed weaning may produce infantile rickets (Dunnigan *et al.* 1982; Edidin *et al.*, 1980; Greer *et al.*, 1982) in contrast to previous claims that breast feeding protects against rickets (Lakdawala and Widdowson 1977). It has been suggested that the water-soluble form of vitamin D in human milk is not antirachitic in the rat and may therefore be metabolically inactive in man (Leerbeck and Sondergaard, 1980). Bovine milk has low vitamin D_3 content. Oral vitamin D supplementation is therefore essential during infancy, and only by routine use in Western countries have most cases of infantile rickets been eliminated.

An interesting hypothesis on the correlation between dietary constituents (other than vitamin D_2) and calciferol deficiency, has been suggested by epidemiological studies on the prevalence of rickets and osteomalacia in the Far and Middle East, in the United Kingdom among Asian immigrants, in Europe during or after the First and Second World Wars, and in Europe and the United States in a small number of food faddists (Dunnigan *et al.*, 1982; Vaishnava, 1975; Reinhold, 1971; Chick *et al.*, 1923; Robertson *et al.*, 1981; Edidin *et al.*, 1980; Dent and Smith, 1969; Roberts *et al.*, 1979). Common nutritional denominators to these outbreaks of calciferol deficiency have been one or more of the following: vegetarian diets consisting almost entirely of bread and vegetables, diets with high extraction (unprocessed) cereals, and diets with high levels of fiber. Though such diets are known to be vitamin D deficient, this deficiency does not seem to be the only etiological factor. In a retrospective epidemiological study of an outbreak of rickets in Ireland in the 1940s (Robertson *et al.*, 1981), the only significant variable over the years surveyed was an increase in flour extraction rate from 70 to 100%, coinciding with the increased prevalence of rickets. The incidence of rickets subsided as the extraction rate was reduced. Thus, high extraction cereals may be rachitogenic independent of other dietary constituents. High extraction wheat meal flour untreated with yeast, which is commonly used in Asian diets, is high in phytate which binds calcium in the gut and may create a state of calcium deficiency. However, calcium deficiency alone would not cause low 25(OH)D levels, a common observation in Asian immigrants in the United Kingdom with clinical or biochemical rickets (Gupta *et al.*, 1974). Reinhold (1976) suggested that wheat fiber may combine with bile acids to create a less absorbable complex that may bind calciferol metabolites disrupting the enterohepatic recirculation (see below), leading finally to a net loss through the gut of calciferol metabolites produced in the skin. This theory, though attractive, lacks convincing experimental support.

ii. Gastrointestinal and hepatobiliary diseases. Calciferol deficiency has been reported with a large spectrum of gastrointestinal abnormalities, with or without steatorrhoea. Osteomalacia or rickets with low concentrations of 25(OH)D in plasma may develop (1) many years after partial gastrectomy, particularly the Billroth II type (gastrojejunostomy) (Morgan *et al.*, 1965; Eddy, 1971); (2) in malabsorption syndromes caused by small intestinal dysfunctions such as coeliac disease (Moss *et al.*, 1965), Crohn's disease (Arnaud *et al.*, 1977), and absorptive deficiency after intestinal bypass surgery (Compston and Creamer, 1977; Parfitt *et al.*, 1978); (3) in chronic pancreatic insufficiency (Prost *et al.*, 1975); and (4) in hepatobiliary disturbances ranging from congenital biliary atresia in infants (Kobayashi *et al.*, 1974) to primary biliary cirrhosis, chronic ascending cholangitis, and chronic active hepatitis in adults (Atkinson et al., 1966; Compston and Thompson, 1977). In obstructive liver diseases malabsorption of 25(OH)D has been observed (Compston and Thompson, 1977). The contribution of malabsorption of dietary vitamin D to the calciferol deficiency in these syndromes is not known, especially since the role of dietary sources in calciferol status seems minimal. On the other hand, gut and hepatobiliary abnormalities may interfere with a well-documented enterohepatic recirculation of calciferol metabolites (Goldsmith, 1982), leading to decreased intestinal reabsorption and accelerated loss of vitamin D metabolites (see discussion below). The possibility of a defective small intestinal response to $1,25(OH)_2D$, due to anatomical and/or functional changes in gut diseases, was suggested (Stamp, 1982), but seems unlikely in view of the usually good response to parenteral treatment with "physiological" doses of the hormone (Dent and Stamp, 1970). It must be emphasized that osteomalacia is not the only bone disease associated with gastrointestinal and hepatobiliary abnormalities. Multiple deficiencies, in particular calcium malabsorption and malnutrition, may also lead to the development of osteoporosis (Atkinson et al., 1966).

b. Deficient Production of Calciferol and Its Metabolites. i. Deficient production of 7-dehydrocholesterol (7-DHC). Although there are no known diseases with deficient 7-DHC production in skin, several lines of evidence suggest that 7-DHC in skin may be under $1,25(OH)_2D$ regulation through a specific intracellular receptor, and therefore may be a potential site for abnormalities. Both in rat skin in vivo (Esvelt et al., 1980) and in human cultured keratinocytes in vitro (Holick et al., 1982), $1,25(OH)_2D_3$ caused a measurable increase in 7-DHC content. High-affinity cytosolic binders for $1,25(OH)_2D_3$ have been demonstrated in rat skin (Simpson and DeLuca, 1980) as well as in human keratinocytes (Feldman et al., 1980; Holick et al., 1982). In human keratinocytes cultured from a patient with end-organ resistance to $1,25(OH)_2D_3$, no high-affinity cytosol binding of $1,25(OH)_2D_3$ was detected. In the same cells, 7-DHC production in the basal state was lower than in normal keratinocytes and no induction of 7-DHC production by $1,25(OH)_2D_3$ was recorded (Holick et al., 1982). In several other patients with end-organ resistance to $1,25(OH)_2D$, in whose cultured keratinocytes production of 7-DHC was not studied, serum 25(OH)D levels were in the normal range in the pretreatment phase (see discussion below). Therefore, there is no evidence that $1,25(OH)_2D$ is an important modulator of 7-DHC production in human skin in vivo.

ii. Deficient production of 25-hydroxyvitamin D. Neither genetic nor acquired defects in hepatic vitamin D-25-hydroxylase activity have been proven to cause pathologic calciferol deficiency. In a single case report, Zerwekh and associates (1979) described a patient with end-organ resistance to $1,25(OH)_2D$ (see discussion below) and proposed an additional abnormality in vitamin D-25-hydroxylase. This was based on serum concentration of 25(OH)D in the lower normal range 3 weeks after reported intake of high doses of vitamin D_2, and on complete clinical and biochemical remission when given high doses of $25(OH)D_3$ (20–50 µg/day) without further increase in the already elevated serum $1,25(OH)_2D$ levels. Since therapy with $25(OH)D_3$ did not ameliorate the resistance to $1,25(OH)_2D$, a putative deficiency in 25(OH)D production could not be considered the cause of the calciferol deficiency state.

Hillman et al. (1979, 1982) have shown that more than 50% of very premature infants (mean gestation 30.1 weeks and mean birthweight 1176 g) can neither maintain normal serum 25(OH)D concentrations nor correct the low concentrations before 9–12 weeks of age, even when treated with 400 IU of vitamin D daily. It has been postulated that these low serum values of 25(OH)D may represent a decreased ability to absorb vitamin D in prematurity and/or a decreased ability of the premature liver to hydroxylate vitamin D to 25(OH)D. Recently, Hillman and Haddad (1983) reported that concentrations of the specific vitamin D binding protein (DBP) were low in cord blood of premature infants, remained low for the first 9 weeks of life, and increased significantly at 12 weeks of age. Serum DBP levels were normal in full-term babies (Haddad and Walgate, 1976a). Thus, the question of a relative deficiency in vitamin D-25-hydroxylation or a relative deficiency of plasma DBP concentrations in prematurity is still unsolved.

In chronic liver diseases, plasma concentrations of 25(OH)D are often low (Haddad and Chyu, 1971; Compston and Thompson, 1977). The possibility of defective hepatic 25-hydroxylase activity has been raised, but a number of studies tend to exclude it (Kooh et al., 1979; Krawitt et al., 1977). It seems rather that profound malabsorption of calciferol metabolites is the main contributing factor (Compston and Thompson, 1977), and rickets or osteomalacia associated with hepatocellular disease may respond to physiological amounts of vitamin D if given parenterally (Dent and Stamp, 1970).

iii. Deficient production of 1,25-dihydroxycalciferol with normal levels of 25(OH)D. (a) Hereditary 25-hydroxyvitamin D-1-hydroxylase deficiency. In 1961, Prader et al. described two young children who showed all the usual clinical, radiological, and biochemical features of vitamin D deficiency despite adequate vitamin D intake. Complete remission was dependent on continuous therapy with high doses of vitamin D. The syndrome has been named pseudovitamin D deficiency or vitamin D dependency (DD). The disease manifests itself before 2 years of age and often during the first 6 months of life. Family studies have revealed this to be a genetic disorder with a pattern suggestive of autosomal recessive inheritance (Scriver *et al.*, 1982). Although there are no direct enzymatic measurements to prove a defective 1-hydroxylase activity, there are several indirect observations to support this etiology. First, while massive doses of vitamin D and 25(OH)D (1000–3000 mg/day and 200–900 mg/day, respectively, 100–300 times the normal "physiological" dose) are required to maintain remission of rickets in DD, 0.25–1.0 µg/day of $1,25(OH)_2D_3$ (a normal physiological dose) or of 1α-hydroxyvitamin D_3 (a synthetic analog of $1,25(OH)_2D_3$) are sufficient to maintain the same effect (Fraser *et al.*, 1973; Reade *et al.*, 1975; Balsan *et al.*, 1979). Second, the content of $1,25(OH)_2D$ in blood was very low in several studies of children with DD (Scriver *et al.*, 1978; Chesney *et al.*, 1980a). The low but detectable levels may represent residual enzyme activity or spurious values due to methodological problems. Finally, the concentration of 25(OH)D was normal or markedly elevated in patients treated with high doses of vitamin D or 25(OH)D (Scriver *et al.*, 1982). Taken together, these observations support the thesis that many patients with DD have an hereditary defect in 25(OH)D-1-hydroxylase activity. The benificial therapeutic effect, in patients with DD, of high circulating amounts of 25(OH)D while $1,25(OH)_2D$ concentrations remained low (Chesney *et al.*, 1980b) has several hypothetical explanations: a metabolite of 25(OH)D [for example 5,6-*trans*-25(OH)D] may act directly on target tissues; alternatively, 25(OH)D at high concentrations may activate the specific intracellular receptor for $1,25(OH)_2D$, whose affinity for 25(OH)D is lower by about two orders of magnitude than for $1,25(OH)_2D$ (see Section II,C,3,c).

A similar syndrome has been studied in a mutant strain of pigs (Harmeyer and Plonait, 1967; Harmeyer *et al.*, 1977; Wilke *et al.*, 1979). The mode of inheritance, as well as the clinical, radiological, and biochemical picture, are similar to the human disease. The homozygous animal develops hypocalcemia, hypophosphatemia, secondary hyperparathyroidism, and severe rickets within 6 weeks of birth, and the condition is fatal by 3–4 months of age if untreated. High doses of vitamin D can produce a remission of the disease. This animal model should provide the opportunity for a direct study of the defective 1-hydroxylase activity in renal tissue.

X-Linked hypophosphatemic rickets (XLH), characterized by persistant postnatal hypophosphatemia, essentially normal concentrations of calcium and parathyroid hormone in serum, early onset rickets, and growth retardation (Scriver et al., 1982), was described initially by Albright et al. (1937). It is an inborn error of phosphate transport due to a primary defect in renal tubular phosphate reabsorption (Glorieux and Scriver, 1972). Circulating amounts of 1,25(OH)$_2$D in XLH were reported to be low or in the normal range (Haussler and McCain, 1977; Scriver et al., 1978). However, even normal concentrations of 1,25(OH)$_2$D may be inappropriately low for the state of phosphate depletion (Drezner et al., 1980), because hypophosphatemia normally enhances 1,25(OH)$_2$D production (see Section II,A,2). Lyles and Drezner (1982) studied the effect of intravenous parathyroid hormone stimulation on 1,25(OH)$_2$D in serum in patients with XLH and in normal controls and found an increase of only about 70% in the former group as compared to 220% in the normals. The diminished 1,25(OH)$_2$D response in the XLH patients occurred even though each group showed equivalent changes in urinary 3',5'-cyclic adenosine monophosphate (cAMP) excretion and tubular phosphate reabsorption. The X-linked hypophosphatemic (hyp) mouse shows a disorder that in its mode of inheritance, clinical features, and biochemistry resembles the human disease (Eicher et al., 1976). In these animals, there is a defective response of 1,25(OH)$_2$D$_3$ production to hypophosphatemia (Meyer et al., 1980), but a normal 1-hydroxylase response to low calcium challenge in vivo (Meyer et al., 1982). Based on these observations, both in man and in the hyp mouse, the regulation of 1,25(OH)$_2$D is defective in XLH. It is not yet clear if the abnormality in vitamin D metabolism is primary or secondary to the renal defect in phosphate handling. It must be emphasized that an altered 1-hydroxylase activity is not the sole deficiency underlying the pathogenesis of this disease. 1,25(OH)$_2$D$_3$ therapy does not correct the renal phosphate leak in XLH (Costa et al., 1981; Glorieux et al., 1980). The observations of inadequate production of 1,25(OH)$_2$D in XLH have clinical importance. The optimal therapeutic response may be dependent on the combined administration of phosphate supplementation and 1,25(OH)$_2$D$_3$ or 1α(OH)D$_3$ (Glorieux et al., 1980; Costa et al., 1981; Rasmussen et al., 1981). Treatment with massive doses of inorganic phosphate in XLH raises serum phosphate, stimulates linear growth rate, and improves calcification of cartilage in the growth plate (Glorieux et al., 1972, 1980). On the other hand, this form of therapy caused secondary hyperparathyroidism with additional drain of body phosphate and increased bone resorption, and failed to evoke an increase in 1,25(OH)$_2$D levels or to induce mineralization of trabecular bone (Glorieux et al., 1972, 1980; Chesney et al., 1980b; Costa et al., 1981). There are conflicting reports on the clinical effects of 1,25(OH)$_2$D$_3$ or 1α(OH)D$_3$ alone in

XLH. While in a small number of patients a beneficial effect was observed (Drezner *et al.*, 1980; Seino *et al.*, 1980), others showed an inadequate effect on growth rate or on the biochemical and radiological manifestations of rickets (Rasmussen *et al.*, 1981; Glorieux *et al.*, 1972). Combined treatment with phosphate and 1-hydroxylated cholecalciferol metabolites in children with XLH increased linear growth rate, improved mineralization of the growth plate and trabecular bone (as judged by histomorphometric studies of bone biopsies), and caused healing of rickets by biochemical and radiological criteria (Glorieux *et al.*, 1980; Rasmussen *et al.*, 1981). There has been insufficient time to assess possible deleterious effects of this therapy which can cause simultaneous rises in urinary excretion rates for phosphorus and calcium.

(b) Acquired 25-hydroxyvitamin D-1-hydroxylase deficiencies. The kidney is central in the calciferol endocrine system, being the principal tissue that produces and secretes $1,25(OH)_2D$ (see Sections II,A,2 and 3). Any disease that causes progressive functional and antomical derangement of the kidney parenchyma will eventually lead to deficient production of $1,25(OH)_2D$. As the 1-hydroxylase system is localized in the proximal tubule, any abnormality affecting primarily this region of the nephron will cause $1,25(OH)_2D$ deficiency at an earlier stage than primary glomerular disease (see below). The ultimate result of a progressive renal disease with chronic failure will obviously be the same.

Numerous hereditary or acquired diseases, a complete list of which is beyond the scope of this review, are localized initially in the renal tubule (Stamp, 1982). Hereditary or acquired Fanconi syndrome, defined as a primary or secondary lesion of the proximal renal tubule leading to multiple tubular defects such as aminoaciduria, glucosuria, hypophosphatemia, and renal tubular acidosis, is frequently associated with rickets or osteomalacia (DeToni, 1933; Fanconi, 1936). While hypophosphatemia (as discussed before) and acidosis are probably the main contributors to the development of the disease, defects in vitamin D metabolism deserve further studies.

Heavy metals such as cadmium, mercury, copper, and lead are toxic to the kidney (Morgan *et al.*, 1962; Clarkson and Kench, 1956; Adams *et al.*, 1969). Long-term cadmium exposure causes a disease characterized by osteomalacia and adult Fanconi syndrome with relatively mild impairment of glomerular function (Adams *et al.*, 1969). The disease may appear as a sporadic or endemic form, Itai-Itai býo or "ouch-ouch" disease in Japan (Emmerson, 1970; Nogawa *et al.*, 1975). The interrelationship between heavy metals and mineral metabolism is complex. Cadmium effectively displaces calcium from the vitamin D-dependent calcium binding protein (Wasserman et al., 1974), and lead competes with calcium for binding sites on mucosal proteins in the intestine (Barton et al., 1978). Heavy metals, as well as sodium maleate [toxicity produces Fanconi syndrome (Berliner et al., 1950)] interfere with sulfhydryl-requiring enzymes. Some heavy metals and sodium maleate may affect transport systems and the membrane permeability of renal tubular cells (Bergeron et al., 1976; Gonick et al., 1976). Acute administration of maleic acid to rats impaired the renal capacity to convert 25(OH)D$_3$ to 1,25(OH)$_2$D$_3$ in vivo (Brewer et al., 1977), and increased lead levels in children were associated with low concentrations of 1,25(OH)$_2$D (Rosen et al., 1980). These observations suggest that in some instances of heavy metal poisoning and/or acquired Fanconi syndrome, a deficient production of active calciferol metabolites is one of the proximal events leading to disturbances in mineral metabolism.

Chronic hyperchloremic acidosis caused by renal tubular disturbances represents another heterogeneous group of hereditary and acquired defects accompanied by disturbances in mineral metabolism (Stamp, 1982). In contrast to the bone disease of chronic renal failure, chronic acidosis may lead to osteomalacia even when the glomerular filtration rate is normal. The questions, is there a primary defect in vitamin D metabolism in these states, and if so, is the defect caused by acidosis per se or is it secondary to the primary tubular defect, are unsettled. In rats and chicks, acute systemic acidosis caused impaired conversion of 25(OH)D$_3$ to 1,25(OH)$_2$D$_3$ (Lee et al., 1977; Sauveur et al., 1977). In two patients with chronic metabolic acidosis and osteomalacia consequent to urinary tract diversion, good clinical, biochemical, and histological responses were seen upon treatment with alkali alone and no vitamin D supplements (Cunningham et al., 1982). Similar observations were obtained in earlier studies (Richards et al., 1972; McSherry and Morris, 1978). On the other hand, in a study on patients with different forms of renal tubular acidosis, the only patients showing radiological evidence of rickets were those with type 2 or the proximal tubular form of renal tubular acidosis (Brenner et al., 1982). As mentioned above, the proximal tubule is the segment of the nephron containing the 1-hydroxylase.

Hypophosphatemic osteomalacia can occur with benign mesenchymal tumors as well as with sarcomata and cancers of prostate and breast (Linovitz et al., 1976; Bhattacharyya and DeLuca, 1974; Lyles et al., 1980). The biochemical abnormalities are hypophosphatemia, low renal tubular phosphate reabsorption, sometimes mild hypocalcemia, normal parathyroid hormone concentrations, normal serum 25-(OH)D, low 1,25(OH)$_2$D, intestinal malabsorption of calcium and phosphorus, and bone histology typical of osteomalacia (Drezner et al., 1982). The causative relationship between some of the tumors and the clinical and biochemical picture was supported by several lines of evidence: (1) complete and rapid clinical, biochemical, and histological cure following resection of the tumor (Drezner and Feinglos, 1977); (2) saline extracts of tumors produced phosphaturia in experimental animals (Drezner et al., 1982; Aschinberg, et al 1977); (3) tumor tissue transplanted into athymic nude mice produced a similar syndrome in the animal (Drezner et al., 1982). The low concentrations of 1,25(OH)$_2$D in the face of severe hypophosphatemia (see above) suggest an acquired defect in the 1-hydroxylase (Drezner et al., 1982). Direct evidence of decreased renal 1-hydroxylase activity was recently obtained in the heterotransplant-animal model. Renal 1-hydroxylase activity in hypophosphatemic tumor-bearing mice was significantly lower than that in either normal mice or tumor-bearing mice without hypophosphatemia (Drezner et al., 1982). It is clear, however, that altered calciferol metabolism is not the sole abnormality underlying this syndrome. The extreme phosphaturia and occasional glycosuria and/or aminoaciduria with usually normal parathyroid hormone secretion indicate multiple alterations in proximal tubular function. Whether the tumor production of phosphaturic factor(s) and the defect in vitamin D metabolism are interrelated or represent separate pathophysiological mechanisms is unclear.

An interesting syndrome with a possible deficient action of calciferols was described recently in infants and adults receiving long-term total parenteral nutrition (Klein et al., 1981; Shike et al., 1981). This is a unique situation, because the intestine, a major target tissue for vitamin D action and an organ involved in mineral homeostasis, has been bypassed by virtue of the intravenous provision of all nutrients including calcium, phosphorus, and vitamin D. The syndrome is characterized by bone pain, patchy osteomalacia, or rickets in infants, and reduced bone metabolism as judged histologically. Calcium, phosphorus, and PTH concentrations are usually normal although transient hypercalcemia occurs in some patients. 25(OH)D and 24,25(OH)$_2$D are normal while 1,25(OH)$_2$D concentrations are reduced in serum (Shike et al., 1981; Klein et al., 1981). Complete remission is achieved upon discontinuation of total parenteral nutrition (Klein et al., 1981). The etiology of the syndrome is unclear. Shike et al. (1981) reported that clinical and biochemical improvement was achieved by omitting vitamin D$_2$ from the parenteral solutions. On the other hand,

Klein *et al.* (1982) claimed that in children administration of 25,000 IU of vitamin D_2 intramuscularly each month, in addition to 1000 IU of vitamin D_2 included per liter of the iv nutrient solution, will prevent or cure the disease. In a related clinical trial, Lemann *et al.* (1982) reported that serum $1,25(OH)_2D$ concentrations fell rapidly in healthy subjects given a liquid formula adequate in minerals. The decline in serum $1,25-(OH)_2D$ appeared to be independent of changes in serum calcium, phosphorus, and parathyroid hormone. Similar observations were made in patients on total parenteral nutrition (Klein *et al.*, 1981). Lemann *et al.* (1982) speculated that liquid diets or total parenteral nutrition suppress the activity of an hypothetical intestinal humoral signal involved in the regulation of $1,25(OH)_2D$ synthesis.

Defective production of $1,25(OH)_2D$ may result from defective production or action of PTH. Thus, in hypoparathyroidism (primary or secondary) and pseudohypoparathyroidism (target tissue resistance to PTH), cAMP-regulated 1-hydroxylase activity is inadequate and $1,25(OH)_2D$ production is decreased (Norman *et al.*, 1982; Fraser, 1980; Section II,A,2,b). The accompanying hyperphosphatemia may be an additional contributory factor in suppressing 1-hydroxylase activity (see above).

The role, if any, of deficient calciferol metabolism in postmenopausal and senile osteoporosis is unknown. In pure osteoporosis, defined as decreased bone content per unit volume, there is by definition no histologic sign of osteomalacia. Decreased intestinal absorption of calcium is well documented in a significant fraction of patients with osteoporosis (Nordin *et al.*, 1979; Gallagher *et al.*, 1979), but reports on serum concentration of $1,25(OH)_2D$ vary from low to normal (Haussler *et al.*, 1979; Bishop *et al.*, 1980; Riggs *et al.*, 1981). It has been argued that even "normal" concentration may be inappropriate considering the low values of calcium absorption from the gut (Riggs *et al.*, 1982). The responsiveness of the 25-hydroxyvitamin D-1-hydroxylase system to diverse stimuli (secretory reserve) has been tested in osteoporotic or postmenopausal women by low-calcium diets, parathyroid extract injection (Riggs *et al.*, 1981), or 24-hour infusion of synthetic human parathyroid fragment (1–34) (Slovik *et al.*, 1981). Nordin *et al.* (1981) and Slovik *et al.* (1981) reported normal amounts of basal $1,25(OH)_2D$ but no response to "physiological" stimuli; Riggs *et al.* (1981) documented a similar increase in serum $1,25(OH)_2D$ in patients and age matched controls. The conflicting results may reflect differences in the techniques used or in the patient populations. Similar controversy exists over the effect of treatment with $1,25(OH)_2D_3$ or $1\alpha(OH)D_3$ in patients with osteoporosis (Gallagher *et al.*, 1982; Christiansen, 1982).

Any advanced kidney disease eventually decreases $1,25(OH)_2D$ production. A significant reduction in serum $1,25(OH)_2D$ is found in patients with reduced glomerular filtration rates (30 ml/minute) though changes may occur at an earlier stage (Haussler et $al.$, 1979). One causative mechanism underlying the deficient production of calciferol metabolites by the kidney in chronic renal disease is the destruction of functional tissue, but additional mediators may be hyperphosphatemia and metabolic acidosis that commonly accompany chronic kidney failure (see above).

$iv.$ $Deficient$ $production$ of $24,25$-$dihydroxycalciferol.$ One reported case may represent hereditary deficiency of 25-hydroxyvitamin D-24-hydroxylase as the cause of deficient calciferol action (Liberman et $al.$, 1980). A patient with ectodermal anomalies, early onset rickets, hypocalcemia, and hyperphosphatemia was described. Concentration of $25(OH)D$ was normal, $1,25(OH)_2D$ was markedly elevated, and $24,25(OH)_2D$ was below the detection limit (0.39 ng/ml). Serum calcium increased and serum phosphorus decreased toward normal upon treatment with $24,25(OH)_2D_3$ but not with vitamin D or $1,25(OH)_2D_3$.

In chronic renal failure, serum concentrations of $24,25(OH)_2D$ are very low, supposedly due to the destruction of functional kidney tissue (Zerwekh et $al.$, 1982). The possibility of extrarenal production of $24,25(OH)_2D$ as well as the question of a physiological role for this metabolite were discussed in Section II.

2. Increased Catabolism of Calciferol Metabolites

$a.$ $Urinary$ $Excretion$ of $Calciferol$ $Metabolites.$ Serum concentrations of $25(OH)D$, $1,25(OH)_2D$, and $24,25(OH)_2D$ are low among patients with nephrotic syndrome, a kidney disease characterized by proteinuria (Goldstein et $al.$, 1981). The reduction in serum calciferol concentrations is inversely related to the magnitude of proteinuria and directly related to the reduction of serum albumin concentration (Goldstein et $al.$, 1981). In nephrotic syndrome, the glomeruli become abnormally permeable, thus accounting for the increased loss of macromolecules like albumin. Sato et $al.$ (1982) directly measured urinary $25(OH)D$ excretion in healthy subjects and patients with nephrotic syndrome and observed the following: (1) a mean decrease of about 50% of serum $25(OH)D$ in patients with nephrotic syndrome; (2) an increase of about 20-fold in the mean urinary excretion of $25(OH)D$ in nephrotic patients as compared to normals (3.7 ± 3.5 and 0.17 ± 0.15 nmol/day, respectively); (3) urinary excretion of $25(OH)D$ correlated directly with the severity of proteinuria; (4) the $25(OH)D$ in the urine of the patients, unlike in normal subjects, was unconjugated. It was concluded that reduced concentrations of bioactive calciferol metabolites in patients with nephrotic syndrome result mainly from urinary losses most probably due to abnormally increased renal clearance of DBP. Renal excretion of other important metabolites [such as D and $1,25(OH)_2D$] has not yet been characterized.

   b. *Enterohepatic Recirculation of Calciferol and Its Metabolites.* Vitamin D and its metabolites undergo enterohepatic recirculation (Goldsmith, 1982). Avioli *et al.* (1967) reported that after injection of [^{3}H]vitamin D into man, 3–6% of radioactivity appeared in the bile over 48 hours. About 50% of the radioactivity in the bile represented conjugated vitamin D metabolites. Arnaud *et al.* (1975), in tests with radioactive $25(OH)D_3$ in man, showed that one-third of the injected radioactivity appeared in the duodenum distal to the ampulla of Vater within 24 hours of injection, but only 3% was excreted in the feces during the same period, suggesting that 90% of the amount secreted was reabsorbed. Analysis of duodenal aspirates revealed that only a small fraction of the radioactivity is extractable by organic solvents, but as much as 40% could be extracted after glucuronidase–sulfatase treatment. Kumar and associates (Kumar, 1980; Wiesner *et al.*, 1980; Kumar *et al.*, 1980) studied the enterohepatic recirculation of $1,25(OH)_2D_3$ and $24,25(OH)_2D_3$ in rats and man, and observed similar qualitative results in both species. [^{3}H]$1,25(OH)_2D_3$ and [^{3}H]$24,25(OH)_2D_3$ injected separately, intravenously, to normal human subjects yielded cumulative means of radioactivity in the duodenal aspirate of about 16 and 12% of injected dose, respectively, within the first 6 hours; 24-hour mean fecal excretion of the isotope was about 27 and 14% of the injected dose for the two calciferol metabolites, respectively. Based on these data and direct measurements of radioactivity in the jejunum, the authors calculated that more than half of the radioactivity secreted through the bile into the duodenum was reabsorbed. These investigators observed that both $1,25(OH)_2D_3$ and $24,25(OH)_2D_3$ were excreted in bile as polar products, and, at least in part, are glucuronides of the parent sterol as determined by mass spectrometry for one such metabolite of $1,25(OH)_2D_3$ (Kumar, 1982). By perfusing isolated rat livers with labeled $1,25(OH)_2D_3$ and demonstrating secretion within 30 minutes of a polar metabolite of $1,25(OH)_2D_3$, Kumar *et al.* (1981a) were able to show that at least one of the polar metabolites of $1,25(OH)_2D_3$ is produced in the liver. The biological activity of the conjugated metabolite is unknown, but it was shown that vitamin D_3 and D_2 3-glucosiduronate were able to increase intestinal calcium transport and bone calcium mobilization when adminstered to vitamin D-deficient rats (Nagubandi *et al.*, 1980). These compounds were inactive, however, when introduced directly into the medium of rat duodenal organ culture. Thus, it was suggested that vitamin D 3-glucosiduronate must be hydrolyzed in order to produce a biological effect. It is conceivable that the polar metabolites of $25(OH)D_3$ and $1,25(OH)_2D_3$ could be reutilized as well. The hepatobiliary recirculation of vitamin D and its major known metabolites is a high volume pathway. Disturbance in excretion and reutilization of vitamin D in this active recirculation, as in liver and intestinal disorders (see above), and by the administration of drugs as cholestyramine (Compston and Thompson, 1977), may lead to calciferol deficiency states.

    c. Enzymatic Catabolism of Calciferol Metabolites. Aside from $25(OH)D$, $1,25(OH)_2D$, and $24,25(OH)_2D$ there are to date 17 known chemically characterized metabolites of vitamin D of which 16 are produced under *in vivo* conditions (Norman *et al.*, 1982) and additional metabolites are being identified at an increasing rate. Assayed at physiological concentrations for intestinal calcium transport or bone calcium mobilization, none of these 17 metabolites, with the exception of 1,24,25-trihydroxyvitamin D_3, is biologically active. Thus, most of these compounds reflect processes of inactivation of the biologically active calciferol metabolites. It appears that the principal form of inactivation of both $1,25(OH)_2D_3$ and $24,25(OH)_2D_3$ is by side chain oxidation (Kumar *et al.*, 1976) to calcitroic acid (Esvelt *et al.*, 1979) in the intestine and/or liver. Circulating $1,25(OH)_2D_3$ displays a short half-life; therefore, any change in the activity of enzymes that modulate the metabolic inactivation of this bioactive metabolite may affect its half-life and biological activity. Of special interest is the recent observation that in addition to the kidney some of these enzymes are present in the intestine (Ohnuma and Norman, 1981; Norman *et al.*, 1982), thus raising a possibility of metabolic control at the target organ level.

    There are not, as yet, any proven states of calciferol deficiency due to enhanced inactivation of bioactive vitamin D metabolites, but it is conceivable that such situations will be delineated in the future. Such a possibility might be the occasional osteomalacia or rickets induced by anticonvulsant drugs (Dent *et al.*, 1970). The incidence of the disease varies according to the criteria used, hypocalcemia, elevated serum alkaline phosphatase, decreased bone mass, low serum levels of $25(OH)D$, or histological confirmation of osteomalacia in bone biopsy (Hahn *et al.*, 1975; Lifschitz and MacLaren, 1973; Winnacker *et al.*, 1977; Mosekilde *et al.*, 1977). Not all investigators accept this theory; some argue that the disease is caused by simple nutritional deficiency due to institutionalization and limited exposure to sunlight rather than a specific effect of drugs (Livingstone *et al.*, 1973). Concentrations of 25(OH)D have been reported to be low on an absolute basis as well as relative to dietary vitamin D intake (Stamp et al., 1972; Hahn et al., 1975). Anticonvulsant drugs can induce hepatic microsomal mixed function oxidases involving the cytochrome P-450 system (Kuntzman, 1969). These enzyme systems through hydroxylation, conjugation, and transfer reactions play an important role in the catabolism of numerous drugs and metabolites including steroid hormones. It was postulated that osteomalacia was produced by induction of enzymes that metabolize vitamin D through pathways other than 25-hydroxylation (Dent et al., 1970). Experimental studies appeared to confirm a modification of hepatic metabolism of vitamin D in vitro (Hahn et al., 1972), experimental rickets were produced by diphenylhydantoin in rats (Harris et al., 1978), and a shorter serum half-life of labeled vitamin D_3 and $25(OH)D_3$ was observed in patients given anticonvulsant drugs (Hahn et al., 1972). Others however, did not detect any abnormality in the formation or the half-life of labeled $25(OH)D_3$ in plasma of patients taking these drugs (Mawer, 1982). In patients given anticonvulsant treatment serum concentrations of $1,25(OH)_2D$ were normal (Jubiz et al., 1977) or low (Christensen et al., 1981). The mechanism by which anticonvulsant drugs may induce calciferol deficiency is not clear; an attractive hypothesis might be an effect on the enzymatic catabolic systems of the bioactive calciferols systemically and at the target organ level (Corradino 1976; Hahn et al., 1978).

Both the chicken and a New World monkey exhibit selective impairment of response to vitamin D_2. In the chicken this impairment has been attributed to selectively low affinity of DBP for $25(OH)D_2$ (Belsey et al., 1974a); this may increase the clearance rate of $25(OH)D_2$. The chicken and, to a lesser degree, the pig discriminate against D_2; in contrast the rat discriminates against D_3 (Horst et al., 1982a).

B. INCREASED CIRCULATING LEVELS OF 1,25-DIHYDROXYCALCIFEROL

1. No Abnormality in Target Cells

a. Calcium Deficiency. Although an adequate intake of calcium is required for normal skeletal growth and mineralization, the dietary requirement for calcium is hard to define (Walker, 1972) and the effects of calcium deficiency on bone metabolism remain uncertain. In children, calcium deficiency occasionally may cause rickets (Maltz et al., 1970; Kooh et al., 1977). The child described by Kooh et al. (1977) developed all the biochemical and radiological signs of rickets during a phase of rapid growth while ingesting a low calcium diet but taking adequate amounts of vitamin D as judged by normal concentration of 25(OH)D in plasma. Rapid healing of rickets was achieved by adequate amounts of calcium alone even when dietary vitamin D and sunlight were eliminated during the therapeutic trial. Recently, Pettifor and co-workers (1978, 1979, 1981) described a group of children between the ages of 4 and 14 years from a rural community in South Africa. All showed severe bone deformities resembling rickets with no overt evidence of malnutrition. Serum analysis revealed mild hypocalcemia or normocalcemia, and evidence of secondary hyperparathyroidism. Bone histomorphometric studies on an iliac crest biopsy from three children revealed severe osteomalacia (Marie *et al.*, 1982). All patients examined showed normal 25(OH)D but elevated 1,25(OH)$_2$D concentrations in serum, thus excluding vitamin D deficiency or a defect in 1,25(OH)D production as the causative mechanism. All cases came from a rural community where dietary calcium intake was very low (125 mg/day) with adequate dietary phosphorus (Pettifor *et al.*, 1981). On administration of adequate dietary calcium alone, the radiological and histological lesions healed, and serum alkaline phosphatase, calcium, iPTH, and 1,25(OH)$_2$D returned to normal. It was concluded that severe calcium deficiency in children can cause osteomalacia. The elevated concentration of 1,25(OH)$_2$D represents a physiological compensatory mechanism. There is, however, a limitation in gastrointestinal response to 1,25(OH)$_2$D due to severe dietary calcium deficiency.

b. Phosphate Deficiency. Experimental phosphate deficiency is known to produce rickets in animals. In man, phosphate deficiency is rare due to the high phosphate content of the diet. However, excessive use of antacids such as aluminium hydroxide gels, which render phosphate nonabsorbable in the gut, may produce phosphate deficiency and in rare cases osteomalacia (Dent and Winter, 1974; Cooke *et al.*, 1978). Experimental phosphate depletion in humans leads to enhanced turnover of radiolabeled 25(OH)D$_3$, increased plasma content of 1,25(OH)$_2$D (Dominguez *et al.*, 1976; Gray *et al.*, 1977), increased net calcium absorption from the gut, a slight fall in serum iPTH, no change in serum calcium, and hypercalciuria.

c. Hungry Bones Syndrome. Patients with severe hyperparathyroid bone disease (osteitis fibrosa cystica) may show, after the removal of the parathyroid adenoma, severe hypocalcemia requiring suprapharmacological doses of 1,25(OH)$_2$D and calcium to correct the hypocalcemia (Dent, 1962; Gonzalez-Villapando *et al.*, 1980). The failure to correct low serum calcium with high 1,25(OH)$_2$D may represent the gap between the demands of an undermineralized bone (hence the name hungry bones), and the supply, limited by the availability of calcium in the intestine and at bone-resorption sites.

2. Abnormalities in Target Cells

a. *Hereditary.* Since 1978 a small number of cases have been reported with features of calciferol deficiency responsive (if at all) only to elevated circulating concentrations of $1,25(OH)_2D$ (Marx, 1983). The features of this group, other than resistance to $1,25(OH)_2D$, are those of vitamin D dependency (including patterns suggestive of autosomal recessive transmission), and the term vitamin D dependency type II is commonly applied.

Special features in certain kindreds will be mentioned briefly. Affected members in half of the kindreds have exhibited diminished or absent hair over the entire body. Kindreds with alopecia generally show the most severe grades of disease by the criteria of earlier age of onset and greater amount of $1,25(OH)_2D$ required for treatment of hypocalcemia (Marx, 1983); alopecia has not been a feature in other states with deficient calciferol action. Some patients have shown satisfactory responses of hypocalcemia and rickets to measures that sustained high $1,25(OH)_2D$ levels; alopecia, however, has not improved with otherwise satisfactory therapy. At least one patient showed no response to measures that sustained $1,25(OH)_2D_3$ concentrations at 100-fold normal for many months (Liberman *et al.*, 1982). While this clinical heterogeneity suggests a spectrum of underlying molecular defects, this has not been analyzed directly because of the ethical and technical problems in obtaining specimens of target tissue (intestinal mucosa) from human beings.

The recognition of a widespread organ distribution of the effector system for $1,25(OH)_2D$ (Section II,C) has led to evaluation of the biology of this disorder through study of fibroblasts cultured from skin. Initial studies have shown at least four types of cellular defect (Table VI): undetectable receptors for $1,25(OH)_2D$ in cell extracts, receptors that are detectable but quantitatively deficient, receptors that exhibit normal numbers and affinity but deficient nuclear translocation of $1,25(OH)_2D_3$, and receptors that are normal at least with regard to number, affinity, and nuclear translocation capability *in vitro*.

Efforts to correlate the heterogeneous molecular defects with the heterogeneous clinical features have been largely unsuccessful. Thus alopecia has been observed with each of the above four types of defect, and body hair has been normal with the nuclear translocation defect and with the receptor positive defect. $1,25(OH)_2D_3$ stimulates activity of 25(OH)D 24-hydroxylase in normal cultured skin fibroblasts, and

TABLE VI

RELATION OF CLINICAL FEATURES TO CELLULAR DEFECTS IN PATIENTS WITH TARGET
RESISTANCE TO 1,25(OH)$_2$D[a]

References	Special clinical features[b]	Capacity for cytosol binding of 1,25(OH)$_2$D (%)	Capacity for nuclear uptake of 1,25(OH)$_2$D (%)
Balsan et al. (1979)		UM[c]	UM
Beer et al. (1981)		UM	UM
Feldman et al. (1982)		UM	UM
Liberman et al. (1982)	No reponse to high 1,25(OH)$_2$D	10	10
Marx et al. (1978)	Normal hair	100	UM
Rosen et al. (1979)		100	UM
Liberman et al. (1980)	Low 24,25(OH)$_2$D	100	100
Griffin et al. (1982)	Normal hair	100	100

[a]Modified from Liberman et al. (1983).

[b]Unless specified, cases exhibited hypocalcemic rickets with alopecia plus response to massive doses of calciferol analogs where given for several months.

[c]UM, Unmeasureable.

this activity is deficient in cells from patients with the receptor-positive (Griffin et al., 1982) and with the receptor-negative (Feldman et al., 1982) variants of vitamin D dependency type II. Application of this analysis in a quantitative manner might provide insight into the variable grades of severity of the disorder in vivo.

b. Acquired. The intestinal mucosa of the fetal rat does not show active transport of calcium in response to 1,25(OH)$_2$D in vitro. This response does not develop until approximately day 14 postpartum and correlates with the appearance of the receptor for 1,25(OH)$_2$D at that time (Halloran and DeLuca, 1981).

Rickets and hypocalcemia with high levels of 1,25(OH)$_2$D occur in some human infants that have survived birth at extremely premature ages (Chesney et al., 1981; Steichen et al., 1981). It is not known if this complex is caused soley by the drain on body calcium supplies imposed by the growing skeleton deprived of the maternal placental pump for calcium (i.e., a variant of "hungry bones"; see Section III,C,1,c), or if it reflects in part immaturity of the intestinal mucosa analogous to that in the neonatal rat (see above).

In vitro, anticonvulsant drugs impair the response of target tissues to calciferols. Duodena from embryonic chicks show impaired calcium transport when cultured with diphenylhydantoin (Corradino, 1976); long bones from fetal rats exhibit impaired calcium release when cultured with diphenylhydantoin and/or phenobarbital (Hahn *et al.,* 1978). The relation of these effects to the syndrome of anticonvulsant-associated osteomalacia (Section III,A,2,c) is uncertain since serum levels of $1,25(OH)_2D$ have been normal (Jubiz et al., 1977) or low (Christensen et al., 1981) in patients receiving anticonvulsants.

REFERENCES

Abe, E., Miyaura, C., Sakagami, H., Takeda, M., Konno, K., Yamazaki, T., Yoshikawa, S., and Suda, T. (1981). Differentiation of mouse myeloid leukemia cells induced by 1a,25-dihydroxyvitamin D_3. *Proc. Natl. Acad. Sci. U.S.A.* **78,** 4990–4994.

Acker, G. M., Garabedian, M., Guillozo, H., Pecquinot, M. A., and Balsan, S. (1982). In vitro formation of 25-hydroxyvitamin D_3 metabolites in endometrium: Dependence on the hormonal status of the rat. *Endocrinology* **111,** 2103–2109.

Adams, R. G., Harrison, J. F., and Scott, P. (1969). The development of cadmium-induced proteinuria, impaired renal function and osteomalacia in alkaline battery workers. *Q. J. Med.* **38,** 425–443.

Adams, T. H., Wong, R. G., and Norman, A. W. (1970). Studies on the mechanism of action of calciferol. II. Effect of the polyene antibiotic, filipin, on vitamin D-mediated calcium transport. *J. Biol. Chem.* **245,** 4432–4442.

Akiba, T., Endou, H., Koseki, C. Sakai, F., Horiuchi, N., and Suda, T. (1980). Localization of 25-hydroxyvitamin D_3-1a-hydroxylase activity in the mammalian kidney. *Biochem. Biophys. Res. Commun.* **94,** 313–318.

Albright, F., Butler, A. M., and Bloomberg, E. (1937). Rickets resistant to vitamin D therapy. *Am. J. Dis. Child.* **54,** 529–547.

Ameenuddin, S., Sunde, M., DeLuca, H. F., Ikekawa, N., and Kobayashi, Y. (1982). 24-Hydroxylation of 25-hydroxyvitamin D_3: Is it required for embryonic development in chicks? *Science* **217,** 451–452.

Arnaud, S. B., Goldsmith, R. S., Lambert, P. S., and Go, V. L. W. (1975). 25-hydroxyvitamin D_3: Evidence of an enterohepatic circulation in man. *Proc. Soc. Exp. Biol. Med.* **149,** 570–572.

Arnaud, S. B., Newcomer, A. D., Hodgson, S. F., Jowsey, J. O., and Go, V. L. W. (1977). Serum 25-hydroxyvitamin D (25-OHD) and the pathogenesis of osteomalacia in patients with non-typical sprue. *Gastroenterology* **72,** 1025.

Aschinberg, L. C., Solomon, L. M., Zeis, P. M., Justice, P., and Rosenthal, I. M. (1977). Vitamin D-resistance rickets associated with epidermal nevus syndrome: Demonstration of a phosphaturie substance in the dermal lesion. *J. Pediatr.* **91,** 56–60.

Atkinson, M., Nordin, B. E. C., and Sherlock, S. (1966). Malabsorption and bone disease in prolonged obstructive jaundice. *Q. J. Med.* **25,** 299–312.

Avioli, L. V., Lee, S. W., McDonald, J. E., Lund, J., and DeLuca, H. F. (1967). Metabolism of vitamin D_3-^3H in human subjects: Distribution in blood, bile, feces and urine. *J. Clin. Invest.* **46,** 983–992.

Balsan, S., Garabedian, M., Lieberherr, M., Gueris, J., and Ulmann, A. (1979). Serum 1,25-dihydroxyvitamin D concentration in two different types of pseudodeficiency rickets. *In* "Vitamin D: Basic Research and Its Clinical Application" (A. W. Norman, K. Schaeffer, D. V. Herrath, H. G. Grigoleit, E. Mawer, T. Suda, H. F. DeLuca and J. W. Coburn, eds.), pp. 1143–1148. de Gruyter, Berlin.

Barbour, G. L., Coburn, J. W., Slatopolsky, E., Norman, A. W., and Horst, R. L. (1981). Hypercalcemia in an anephric patient with sarcoidosis: Evidence for extrarenal generation of 1,25-dihydroxyvitamin D. *N. Engl. J. Med.* **305,** 440–443.

Bar-Shavit, Z., Noff, D., Edelstein, S., Meyer, M., Shibolet, S., and Goldman, R. (1981). 1,25-Dihydroxyvitamin D_3 and the regulation of macrophage function. *Calcif. Tissue Int.* **33,** 673–676.

Barton, J. C., Conrad, M. E., Harrison, L., and Nuby, S. (1978). Effects of calcium on the absorption and retention of lead. *J. Lab. Clin. Med.* **91,** 366–376.

Beer, S., Tieder, M., Kohelet, D., Liberman, U. A., Vure, E., Bar-Joseph, G., Gabizon, D., Borochowitz, V., Varon, M., and Modai, D. (1981). Vitamin-D-resistant rickets with alopecia: A form of end organ resistance to 1,25 dihydroxy vitamin D. *Clin. Endocrinol.* **14,** 395–402.

Belsey, R. E., DeLuca, H. F., and Potts, J. T., Jr. (1974a). Selective binding properties of Vitamin D transport protein in chick plasma in vitro. *Nature* **247,** 208–209.

Belsey, R., Clark, M. B, Bernat, M., Glowacki, J., Holick, M. F., DeLuca, H. F., and Potts, J. T., Jr. (1974b). The physiologic significance of plasma transport of vitamin D and metabolites. *Am. J. Med.* **57,** 50–56.

Bergeron, M., Dubord, L., and Hausser, C. (1976). Membrane permeability as a cause of transport defects in experimental Fanconi syndrome. *J. Clin. Invest.* **57,** 1181–1189.

Bhattacharyya, M., and DeLuca, H. (1974). Subcellular location of rat liver calciferol-25-hydroxylase. *Arch. Biochem. Biophys.* **160,** 58–62.

Berliner, R. W., Kennedy, R. J., and Hilton, J. C. (1950). Effect of maleic acid on renal function. *Proc. Soc. Exp. Biol. Med.* **75,** 791–794.

Bikle, D. D., and Rasmussen, H. (1975). The ionic control of 1,25-dihydroxyvitamin D_3 production in isolated chick renal tubules. *J. Clin. Invest.* **55,** 292–298.

Bikle, D. D., and Rasmussen, H. (1978). A biochemical model for the ionic control of 25-hydroxyvitamin D_3 1a-hydroxylase. *J. Biol. Chem.* **253,** 3042–3048.

Bikle, D. D., Empson, R. N., Jr., Herman, R. H., Morrissey, R. L., and Zolock, D. R. (1977). The effect of 1,25-dihydroxyvitamin D-3 on the distribution of alkaline phosphatase activity along the chick intestinal villus. *Biochim. Biophys. Acta* **499,** 61–66.

Bikle, D. D., Zolock, D. T., Morrisey, R. L., and Herman, R. H. (1978). Independence of 1,25-dihydroxyvitamin D_3-mediated calcium transport from *de novo* RNA and protein synthesis. *J. Biol. Chem.* **253,** 484–488.

Birge, S. J., and Haddad, J. G. (1975). 25-Hydroxycholecalciferol stimulation of muscle metabolism. *J. Clin. Invest.* **56,** 1100–1107.

Birge, S. J., and Miller, R. (1977). The role of phospahte in the action of vitamin D on the intestine. *J. Clin. Invest.* **60,** 980–988.

Bishop, J. E., Norman, A. W., Coburn, J. W., Roberts, P. A., and Henry, H. L. (1980). Studies on the metabolism of calciferol XVI. Determination of the concentration of 25-hydroxyvitamin D, 24,25-dihydroxyvitamin D and 1,25-dihydroxyvitamin D in a single two milliliter plasma sample. *Miner. Electrolyte Metab.* **3,** 181–189.

Bishop, J. E., Hunziker, W., and Norman, A. W. (1982). Evidence for multiple molecular weight forms of the chick intestinal 1,25-dihydroxyvitamin D_3 receptor. *Biochem. Biophys. Res. Commun.* **108,** 140–145.

Bjorkhem, I., and Holmberg, I. (1978). Assay and properties of a mitochondrial 25-hydroxylase active on vitamin D_3. *J. Biol. Chem.* **253,** 842–849.

Bjorkhem, I., and Holmberg, I. (1979). On the 25-hydroxylation of vitamin D_3 in vitro studied with a mass fragmentographic technique. *J. Biol. Chem.,* **254,** 9518–9524.

Bjorkhem, I., Hansson, R., Holmberg, I., and Wikvell, K. (1979). 25-Hydroxylation of vitamin D_3 by a reconstituted system from rat liver microsomes. *Biochem. Biophys. Res. Commun.* **90,** 615–622.

Bjorkhem, I., Holmberg, I., Oftebro, H., and Pedersen, J. L. (1980). Properties of a reconstituted vitamin D_3 25-hydroxylase from rat liver mitochondria. *J. Biol. Chem.* **255,** 5244–5249.

Bonjour, J. P., Preston, C., and Fleisch, H. (1977). Effect of 1,25-dihydroxyvitamin D_3 on the renal handling of P_i in thyroparathyroidectomized rats. *J. Clin. Invest.* **60,** 1419–1428.

Bordin, S., and Petra, P. H. (1980). Immunocytochemical localization of the sex steroid-binding protein of plasma in tissues of the adult monkey *Macaca nemestrina. Proc. Natl. Acad. Sci. U.S.A.* **77,** 5678–5682.

Bouillon, R., Van Baelen, H., Rombauts, W., and DeMoor, P. (1976). The purification and characterization of the human-serum binding protein for 25-hydroxycholecalciferol (Transcalciferin): Identity with group-specific component. *Eur. J. Biochem.* **66,** 285–291.

Bouillon, R., Van Baelen, H., Keng Tan, B., and DeMoor, P. (1980a). The isolation and characterization of the 25-hydroxyvitamin D-binding protein from chick serum. *J. Biol. Chem.* **255,** 10925–10930.

Bouillon, R., Van Baelen, H., and de Moor, P. (1980b). Comparative study of the affinity of the serum vitamin D-binding protein. *J. Steroid Biochem.* **13,** 1029–1034.

Bouillon, R., Van Assche F. A., Van Baelen, H., Heyns, W., and DeMoor, P. (1981). Influence of the vitamin D-binding protein on the serum concentration of 1,25-dihydroxyvitamin D_3: Significance of the free 1,25-dihydroxyvitamin D_3 concentration. *J. Clin. Invest.* **67,** 589–596.

Brenner, R. J., Spring, D. B., Sebastian, A., McSherry E. M., Genant, H. K., Palubinskas, A. J., and Morris, R. C., Jr. (1982). Incidence of radiographically evident bone disease, nephrocalcinosis, and nephrolithiasis in various types of renal tubular acidosis. *N. Engl. J. Med* **307,** 217–221.

Brewer, E. D., Tsai, H. C., Szeto, K. S., and Morris, R. C., Jr. (1977). Maleic acid-induced impaired conversion of 25(OH)D_3 to 1,25(OH)$_2D_3$: Implication for Fanconi's syndrome. *Kidney Int.* **12,** 244–252.

Brickman, A. S., Hartenbower, D. L., Norman, A. W., and Coburn, J. W. (1977). Actions of 1a-hydroxyvitamin D_3 and 1,25-dihydroxyvitamin D_3 on mineral metabolism in man. *Am. J. Clin. Nutr.* **30,** 1064–1069.

Brumbaugh, P. F., and Haussler, M. R. (1973). Nuclear and cytoplasmic receptors for 1α,25-dihydroxycholecalciferol in intestinal mucosa. *Biochem. Biophys. Res. Commun.* **53,** 74–80.

Brumbaugh, P. F., and Haussler, M. R. (1974). 1α,25-Dihydroxycholecalciferol receptors in intestine: II. Temperature-dependent transfer of the hormone to chromatin via a specific cytosol receptor. *J. Biol. Chem.* **249,** 1258–1262.

Brumbaugh, P. F., and Haussler, M. R. (1975a). Specific binding of 1,25-dihydroxycholecalciferol to nuclear components of chick intestine. *J. Biol. Chem.* **250,** 1588–1594.

Brumbaugh, P. F., and Haussler, M. R. (1975b). Nuclear and cytoplasmic binding components for vitamin D binding components. *Life Sci.* **16,** 353–362.

Brumbaugh P. F., Hughes, M. R., and Haussler, M. R. (1975). Cytoplasmic and nuclear binding components for 1α,25-dihydroxyvitamin D_3 in chick parathyroid glands. *Proc. Nat. Acad. Sci. U.S.A.* **72,** 4871–4875.

Brunette, M. G., Chan, M., Ferriere, C., and Roberts, K. D. (1978). Site of 1,25(OH)$_2$vitamin D_3 synthesis in the kidney. *Nature (London)* **276,** 287–289.

Bruns, M. E. H., Fliesher, E. B., and Avioli, L. V. (1977). Control of vitamin D-dependent calcium binding protein in rat intestine by growth and fasting. *J. Biol. Chem.* **252,** 4145–4150.

Canterbury, J. M., Gavellas, G., Bourgoignie, J. J., and Reiss, E. (1980). Metabolic consequences of oral administration of 24,25-dihydroxycholecalciferol to uremic dogs. *J. Clin. Invest.* **65**, 571–576.

Chandler, J. S., Pike, J. W., and Haussler, M. R. (1979). 1,25-Dihydroxyvitamin D_3 receptors in rat kidney cytosol. *Biochem. Biophys. Res. Commun.* **90**, 1057–1063.

Charles, M. A., Martial, J., Zolock, D., Morrissey, R., and Baxter, J. D. (1981). Regulation of calcium-binding protein messenger RNA by 1,25-dihydroxycholecalciferol. *Calcif. Tissue Int.* **33**, 15–18.

Chen, T. L., and DeLuca, H. F. (1973). Receptors for 1,25-dihydroxycholcaleciferol in rat intestine. *J. Biol. Chem.* **248**, 4890–4895.

Chen, T. L., and Feldman, D. (1981). Regulation of 1,25-dihydroxyvitamin D_3 receptors in cultured mouse bone cells: Correlation of receptor concentration with the rate of cell division. *J. Biol. Chem* **256**, 5561–5566.

Chen, T. L., Hirst, M. A., and Feldman, D. (1979). A receptor-like binding macromolecule for 1α,25-dihydroxycholecalciferol in cultured mouse bone cells. *J. Biol. Chem.* **254**, 7491–7494.

Chen, T. L., Cone, C. M., and Feldman, D. (1982). Glucocorticoids cause biphasic changes in the quantity of 1,25$(OH)_2D_3$ receptors in cultured mouse bone cells. 64th Annual Meeting of Endocrine Society, p. 699, (Abstract).

Chesney, R. W., Rosen, J. F., Hamstra, A. J., and DeLuca, H. F. (1980a). Serum 1,25-dihydroxyvitamin D levels in normal children and in vitamin D disorders. *Am. J. Dis. Child.* **134**, 135–139.

Chesney, R. W., Mazess, R. B., Rose, P., Hamstra, A. J., and DeLuca, H. F. (1980b). Supranormal 25-hydroxyvitamin D and subnormal 1,25-dihydroxyvitamin D: Their role in X-linked hypophosphatemic rickets. *Am. J. Dis. Child.* **134**, 140–143.

Chesney, R. W., Hamstra, A. J., and DeLuca, H. F. (1981). Rickets of prematurity. Supranormal levels of serum 1,25-dihydroxyvitamin D. *Am. J. Dis. Child.* **135**, 34–37.

Chick, H., Dalyell, E. J., Hume, E. M., Mackay, H. M. M., and Henderson-Smith, H. (1923). Studies of rickets in Vienna, 1919–1922: Report of the Accessory Food Factors Committee. *Med. Res. Counc. (GB) Spec. Rep. Ser. No. 77.* HMSO, London.

Christakos, S., and Norman, A. W. (1978). Vitamin D_3-induced calcium binding protein in bone tissue. *Science* **202**, 70–71.

Christakos, S., and Norman, A. W. (1979). Studies on the mode of action of calciferol XVIII. Evidence for a specific high affinity binding protein for 1,25-dihydroxyvitamin D_3 in chick kidney and pancreas. *Biochem. Biophys. Res. Commun.* **89**, 56.

Christakos, S., Friedlander, E. J., Frandsen, B. R., and Norman, A. W. (1979). Studies on the mode of action of calciferol. XIII. Development of a radioimmunoassay for vitamin-D-dependent chick intestinal calcium-binding protein and tissue distribution. *Endocrinology* **104**, 1495–1503.

Christakos, S., Brunette, M. G., and Norman, A. W. (1981). Localization of immunoreactive vitamin D-dependent calcium binding protein in chick nephron. *Endocrinology*. **109**, 322–324.

Christensen, C. K., Lund, B., Lund, B. J., Sorensen, O. H., Nielsen, H. E., and Mosekilde L. (1981). Reduced 1,25-dihydroxyvitamin D and 24,25-dihydroxyvitamin D in epileptic patients receiving chronic combined anticonvulsant therapy. *Metab. Bone Dis. Relat. Res.* **3**, 17–22.

Christiansen, C. (1982). Osteoporosis and vitamin D metabolites. A status report. *In* "Vitamin D, Chemical, Biochemical and Clinical Endocrinology of Calcium Metabolism" (A. W. Norman, K. Schaefer, D. V. Herrath, and H. G. Grigoleit, eds.), pp. 915–920. de Gruyter, Berlin.

Christiansen, C., Rodbro, P., Naestoft, J., and Christensen, M. S. (1981). A possible direct effect of 24,25-dihydroxycholecalciferol on the parathyroid gland in patients with chronic renal failure. *Clin. Endocrinol.* **15**, 237–242.

Clark, S. A., Stumpf, W. E., Sar, M., DeLuca, H. F., and Tanaka, Y. (1980). Target cells for 1,25-dihydroxyvitamin D_3 in the pancreas. *Cell Tissue Res.* **209**, 515–520.

Clark, S. A., Stumpf, W. E., and Sar, M. (1981). Effect of 1,25 dihydroxyvitamin D_3 on insulin secretion. *Diabetes* **30**, 382–386.

Clarkson, T. W., and Kench, J. E. (1956). Urinary excretion of amino-acids by men absorbing heavy metals. *Biochem. J.* **62**, 361–372.

Clemens, T. L., Adams, J. A., Henderson, S. L., and Holick, M. F. (1982). Increased skin pigment reduces the capacity of skin to synthesize vitamin D_3. *Lancet* **1**, 74–76.

Cleve, H., and Patutschnick, W. (1979). Neuraminidase treatment reveals sialic acid differences in certain genetic variants of the Gc system (Vitamin-D-binding protein). *Hum. Genet.* **47**, 193–199.

Cloix, J. F., d'Herbigny E., and Ulmann, A. (1980). Renal parathyroid hormone-dependent adenylate cyclase in vitamin D-deficient rats: Inhibition by hydroxylated vitamin D_3 metabolites. *J. Biol. Chem.* **255**, 11280–11283.

Cloix, J. F., Ulmann, A., Monet, J. D., and Funck-Brentano, J. L. (1981). Human parathyroid gland adenylate cyclase activity: Inhibition by 24,25-dihydroxycholecalciferol in vitro. *Clin. Sci.* **60**, 339–341.

Coburn, J. W., and Brautbar, N. (1980). Disease studies in man related to vitamin D. *In* "Vitamin D, Molecular Biology and Clinical Nutrition" (A. W. Norman, ed.), pp. 515–577. Dekker New York.

Colston, K., and Feldman, D. (1982). 1,25-dihydroxyvitamin D_3 receptors and functions in cultured pig kidney cells (LLC PK): Regulation of 24,25-dihydroxyvitamin D_3 production. *J. Biol. Chem.* **257**, 2504–2508.

Colston, K., Hirst, M., and Feldman, D. (1980). Organ distribution of the cytoplasmic 1,25-dihydroxycholecalciferol receptor in various mouse tissues. *Endocrinology* **107**, 1916–1922.

Colston, K., Colston, M. J., and Feldman, D. (1981). 1,25-dihydroxyvitamin D_3 and malignant melanoma: The presence of receptors and inhibition of cell growth in culture. *Endocrinology* **108**, 1083–1085.

Compston, J. E., and Creamer, B. (1977). Plasma levels and intestinal absorption of 25-hydroxyvitamin D in patients with small intestinal resection. *Gut* **18**, 171–175.

Compston, J. E., and Thompson, R. P. H. (1977). Intestinal absorption of 25-hydroxyvitamin D and osteomalacia in primary biliary cirrhosis. *Lancet* **1**, 721–724.

Constans, J., Viau, M., and Boissou, C. (1980). Affinity differences for the 25-OH-D_3 associated with the genetic heterogeneity of the vitamin D-binding protein *FEBS Lett.* **111**, 107–111.

Cooke, N., Teitelbaum, S., and Avioli, L. V. (1978). Antacid induced osteomalacia and nephrolithiasis. *Arch. Intern. Med.* **138**, 1007–1009.

Cooke, N. E., Walgate, J., and Haddad J. G., Jr. (1979). Human serum binding protein for vitamin D and its metabolites II. Specific, high affinity association with a protein in nucleated tissue. *J. Biol. Chem.* **254**, 5965–5971.

Corradino, R. A. (1973). 1,25-dihydroxycholecalciferol: Inhibition of action in organ-cultured intestine by actinomycin D and α-amanitin. *Nature (London)* **243**, 41–43.

Corradino, R. A. (1976). Diphenylhydantoin: Direct inhibition of the vitamin D_3-mediated calcium absorptive mechanism in organ-cultured duodenum. *Biochem. Pharmacol.* **25**, 863–864.

Corradino, R. A., and Wasserman, R. H. (1968). Actinomycin D inhibition of vitamin D_3-induced calcium-binding protein (CaBP) formation in chick duodenal mucosa. *Arch. Bicohem. Biophys.* **126**, 957–960.

Corradino, R. A., Fullmer, C. S., and Wasserman, R. H. (1976). Embryonic chick intestine in organ culture: Stimulation of calcium transport by exogenous vitamin D-induced calcium-binding protein. *Arch. Biochem. Biophys.* **174**, 738–743.

Corvol, M. T., Dumontier, M. F., Garabedian, M., and Rapaport, R. (1978). Vitamin D and cartilage. II. Biological activity of 25-hydroxycholecalciferol and 24,25- and 1,25-dihydroxycholecalciferols on cultured growth plate chondrocytes. *Endocrinology* **102**, 1269–1274.

Corvol, M., Ulmann, A., and Garabedian, M. (1980). Specific nuclear uptake of 24,25-dihydroxycholecalciferol, a vitamin D_3 metabolite biologically active in cartilage. *FEBS Lett.* **116**, 273–276.

Costa, T., Marie, P. J., Scriver, C. R., Cole, D. E. C., Reade, T. M., Nogrady, B., Glorieux, F. H., and Delvin, E. E. (1981). X-linked hypophosphatemia: Effect of calcitriol on renal handling of phosphate serum phosphate and bone mineralization. *J. Clin. Endocrinol. Metab.* **54**, 463–476.

Cunningham, B. M., Fraher, L. J., Clemens, T. L., Revell, P. A., and Papapoulos, S. E. (1982). Chronic acidosis with metabolic bone disease, effect of alkali on bone morphology and vitamin D metabolism. *Am. J. Med.* **73**, 199–204.

Daiger, S. P., Schanfield, S. P., and Cavilli-Sforza, L. L. (1975). Human group specific component (Gc) proteins bind vitamin D and 25-hydroxyvitamin D. *Proc. Natl. Acad. Sci. U.S.A.* **72**, 2076–2080.

Danan, J.-L., DeLorme, A.-C., and Cusinier-Gleizes, P. (1981). Biochemical evidence for a cytoplasmic 1α,25-dihydroxyvitamin D_3 receptor-like protein in rat yolk sac. *J. Biol. Chem.* **256**, 4847–4850.

Dent, C. E. (1962). Some problems of hyperparathyroidism. *Br. Med. J.* **2**, 1419–1425.

Dent, C. E., and Smith, R. (1969). Nutritional osteomalacia. *Q. J. Med.* **38**, 195–209.

Dent, C. E., and Stamp, T. C. B. (1970). Theoretical renal phosphorus threshold in investigation and treatment of osteomalacia. *Lancet* **1**, 857–860.

Dent, C. E., and Winter, C. (1974). Osteomalacia due to phosphate depletion from excess aluminium hydroxide ingestion. *Br. Med. J.* **1**, 551–552.

Dent, C. E., Richens, A., Rowe, D. J. F., and Stamp, T. C. B. (1970). Osteomalacia with anticonvulsant therapy in epilepsy. *Br. Med. J.* **4**, 69–72.

DeToni, G. (1933). Remarks on the relations between renal rickets (renal dwarfism) and renal diabetes. *Acta Paediatr.* **16**, 479–484.

Dokoh, S., Donaldson, C. A., Manon, S. L., Pike, J. W., and Haussler, M. R. (1983). The ovary: A target organ for 1,25-dihydroxyvitamin D_3. *Endocrinology* **112**, 200–206.

Dominquez, J. H., Gray, R. W., and Lemann, J., Jr. (1976). Dietary phosphate deprivation in women and men: Effect on mineral and acid balance, parathyroid hormone and the metabolism of 25-OH-vitamin D. *J. Clin. Endocrinol. Metab.* **43**, 1056–1068.

Drezner, M. K., and Feinglos, M. N. (1977). Osteomalacia due to 1,25-dihydroxycholecalciferol deficiency, associated with a giant cell tumor of bone. *J. Clin. Invest.* **60**, 1046–1053.

Drezner, M. K., Lyles, K. W., Haussler, M. R., and Harrelson, J. M. (1980). Evaluation of a role for 1,25-dihydroxyvitamin D_3 in the pathogenesis and treatment of X-linked hypophosphatemic rickets and osteomalacia. *J. Clin. Invest.* **66**, 1020–1032.

Drezner, M. K., Lobaugh, B., Lyles, K. W., Carey, D. E., Paulson, D. F., and Harrelson, J.

M. (1982). The pathogenesis and treatment of tumor-induced osteomalacia. *In* "Vitamin D, Chemical, Biochemical and Clinical Endocrinology of Calcium Metabolism" (A. W. Norman, K. Schaefer, D. v. Herrath, and H. G. Grigoleit, eds.), pp. 949–954. de Gruyter, Berlin.

Dueland, S., Holmberg, I., Berg, T., and Pedersen, J. L. (1981). Uptake and 25-hydroxylation of vitamin D_3 by isolated rat liver cells. *J. Biol. Chem.* **256,** 10430–10434.

Dunnigan, M. G. (1977). Asian rickets and osteomalacia in Britain. *In* "Child Nutrition and Its Relation to Mental and Physical Development" pp. 43–70. Kellogg Company of Great Britain, Stratford, Manchester.

Dunnigan, M. G., McIntosh, W. B., Ford, J. A., and Robertson, I. (1982). Acquired disorders of vitamin D metabolism. *In* "Calcium Disorders" (D. Heath and S. J. Marx, eds.), pp. 125–149. Butterworth, London.

Eddy, R. L. (1971). Metabolic bone disease after gastrectomy. *Am. J. Med.* **50,** 442–449.

Edidin, D., Levitsky, L. L., Schey, W., Dumbovic, R., and Campos, A. (1980). Resurgence of nutritional rickets associated with breast feeding and special dietary practices. *Pediatrics* **62,** 232–235.

Eicher, E. M., Southard, J. L., Scriver, C. R., and Glorieux, F. H. (1976). Hypophosphatemia: Mouse model for human familial hypophosphatemic (vitamin D-resistant) rickets. *Proc. Nat. Acad. Sci. U.S.A.* **73,** 4667–4671.

Eil, C., and Marx, S. J. (1981). Nuclear uptake of 1,25-dihydroxy[^{3}H]cholecalciferol in dispersed fibroblasts cultured from normal human skin. *Proc. Natl. Acad. Sci. U.S.A.* **78,** 2562–2566.

Eil, C., Liberman, U., Rosen, J. F., and Marx, S. J. (1981). A cellular defect in hereditary vitamin D-dependent rickets type II: Defective nuclear uptake of 1,25-dihydroxyvitamin D in cultured skin fibroblasts. *N. Engl. J. Med.* **304,** 1588–1591.

Eisman, J. A., and DeLuca, H. F. (1977). Intestinal 1,25-dihydroxyvitamin D_3 binding protein: Specificity of binding. *Steroids* **30,** 245–257.

Eisman, J. A., MacIntyre I., Martin T. J., and Moseley J. M. (1979). 1,25-dihydroxyvitamin D in breast cancer cells. *Lancet* **2,** 1335–1336.

Eisman, J. A., MacIntyre, I., Martin, T. J., Frampton, R. J., and King, R. J. B. (1980). Normal and malignant breast tissue is a target organ for 1,25(OH)$_2$ vitamin D_3. *Clin Endocrinol.* **13,** 267–272.

Eisman, J. A., Frampton, R. J., Sher, E., Suva, L. J., and Martin, T. J. (1982). Biochemistry of 1,25-dihydroxyvitamin D_3 receptors in human cancer cells. *In* "Vitamin D: Chemical, Biochemical and Clinical Endocrinology of Calcium" (A. W. Norman, K. Schaefer, J. W. Coburn, H. F. DeLuca, D. Fraser, H. G. Grigoleit, and D. V. Herrath, eds.) pp. 65–71. de Gruyter.

Emmerson, B. T. (1970). "Ouch ouch" disease: The osteomalacia of cadmium nephropathy. *Ann. Intern. Med.* **73,** 854–855.

Endo, H., Kiyoki, M., Kawashima, K., Naruchi, T., and Hashimoto, Y. (1980). Vitamin D_3 metabolites and PTH synergistically stimulate bone formation of chick embryonic femur in vitro. *Nature (London)* **286,** 262–264.

Esvelt, R. P., and DeLuca, H. F. (1981). Calcitroic acid: Biological activity and tissue distribution studies. *Arch. Biochem. Biophys.* **206,** 403–413.

Esvelt, R. P., Schnoes, H. K., and DeLuca, H. F. (1979). Isolation and characterization of 1-hydroxy-23-carboxytetranorvitamin D: A major metabolite of 1,25-dihydroxyvitamin D_3. *Biochemistry* **18,** 3977–3983.

Esvelt, R. P., DeLuca, H. F., Wickmann, J. K., Yoshizawa, S., Zurcher, J., Sar, M., and Stumpf, W. E. (1980). 1,25-dihydroxyvitamin D_3 stimulated increase of 7,8-didehydrocholesterol levels in rat skin. *Biochemistry* **19,** 6158–6161.

Fanconi, G. (1936). Der fruhinfantile nephrotische-glykosuriche Zwergwuchs mit hypophosphatimischer Rachitis. *Jahrb. Kinderheilkd.* **147**, 299–338.

Feldman, D., McCain, T. A., Hirst, M. A., Chen, T. L., and Colston, K. W. (1979). Characterization of a cytoplasmic receptor-like binder for a 1α,25-dihydroxycholecalciferol in rat intestinal mucosa. *J. Biol. Chem.* **254**, 10378–10384.

Feldman, D., Chen, T., Hirst, M., Colston, K., Karasek, M., and Cone, C. (1980). Demonstration of 1,25-dihydroxyvitamin D_3 in human skin biopsies. *J. Clin. Endocrinol. Metab.* **51**, 1463–1465.

Feldman, D., Chen, T., Cone, C., Hirst, M., Shani, S., Benderli, A., and Hochberg, Z. (1982). Vitamin D resistant rickets with alopecia: Cultured skin fibroblasts exhibit defective cytoplasmic receptors and unresponsiveness to 1,25(OH)$_2$D$_3$. *J. Clin. Endocrinol. Metab.* **55**, 1020–1022.

Feldman, S. C., and Christakos, S. (1983). Vitamin D-dependent calcium-binding protein in rat brain: Biochemical and immunocytochemical characterization. *Endocrinology* **112**, 290–302.

Fontaine, O., Matsumoto, T., Goodman, D. B. P., and Rasmussen, H. (1981). Liponomic control of Ca^{++} transport: Relationship to mechanism of action of 1,25-dihydroxyvitamin D_3. *Proc. Natl. Acad. Sci. U.S.A.* **78**, 1751–1754.

Ford, J. A., McIntosh, W. B., Butterfield, R., Preece, M. A., Pietrek, J., Arrowsmith, W. A., Arthurton, M. W., Turner, W., O'Riordan, J. L. H., and Dunnigan, M. G. (1976). Clinical and subclinical vitamin D deficiency in Bradford children. *Arch. Dis. Child.* **51**, 939–943.

Franceschi, R. T., and DeLuca, M. F. (1979). Aggregation properties of the 1,25-dihydroxyvitamin D_3 receptor from chick intestinal cytosol. *J. Biol. Chem.* **254**, 11629–11635.

Franceschi, R. T., and DeLuca, H. F. (1981). The effect of inhibitors of protein and RNA synthesis on 1α,25-dihydroxyvitamin D_3-dependent calcium uptake in cultured embryonic duodenum. *J. Biol. Chem.* **256**, 3848–3852.

Fraser, D. R. (1980). Regulation of the metabolism of vitamin D. *Physiol. Rev.* **60**, 551–613.

Fraser, D., Kooh, S. W., Kind, H. P., Holick, M. F., Tanaka, Y., and DeLuca, H. F. (1973). Pathogenesis of hereditary vitamin-D-dependent rickets: An inborn error of vitamin D metabolism involving defective conversion of 15-hydroxyvitamin D to 1,25-dehydroxyvitamin D. *N. Engl. J. Med.* **289**, 817–822.

Freake, H. C., Spanos, E., Eisman, J. A., Galasko, C. S. B., Martin, T. J., and MacIntyre, I. (1980). Specific binding of 1,25-dihydroxyvitamin D_3 in the VX$_2$ carcinoma. *Biochem. Biophys. Res. Commun.* **97**, 1505–1511.

Freake, H. C., Marcocci, C., Iwasaki, J., and MacIntyre, I. (1981). 1,25-Dihydroxyvitamin D_3 specifically binds to a human breast cancer cell line (T47D) and stimulates growth. *Biochem. Biophys. Res. Commun.* **101**, 1131–1138.

Freedman, R. A., Weiser, M. M., and Isselbacher, K. J. (1977). Calcium translocation by Golgi and lateral-basal membrane vesicles from rat intestine: Decrease in vitamin D-deficient rats. *Proc. Natl. Acad. Sci. U.S.A.* **74**, 3612–3616.

Fukushima, M., Nishii, Y., Suzuki, M., and Suda, T. (1978). Comparative studies on the 25-hydroxylations of cholecalciferol and 1a-hydroxycholecalciferol in perfused rat liver. *Biochem. J.,* **170**, 495–502.

Fullmer, C. S., and Wasserman, R. H. (1973). Bovine intestinal calcium binding proteins: Purification and some properties. *Biochim. Biophys. Acta* **317**, 172–186.

Gallagher, J. C., Riggs, B. L., Eisman, J., Hamstra, A., Arnaud, S. B., and DeLuca, H. F. (1979). Intestinal calcium absorption and serum vitamin D metabolites in normal subjects and osteoporotic patients: Effect of age and dietary calcium. *J. Clin. Invest.* **64**, 729–736.

Gallagher, J. C., Jerpbak, C. M., Jee, W. S. S., Johnson, K. A., DeLuca, A. F., and Riggs, B. L. (1982). 1,25-dihydroxyvitamin D_3: Short-and-long-term effects on bone and calcium metabolism in patients with postmenopausal osteoporosis. *Proc. Natl. Acad. Sci. U.S.A.* **79**, 3325–3329.

Garabedian, M., Bailly du Bois, M., Corvol, M. T., Pezant, E., and Balsan, S. (1978). Vitamin D and cartilage. I. In vitro metabolism of 25-hydroxycholecalciferol by cartilage. *Endocrinology* **102**, 1262–1268.

Glorieux, F., and Scriver, C. R. (1972). Loss of a parathyroid hormone-sensitive component of phosphate transport in X-linked hypophosphatemia. *Science* **175**, 997–1000.

Glorieux, F. H., Scriver, C. R., Reade, T. M., Goldman, H., and Roseborough, A. (1972). Use of phosphate and vitamin D to prevent dwarfism and rickets in X-linked hypophosphatemia. *N. Engl. J. Med.* **287**, 481–487.

Glorieux, F. H., Scriver, C. R., Holick, M. F., and DeLuca, H. F. (1973). X-linked hypophosphataemic rickets: Inadequate therapeutic response to 1-25-dihydroxy-cholecalciferol. *Lancet* **2**, 287–289.

Glorieux, F. H., Marie, P. J., Pettifor, J. M., and Delvin, E. E. (1980). Bone response to phosphate salts, ergocalciferol, and calcitriol in hypophosphatemic vitamin D-resistant rickets. *N. Engl. J. Med.* **303**, 1023–1031.

Goldsmith, R. S. (1982). Enterohepatic cyling of vitamin D and its metabolites. *Miner. Electrolyte Metab.* **8**, 289–292.

Goldstein, D. A., Holdimann, B., Sherman, D., Norman, A. W., and Massry, S. G. (1981). Vitamin D metabolites and calcium metabolism in patients with nephrotic syndrome and normal renal function. *J. Clin. Endocrinol. Metab.* **52**, 116–121.

Gonick, H., Indraprasit, S., and Neustein, H. (1976). Cadmium-induced experimental Fanconi syndrome. *Curr. Probl. Clin. Biochem.* **4**, 111–118.

Gonzalez-Villapando, C., Porath, A., Berelowitz, M., Marshall, L., and Favus, M. J. (1980). Vitamin D metabolism during recovery from severe osteitis fibrosa cystica of primary hyperparathyroidism. *J. Clin. Endocrinol. Metab.* **51**, 1180–1183.

Gray, R. W., Wilz, D. R., Caldas, A. E., and Lemann J., Jr. (1977). The importance of phosphate in regulating plasma 1,25-$(OH)_2$-vitamin D levels in humans: Studies in healthy subjects, in calcium-stone formers and in patients with primary hyperparathyroidism. *J. Clin. Endocrinol. Metab.* **45**, 299–306.

Greer, F. R., Searcy, J. E., Levin, R. S., Steichen, J. J., Steichen-Asche, P. S., and Tsang, R. C. (1982). Bone mineral content and serum 25-hydroxyvitamin D concentrations in breast-fed infants with and without supplemental vitamin D: One year follow up. *J. Pediatr.* **100**, 919–922.

Griffin, J. E., Chandler, J. S., Haussler, M. R., and Zerwekh, J. E. (1982). Receptor-positive resistance to 1,25-dihydroxyvitamin D_3: A new cause of osteomalacia associated with impaired induction of 24-hydroxylase in fibroblasts. *Clin. Res.* **30**, 524A.

Grody, W. W., Schraeder, W. J., and O'Malley, B. W. (1982). Activation, transformation, and subunit structure of steroid hormone receptors. *Endocrinol. Rev.* **3**, 141–163.

Gupta, M. M., Round, J. M., and Stamp, T. C. B. (1974). Spontaneous cure of vitamin D deficiency in Asians during summer. *Lancet* **1**, 586–588.

Haddad, J. (1982). Human serum binding protein for vitamin D and its metabolites (DBP): Evidence that actin is the DBP binding component in human skeletal muscle. *Arch. Biochem. Biophys.* **213**, 538–544.

Haddad, J. G., and Birge, S. J. (1975). Widespread, specific binding of 25-hydroxycholecalciferol in rat tissues. *J. Biol. Chem.* **250**, 299–303.

Haddad, J. G., and Chyu, K. J. (1971). Competitive protein-binding radioassay for 25-hydroxy-cholecalciferol *J. Clin. Endocrinol. Metab.* **33**, 992–994.

Haddad, J. G., and Walgate, J. (1976a). Radioimmunoassay of the binding protein for vitamin D and its metabolites in human serum. *J. Clin. Invest.* **58**, 1217–1222.

Haddad, J. G., and Walgate, J. (1976b) 25-hydroxyvitamin D transport in human plasma: isolation and partial characterization of calcifediol-binding protein. *J. Biol. Chem.* **251**, 4803–4809.

Haddad, J. G., Hillman, L., and Rojanasathit, S. (1976). Human serum binding capacity and affinity for 25-hydroxyergocalciferol and 25-hydroxycholecalciferol. *J. Clin. Endocrinol. Metab.* **43**, 86–91.

Haddad, J. G., Fraser, D. R., and Lawson, D. E. M. (1981). Vitamin D plasma binding protein: Turnover and fate in the rabbit. *J. Clin. Invest.* **67**, 1550–1560.

Hahn, T. J., Birge, S. J., Scharp, C. R., and Avioli, L. V. (1972). Phenobarbital-induced alterations in vitamin D metabolism. *J. Clin. Invest.* **51**, 741–748.

Hahn, T. J., Hendin, B. A., Scharp, C. R., Boisseau, V. C., and Haddad, J. G. (1975). Serum 25-hydroxycalciferol levels and bone mass in children on chronic anticonvulsant therapy. *N. Engl. J. Med.* **292**, 550–554.

Hahn, T. J., Scharp, C. R., Richardson, C. A., Halstead, L. R., Kahn, A. J., and Teitlebaum, S. L. (1978). Interaction of diphenylhydantoin (phenytoin) and phenobarbital with hormonal mediation of fetal rat bone resorption in vitro. *J. Clin. Invest.* **62**, 406–414.

Hallick, R. B., and DeLuca, H. F. (1969). Vitamin D_3-stimulated template activity of chromatin. *Proc. Natl. Acad. Sci. U.S.A.* **63**, 528–531.

Halloran, B. P. and DeLuca, H. F. (1981). Intestinal calcium transport: Evidence for two distinct mechanisms of action of $1,25(OH)_2D_3$. *Arch. Biochem. Biophys.* **208**, 477–486.

Halloran, B. P., and DeLuca, H. F. (1982). Appearance of the intestinal cytosolic receptor for 1,25-dihydroxyvitamin D_3 during neonatal development in the rat. *J. Biol. Chem.* **256**, 7338–7342.

Halloran, B. P., DeLuca, H. F., and Vincenzi, F. F. (1980). $(Ca^{2+} + Mg^{2+})$ ATPase and calmodulin activity of red red-blood cells: Lack of dependence on vitamin D. *FEBS Lett.* **114**, 89–92.

Halloran, B. P., DeLuca, H. F., Barthell, E., Yamada, S., Ohmori, M., and Takayama, H. (1981). An examination of the importance of 24-hydroxylation to the function of vitamin D during early development. *Endocrinology* **108**, 2067–2071.

Harmeyer, J., and Plonait, H. (1967). Generalisierte Hyperaminoacidurie mit erblicher Rachitis bei Schweinen. *Helv. Paediatr. Acta* **22**, 216–229.

Harmeyer, J., Grabe, C. V., and Martens, H. (1977). Effect of metabolites and analogues of vitamin D_3 in hereditary pseudo-vitamin D deficiency of pigs. *In* "Vitamin D, Biochemical, Chemical, and Clinical Aspects Related to Calcium Metabolism" (A. W. Norman, K. Schaefer, J. W. Coburn, H. F. DeLuca, D. Fraser, H. G. Grigoleit, and D. v. Herrat, eds.), pp. 785–788. de Gruyter, Berlin.

Harris, M., Rowe, D. J. F., and Daroy, A. J. (1978). Anticonvulsant osteomalacia induced in the rat by diphenylhydantoin. *Calcif. Tissue Res.* **25**, 13–18.

Haussler, M. R., and McCain, T. A. (1977). Basic and clinical concepts related to vitamin D metabolism and action. *N. Engl. J. Med.* **297**, 974–983 and 1041–1050.

Haussler, M. R., Nagode, L. A., and Rasmussen, H. (1970). Induction of intestinal brush border alkaline phosphatase by vitamin D and identity with Ca-ATPase. *Nature (London)* **228**, 1199–1201.

Haussler, M. R., Drezner, M. K., Pike, J. W., Chandler, J. S., and Hagan, L. A. (1979).

Assay of 1,25-dihydroxyvitamin D and other active vitamin D metabolites in serum: Application to animals and humans. *In* "Vitamin D. Basic Research and Clinical Application" (A. W. Norman, Schaeffer, K. D. v. Herrath, H. G. Grigoleit, E. Mawer, T. Suda, H. F. DeLuca, and J. W. Coburn, eds.), pp. 186–196. de Gruyter, Berlin.

Haussler, M. R., Manolagas, S. C., and Deftos, L. J. (1980). Evidence for a 1,25-dihydroxyvitamin D_3-dependent calcium uptake in cultured embryonic duodenum. *J. Biol. Chem.* **256**, 3848–3852.

Haussler, M. R., Pike, J. W., Dokoh, S., Chandler, J. S., Chandler, S. K., Donaldson, C. A., and Marion, S. L. (1982). 1,25-Dihydroxyvitamin D receptor in cultured cell lines: Occurrence, subcellular distribution and relationship to bioresponses. *In* "Vitamin D: Chemical, Biochemical and Clinical Endocrinology of Calcium Metabolism" Ed (A. W. Norman, K. Schaefer, D. v. Herrath, and H. G. Grigoleit, eds.), pp. 109–113. de Gruyter, Berlin. 109–113.

Henry, H. L. (1979). Regulation of the hydroxylation of 25-hydroxyvitamin D_3 in vivo and in primary cultures of chick kidney cells. *J. Biol. Chem.* **254**, 2722–2729.

Henry, H. L. (1981). Insulin permits parathyroid hormone stimulation of 1,25-dihydroxyvitamin D_3 production in cultured kidney cells. *Endocrinology* **108**, 733–735.

Henry, H. L. and Norman, A. W. (1978). Vitamin D: Two dihydroxylated metabolites are required for normal chicken egg hatchability. *Science* **201**, 835–837.

Henry, H. L., Midgett, R. J., and Norman, A. W. (1974). Regulation of 25-hydroxyvitamin D_3-1-hydroxylase in vivo. *J. Biol. Chem.* **249**, 7584–7592

Henry, H. L., Taylor, A. N., and Norman, A. W. (1977). Response of chick parathyroid glands to the vitamin D metabolites, 1,25-dihydroxycholecalciferol and 24,25-dihydroxycholecalciferol. *J. Nutr.* **107**, 1918–1926.

Hermsdorf, C. L., and Bronner, F. (1975). Vitamin D-dependent calcium binding protein from rat kidney. *Biochim. Biophys. Acta* **379**, 553–561.

Hillman, L. S., and Haddad, J. G. (1983). Serial analyses of serum vitamin D-binding protein in preterm infants from birth to postconceptual maturity. *J. Clin. Endocrinol. Metab.* **51**, 189–191.

Hillman, L. S., Noff, N., Martin, L. A., and Haddad, J. G. (1979). Serum 25-hydroxyvitamin D (25-OHD) deficiency in premature infants. *Pediatr. Res.* **13**, 475.

Hillman, L., Salmons, S., and Fiore B. (1982). Treatment trials of higher dose vitamin D and 25-hydroxycholecalciferol in premature infants. *In* "Vitamin D, Chemical, Biochemical and Clinical Endocrinology of Calcium Metabolism" (A. W. Norman, K. Schaefer, D. v. Herrath, and H. G. Grigoleit, eds.), pp. 781–783. de Gruyter, Berlin.

Hirst, M. A., and Feldman, D. (1981). Glucocorticoids down regulate the number of 1,25-dihydroxyvitamin D_3 receptors in mouse intestine. *Biochem. Biophys. Res. Commun.* **105**, 1590–1596.

Hitchman, A. J. W., Kerr, M. K., and Harrison, J. E. (1973). The purification of pig vitamin D induced intestinal calcium binding protein. *Arch. Biochem. Biophys.* **155**, 221–222.

Hiwatashi, A., Nishii, Y., and Ichikawa, Y. (1982). Purification of cytochrome P-450-D1a (25-hydroxyvitamin D_3-1a-hydroxylase) of bovine kidney mitochondria. *Biochem. Biophys. Res. Commun.* **105**, 320–327.

Hobden, A. N., Harding, M., and Lawson, D. E. M. (1980). 1,25-dihydroxycholecalciferol stimulation of a mitochondrial protein in chick intestinal cells. *Nature (London)* **288**, 718–720.

Hodgkinson, A., Marshall, D. H., and Nordin, B. E. C. (1979). Vitamin D and magnesium absorption in man. *Clin. Sci.* **57**, 121–123.

Holdsworth, E. S. (1970). The effect of vitamin D on enzyme activities in the mucosal cells of the chick small intestine. *J. Membr. Biol.* **3**, 43–53.

Holick M. F., Garabedian, M., Schnoes, H. K., and DeLuca, H. F. (1975). Relationship of 25-hydroxyvitamin D_3 side chain structure to biologic activity. *J. Biol. Chem.* **250**, 226–230.

Holick, M. F., Adams, J. S., Clemens, T. L., MacLaughlin, J., Horiuchi, N., Smith, E., Holick, S. A., Nolan J., and Hanaifan, N. (1982). Photoendocrinology of vitamin D: The past, present and future. *In* "Vitamin D, Chemical, Biochemical and Clinical Endocrinology of Calcium Metabolism" (A. W. Norman, K. Schaefer, D. v. Herrath, and H. G. Grigoleit, eds.), pp. 1151–1156. de Gruyter, Berlin.

Holtrop, M. E., Cox, K. A., Clark, M. B., Holick, M. F., and Anast, C. S. (1981). 1,25-Dihydroxycholecalciferol stimulates osteoclasts in rat bones in the absence of parathyroid hormone. *Endocrinology* **108**, 2293–2301.

Horiuchi, N., Suda, T., Takahashi, H., Shimizawa, E., and Ogata, E. (1977). In vivo evidence for the intermediary role of $3',5'$-cyclic AMP in parathyorid hormone-induced stimulation of 1a,25-dihydroxyvitamin D_3 synthesis in rats. *Endocrinology* **101**, 969–974.

Horst, R. L. (1979). 25-OHD$_3$-26,23-lactone: A metabolite of vitamin D_3 that is 5 times more potent than 25-OHD$_3$ in the rat plasma competitive protein binding radioassay. *Biochem. Biophys. Res. Commun.* **89**, 286–293.

Horst, R. L., Napoli, J. L., and Littledike, E. T. (1982a). Discrimination in the metabolism of orally dosed ergocalciferol and cholecalciferol by the pig, rat, and chick. *Biochem. J.* **204**, 185–189.

Horst, R. L., Reinhardt, T. A., and Napoli, J. L. (1982b), 23-keto-25-hydroxyvitamin D_3 and 23-keto-1,25-dihydroxyvitamin D_3: Two new vitamin D_3 metabolites with high affinity for the 1,25-dihydroxyvitamin D_3 receptor. *Biochem. Biophys. Res. Commun.* **107**, 1319–1325.

Howard, G. A., Turner, R. T., Sherrard, D. J., and Baylink, D. J. (1981). Human bone cells in culture metabolize 25-hydroxyvitamin D_3 to 1,25-dihydroxyvitamin D_3 and 24,25-dihydroxyvitamin D_3. *J. Biol. Chem.* **256**, 7738–7740.

Howe, C. L., Keller, T. C. S., III, Mooseker, M. S., and Wasserman, R. H. (1982). Analysis of cytoskeletal proteins and Ca^{2+}-dependent regulation of structure in intestinal brush borders from rachitic chicks. *Proc. Natl. Acad. Sci. U.S.A.* **79**, 1134–1138.

Hughes, M. R., and Haussler, M. R. (1978), 1α,25-Dihydroxyvitamin D_3 receptors in parathyroid glands: Preliminary characterization of cytoplasmic and nuclear binding components. *J. Biol. Chem.* **253**, 1065–1073.

Hugi, K., Bonjour, J. P., and Fleisch, H. (1979). Renal handling of calcium: Influence of parathyroid hormone and 1,25-dihydroxyvitamin D_3. *Am. J. Physiol.* **236**, F349–F356.

Hunziker, W., Walters, M. R., Bishop, J. E., and Norman, A. W. (1982). Effect of vitamin D status on the equilibrium between occupied and unoccupied 1,25-dihydroxyvitamin D intestinal receptors in the chick. *J. Clin. Invest.* **69**, 826–834.

Imawari, M., Kida, K., and Goodman, D. S. (1976). The transport of vitamin D and its 25-hydroxy metabolite in human plasma: Isolation and partial characterization of vitamin D and 25-hydroxyvitamin D binding protein. *J. Clin. Invest.* **58**, 514–523.

Imawari, M., Matsuzaki, Y., Mitamura, K., and Osuga, T. (1982). Synthesis of serum and cytosol vitamin D-binding proteins by rat liver and kidney. *J. Biol. Chem.* **257**, 8153–8157.

Jones, G., Byrnes, B., Palma, F., Segev, D., and Mazur, Y. (1980a). Displacement potency of vitamin D_2 analogs in competitive protein-binding assays for 25-hydroxyvitamin

D3, 24,25-dihydroxyvitamin D3, and 1,25-dihydroxyvitamin D3. *J. Clin. Endo-crinol. Metab.* **50,** 773–776.

Jones, G., Schnoes, H. K., Levan, L., and DeLuca, H. F. (1980b). Isolation and identification of 24-hydroxyvitamin D_2 and 24,25-dihydroxyvitamin D_2. *Arch. Biochem. Biophys.* **202,** 450–457.

Jubiz, W., Haussler, M. R., and McCain, T. A. (1977). 1,25-dihydroxyvitamin D levels in patients receiving anticonvulsant drugs. *J. Clin. Endocrinol. Metab.* **44,** 617–621.

Kawakami, M., Imawari, M., and Goodman, D. S. (1979). Quantitative studies of the interaction of cholecalciferol (vitamin D_3) and its metabolites with different genetic variants of the serum binding protein for these sterols. *Biochem. J.* **179,** 413–423.

Kawashima, H., and Kurokawa, K. (1982). Localization of receptors for 1,25-dihydroxy-vitamin D_3 along the rat nephron: Direct evidence for presence of the receptors in both proximal and distal nephron. *J. Biol. Chem.* **257,** 13428–13432.

Kawashima, H., Torikai, S., and Kurokawa, K. (1981a). Localization of 25-hydroxyvita-min D_3 1a-hydroxylase and 24-hydroxylase along the rat nephron. *Proc. Natl. Acad. Sci. U.S.A.* **78,** 1199–1203.

Kawashima, H., Torikai, S., and Kurokawa, K. (1981b). Calcitonin selectively stimulates 25-hydroxyvitamin D_3-1a-hydroxylase in proximal straight tubule of rat kidney. *Nature (London)* **291,** 327–329.

Kawashima, H., Kraut, J. A., and Kurokawa, K. (1982). Metabolic acidosis suppresses 25-hydroxyvitamin D_3-1a-hydroxylase in the rat kidney. *J. Clin. Invest.* **70,** 135–140.

Kent, G. N., Jilka, R. L., and Cohn, D. V. (1980). Homologous and heterologous control of bone cell adenosine 3′,5′-monophosphate response to hormones by parathormone, prostaglandin E2, calcitonin, and 1,25-dihydroxycholecalciferol. *Endocrinology* **107,** 1474–1481.

Klein, G. L., Horst, R. L., Norman, A. W., Ament, M. E., Slatopolsky, E., and Coburn, J. W. (1981). Reduced serum levels of 1,25-dihydroxyvitamin D during long-term total parenteral nutrition. *Ann. Intern. Med.* **94,** 638–643.

Klein, G. L., Ament, M. E., Norman, A. W., and Coburn, J. W. (1982). Metabolic bone disease associated with total parenteral nutrition in children. *In* "Vitamin D: Chemical, Biochemical and Clinical Endocrinology of Calcium Metabolism" (A. W. Norman, K. Schaefer, D. v. Herrath, and H. G. Grigoleit, eds.), pp. 981. de Gruyter, Berlin.

Kobayashi, A., Kawai, S., Utsunomiya, T., and Ohbe, Y. (1974). Bone disease in infants and children with hepatobiliary disease. *Arch. Dis. Child.* **49,** 641–646.

Kooh, S. W., Fraser, D., Reilly, B. J., Hamilton, J. R., Gall, D. G., and Bell, L. (1977). Rickets due to calcium deficiency. *N. Engl. J. Med.* **297,** 1264–1266.

Kooh, S. W., Jones, G., Reilly, B. J., and Fraser, D. (1979). Pathogenesis of rickets in hepatobiliary disease in children. *J. Paediatr.* **94,** 870–874.

Krawitt, E. L., Grundman, M. J., and Mawer, E. B. (1977). Absorption, hydroxylation and excretion of vitamin D_3 in primary biliary cirrhosis. *Lancet* **2,** 1246–1249.

Kream, B. E., Jose, M., Yamada, S., and DeLuca, H. F. (1977a). A specific high-affinity binding macromolecule for 1,25-dihydroxyvitamin D_3 in fetal bone. *Science* **197,** 1086–1088.

Kream, B. E., Yamada, S., Schnoes, H., and DeLuca, H. F. (1977b). Specific cytosol-binding protein for 1,25-dihydroxyvitamin D_3 in rat intestine *J. Biol. Chem.* **252,** 4501–4505.

Kremer, R., and Goltzman, D. (1982). Parathyroid hormone stimulates mammalian renal 25-hydroxyvitamin D_3 1a-hydroxylase in vitro. *Endocrinology* **110,** 294–296.

Kretsinger, R. H., Mann, J. E., and Simmonds, J. G. (1982). Model of facilitated diffusion of calcium by the intestinal calcium binding protein. In "Vitamin D: Chemical, Biochemical and Clinical Endocrinology of Calcium Metabolism" (A. W. Norman, K. Schaefer, D. v. Herrath, and H. G. Grigoleit, eds.), pp. 233–248. Berlin.

Kulkowski, J. A., Chan, T., Martinez, J., and Ghazarian, J. A. (1979). Modulation of 25-hydroxyvitamin D_3-24-hydroxylase by aminophylline: A cytochrome P-450 monooxygenase system. Biochem. Biophys. Res. Commun. 90, 50–57.

Kumar, R. (1980). Enterohepatic physiology of 1,25-dihydroxyvitamin D_3. J. Clin. Invest. 65, 277–284.

Kumar, R. (1982). Enterohepatic physiology of dihydroxylated vitamin D_3 metabolites. In "Vitamin D: Chemical, Biochemical, and Clinical Endocrinology of Calcium Metabolism" (A. W. Norman, K. Schaefer, D. v. Herrath, and H. G. Grigoleit, eds.), pp. 635–640. de Gruyter, Berlin.

Kumar, R., Harnden, D., and DeLuca, H. F. (1976). Metabolism of 1,25-dihydroxyvitamin D_3: Evidence for side-chain oxidation. Biochemistry 15, 2420–2423.

Kumar, R., Schnoes, H. K., and DeLuca, H. F. (1978). Rat intestinal 25-hydroxyvitamin D_3- and 1a,25-dihydroxyvitamin D_3-24-hydroxylase. J. Biol. Chem. 253, 3804–3809.

Kumar, R., Nagubandi, S., and Londowski, J. M. (1980). The enterohepatic physiology of 24,25-dihydroxyvitamin D_3. J. Lab. Clin. Med. 96, 278–284.

Kumar, R., Nagubandi, S., and Londowski, J. M. (1981a). Production of a polar metabolite of 1,25-dihydroxyvitamin D_3 in a rat liver perfusion system. Dig. Dis. Sci. 26, 242–246.

Kumar, R., Nagubandi, S., Jardine, I., Londowski, J. M., and Bollman, S. (1981b). The isolation and identification of 5,6-trans-25-hydroxyvitamin D_3 from the plasma of rats dosed with vitamin D_3. J. Biol. Chem. 256, 9389–9392.

Kuntzman, R. (1969). Drugs and enzyme induction. Annu. Rev. Pharmacol. 9, 21–26.

Lakdawala, D. R., and Widdowson, E. M. (1977). Vitamin D in human milk. Lancet 1, 167–168.

Lambert, P. W., Stern, P. H., Avioli, R. C., Brackett, N. C., Turner, R. T., Greene, A., Fu, I. Y., and Bell, N. H. (1982). Evidence for extrarenal production of 1a,25-dihydroxyvitamin D in man. J. Clin. Invest. 69, 722–725.

Lane, S. M., and Lawson, D. E. M. (1978). Differentiation of the changes in alkaline phosphatase from calcium ion-activated adenosine triphosphatase activities associated with increased calcium absorption in chick intestine. Biochem. J. 174, 1067–1070.

Laouari, D., Pavlovitch, H., Deceneux, G., and Balsan, S. (1980). A vitamin D-dependent calcium binding protein in rat skin. FEBS Lett. 14, 285–289.

Larkins, R. G., Macauley, S. J., and MacIntyre, I. (1975). Inhibitors of protein and RNA synthesis and 1,25-dihydroxycholecalciferol formation in vitro. Mol. Cell. Endocrinol. 2, 193–202.

Lawson, D. E. M. (1979). Dietary vitamin D. Lancet 2, 1021.

Lawson, D. E. M., and Wilson, P. W. (1974). Intranuclear localization and receptor proteins for 1,25-dihydroxycholecalciferol in chick intestine. Biochem. J. 144, 573–583.

Lawson, D. E. M., Paul, A. A., Black, A. E., Cole, T. J., Mandal, A. R., and Davie, M. (1979). Relative contributions of diet and sunlight to vitamin D status in the elderly. Br. Med. J. 2, 303–305.

Lee, S. W., Russel, J., and Arioli, L. V. (1977). 25-hydroxy-cholecalciferol to 1,25-dihydroxycholecalciferol: Conversion impaired by systemic metabolic acidosis. Science 195, 994–996.

Leerbeck, E., and Sondergaard, H. (1980). The total content of vitamin D in human milk and cows' milk. *Br. J. Nutr.* **44,** 7–12.

Lemann, J., Jr., Adams, N. D., and Gray, R. W. (1982). Liquid formula diets reduced serum 1,25-$(OH)_2$-vitamin D concentrations in humans. *In* "Vitamin D: Chemical, Biochemical and Clinical Endocrinology of Calcium Metabolism" (A. W. Norman, K. Schaefer, D. v. Herrath, and H. G. Grigoleit, eds.), pp. 669–675. de Gruyter, Berlin.

Liang, C. T., Barnes, J., Balakir, R., Cheng, L., and Sacktor, B. (1982). In vitro stimulation of phosphate uptake in isolated chick renal cells by 1,25-dihydroxycholecalciferol. *Proc. Natl. Acad. Sci. U.S.A.* **79,** 3532–3536.

Liberman, U. A., Samuel R., Halabe A., Kauli, R., Edelstein, S., Weisman, Y., Papapoulos, S. Clemens, T. L., Fraher, L. J., and O'Riordan, J. L. H. (1980). End-organ resistance to 1,25-dihydroxycholecalciferol. *Lancet* **1,** 504–507.

Liberman, U. A., Balsan S., and Marx, S. J. (1982). True resistance to 1,25-dihydroxyvitamin D—cellular basis and implication of a new congenital syndrome. 64th Annual Meeting of Endocrine Society, p. 214. (Abstract).

Liberman, U. A., Eil, C., and Marx, S. J. (1983). Resistance to 1,25-dihydroxyvitamin D: Association with heterogeneous defects in cultured skin fibroblasts. *J. Clin. Invest.* **71,** 192–200.

Lieberherr, M., Garabedian, M., Guillozo, H., Thil, C. L., and Balsan, S. (1980). In vitro effects of vitamin D_3 metabolites on rat calveria cAMP content. *Calcif. Tissue Int.* **30,** 209–216.

Lifschitz, F., and MacLaren, N. K. (1973). Vitamin D-dependent rickets in institutionalized, mentally-retarded children receiving long-term anticonvulsant therapy. 1. A survey of 288 patients. *J. Pediatr.* **83,** 612–620.

Linovitz, R. J., Resnick, D., Keissling, P., Kondon, J. J., Sehler, B., Nejdl, R. J., Rowe, J. H., and Deftos, L. J. (1976). Tumor-induced osteomalacia and rickets: A surgically curable syndrome. *J. Bone Jt. Surg. (Am.)* **58A,** 419–423.

Littledike, E. T., and Horst, R. L. (1982). Metabolism of vitamin D_3 in nephrectomized pigs given pharmacological amounts of vitamin D_3. *Endocrinology* **111,** 2008–2013.

Livingstone, S., Berman, W., and Pauli, L. L. (1973). Anticonvulsant drugs and vitamin D metabolism. *JAMA* **224,** 1634–1635.

Loomis, W. F. (1970). Rickets. *Sci. Am.* **223,** 77–91.

Lyles, K. W., and Drezner, M. K. (1982). Parathyroid hormone effects on serum 1,25-dihydroxyvitamin D levels in patients with X-linked hypophosphatemic rickets: Evidence for abnormal 25-hydroxyvitamin D-1-hydroxylase activity. *J. Clin. Endocrinol. Metab.* **54,** 638–644.

Lyles, K. W., Berry, W. R., Haussler, M., Harrelson, J. M., and Drezner, M. K. (1980). Hypophosphatemic osteomalacia: Association with prostatic carcinoma. *Ann. Intern. Med.* **93,** 275–278.

McSherry, E., and Morris, R. C. (1978). Attainment and maintenance of normal stature with alkali therapy in infants and children with classic renal tubular acidosis. *J. Clin. Invest.* **61,** 509–527.

Madhok, T. C., and DeLuca, H. F. (1979). Characteristics of the rat liver microsomal enzyme system converting cholecalciferol into 25-hydroxycholecalciferol: Evidence for the participation of cytochrome P-450. *Biochem. J.* **184,** 491–499.

Majeska, R. J., and Rodan, G. A. (1982). The effect of 1,25$(OH)_2D_3$ on alkaline phosphatase in osteoblastic osteosarcoma cells. *J. Biol. Chem.* **257,** 3362–3365.

Mallon, J. P., Matuszewski, D. S., Baggiolini, E. G., Partridge, J. J., and Uskokovic, M. R. (1981). Effect of 1α,25-dihydroxycholecalciferol analogs on bone resorption *in vitro. J. Steroid Biochem.* **14,** 549–602.

Maltz, H. E., Fish, M. B., and Holliday, M. A. (1970). Calcium deficiency rickets and the renal response to calcium infusion. *Pediatrics* **46**, 865–870.

Manolagas, S. C., and Deftos, L. J. (1980a). Studies of the internalization of vitamin D_3 metabolites by cultured osteogenic sarcoma cells and their application to a non-chromatographic cytoreceptor assay for 1,25-dihydroxyvitamin D_3. *Biochem. Biophys. Res. Commun.* **95**, 596–602.

Manolagas, S. C., and Deftos, L. J. (1980b). Cytoreceptor assay for 1,25-dihydroxyvitamin D_3: A novel radiometric method based on binding of the hormone to intracellular receptors in vitro. *Lancet* **2**, 401–402.

Manolagas, S. C., Anderson, D. C., and Lamb, G. A. (1976). Glucocorticoids regulate the concentration of 1,25-dihydroxycholecalciferol receptors in bone. *Nature (London)* **277**, 314–316.

Manolagas, S., Haussler, M. R., and Deftos, L. J., (1980). 1,25-dihydroxyvitamin D_3 receptor-like macromolecule in rat osteogenic sarcoma cell lines. *J. Biol. Chem.* **255**, 4414–4417.

Manolagas, S. C., Abare, J., Tolley, J., Meler, D., Howard, J., Burton, D., and Deftos, L. J. (1981). Glucocorticoids and calcium increase the concentration of 1,25-dihydroxy D_3 receptor of cultured osteogenic sarcoma cells. Third Annual Meeting American Society Bone and Mineral Research, p. 8. (Abstract).

Marcocci, C., Freake, H. C., Iwasaki, J., Lopez, E., and MacIntyre, I. (1982). Demonstration and organ distribution of the 1,25-dihydroxyvitamin D_3-binding protein in fish *(A. anguilla) Endocrinology* **110**, 1347–1350.

Marcus, R., Orner, F. B., and Brickman, A. S. (1980). Effects in vivo of vitamin D metabolites and 17B-estradiol on parathyroid hormone-dependent formation of adenosine $3',5'$-monophosphate in rat bone. *Endocrinology* **107**, 1593–1599.

Marie, P. J., Pettifor, J. M., Ross, F. P., and Glorieux, F. H. (1982). Histological osteomalacia due to dietary calcium deficiency in children. *N. Engl. J. Med.* **307**, 584–588.

Martin, D. C., Melancon, M. J., and DeLuca, M. F. (1969). Vitamin D stimulated calcium-dependent adenosine triphosphatase from brush borders of rat small intestine. *Biochem. Biophys. Res. Commun.* **35**, 819–823.

Marx, S. J. (1983). Resistance to vitamin D. *In* "Vitamin D Metabolism: Basic and Clinical Aspects" (R. Kumar, ed.). Nijhoff, The Hague. In press.

Marx, S. J., Spiegel, A. M., Brown, E. M., Gardner, D. G., Downs, R. W., Jr., Attie, M., Hamstra, A. J., and DeLuca, H. F. (1978). A familial syndrome of decrease in sensitivity to 1,25-dihydroxyvitamin D. *J. Clin. Endocrinol. Metab.* **47**, 1303–1310.

Massoro, E. R., Simpson, R. U., and DeLuca, H. F. (1982). Stimulation of specific 1,25-dihydroxyvitamin D_3 binding protein in cultured postnatal rat intestine by hydrocortisone. J. Biol. Chem. **257**, 13736–13739.

Matsumoto, T., Fontaine, O., and Rasmussen, H. (1980). Effect of 1,25-dihydroxyvitamin D_3 on phosphate uptake in chick intestinal brush border membrane vesicles. *Biochim. Bipohys. Acta* **599**, 13–23.

Matsumoto, T., Fontaine, O., and Rasmussen, H. (1981). Effect of 1,25-dihydroxyvitamin D_3 on phospholipid metabolism in chick duodenal mucosal cell: Relationship to its mechanism of action. *J. Biol. Chem.* **256**, 3354–3360.

Mawer, E. B. (1982). Patterns of vitamin D metabolism in humans: relation to nutritional status. *In* "Endocrinology of Calcium Metabolism" (J. A. Parsons, ed.), pp. 149–196. Raven, New York.

Melancon, J. F., Jr., and DeLuca, M. F. (1970). Vitamin D stimulation of calcium-dependent adenosine triphosphatase in chick intestinal brush borders. *Biochemistry* **9**, 1658–1664.

Mellon, W. S., Franceschi, R. T., and DeLuca, H. F. (1980). An *in vitro* study of the stability of the chicken intestinal cytosol 1,25-dihydroxyvitamin D_3 specific receptor. *Arch. Biochem. Biophys.* **202**, 83–92.

Merke, J., and Norman, A. W. (1981). Studies on the mode of action of calciferol. XXXII. Evidence for a 24(R),25(OH)$_2$D$_3$ receptor in the parathyroid gland of the rachitic chick. *Biochem. Biophys. Res. Commun.* **100**, 551–558.

Meyer, R. A., Jr., Gray, R. W., and Meyer, M. H. (1980). Abnormal vitamin D metabolism in the X-linked hypophosphatemic mouse. *Endocrinology* **107**, 1577–1581.

Meyer, R. A., Gray, R. W., Roos, B. A., and Kiebzak, G. M. (1982). Increased plasma 1,25-dihydroxyvitamin D after low calcium challenge in X-linked hypophosphatemic mice. *Endocrinology* **111**, 174–177.

Miravet, L., Gueris, J., Redel, J., Norman, A., and Ryckwaert, A. (1981). Action of vitamin D metabolites on PTH secretion in man. *Calcif. Tissue Int.* **33**, 191–194.

Morgan, D. B., Paterson, C. R., Pulvertaft, C. N., Woods, C. G., and Fourman, P. (1965). Search for osteomalacia in 1228 patients after gastrectomy and other operations on the stomach. *Lancet* **2**, 1085–1088.

Morgan, H. G., Steward, W. K., Lowe, K. G., Stowers, J. M., and Johnstone, J. H. (1962). Wilson's disease and the Fanconi syndrome. *Q. J. Med.* **31**, 361–384.

Mezzetti, G., Moruzzi, M. S., and Barbirolli, B. (1981). Evidence for a 1,25-dihydroxycholecalciferol-dependent spermine-binding protein in chick duodenal mucosa. *Biochem. Biophys. Res. Commun.* **102**, 287–294.

Morrisey, R. L., and Roth, D. F. (1974). Purification of human renal calcium binding protein from necropsy specimens. *Proc. Soc. Exp. Biol. Med.* **145**, 699–703.

Morrissey, R. L., Zolock, D. T., Bikle, D. D., Empson, R., N., Jr., and Bucci, T. J. (1978). Intestinal response to 1α,25-dihydroxycholecalciferol: I. RNA polymerase, alkaline phosphatase, calcium and phosphorus uptake in vitro, and in vivo calcium transport and accumulation. *Biochim. Biophys. Acta* **538**, 23–33.

Mosekilde, L., Christensen, M. S., Lund, B., Sorensen, O. H., and Melsen, F. (1977). The interrelationships between serum 25-hydroxycholecalciferol, serum parathyroid hormone and bone changes in anticonvulsant osteomalacia. *Acta Endocrinol.* **84**, 559–565.

Moss, A. J., Waterhouse, C., and Terry, R. (1965). Gluten-sensitive enteropathy with osteomalacia but without steatorrhoea. *N. Engl. J. Med.* **272**, 825–830.

Murdoch, G. H., and Rosenfeld, M. G. (1981). Regulation of pituitary function and prolactin production in the GH4 cell line by vitamin D. *J. Biol. Chem.* **256**, 4050–4055.

Nagubandi, S., Kumar, R., Londowski, J. M., Corradino, R. A., and Tietz, P. S. (1980). Role of vitamin D glucosiduronate in calcium homeostasis. *J. Clin. Invest.* **66**, 1274–1280.

Narbaitz, R., Sar, M., Stumpf, W. E., Huang, S., and DeLuca, H. F. (1981). 1,25-dihydroxyvitamin D_3 target cells in rat mammary gland. *Horm. Res.* **15**, 263–269.

Nko, M., Gruson, M., Gueris, J., Mouktar, M. S., Redel, J., Demignon, J., and Miravet, L. (1982). Effects of vitamin D_3 dihydroxylated metabolites on parathyroid hormone in the rat. *Miner. Electrolyte Metab.* **7**, 67–75.

Nogawa, K., Ishikazi, A., Fukushima, M., Shibata, I., and Hagino, N. (1975). Studies on the women with acquired Fanconi syndrome observed in the Ichi river basin polluted by cadmium. Is this Itai-Itai disease? *Environ. Res.* **10**, 280–307.

Nordin, B. E. C., Peacock, M., Crilly, R. G., and Marshall, D. H. (1979). Calcium absorption and plasma 1,25(OH)$_2$D levels in post-menopausal osteoporosis. *In* "Vitamin D: Basic Rsearch and its Clinical Application" (A. W. Norman, K. Schaefer, D. v. Herrath, H. G. Grigoleit, J. W. Coburn, H. F. DeLuca, E. B. Mawer, and T. Suda, eds.), pp. 99–106. Gruyter, Berlin.

Norman, A. W. (1979). Vitamin D metabolism and calcium absorption. *Am. J. Med.* **67**, 989–998.

Norman, A. W., Mirchoff, A. K., Adams, T. M., and Spielvogel, A. (1970). Studies on the mechanism of action of calciferol. III. Vitamin D mediated increase of intestinal brush border alkaline phosphatase activity. *Biochim. Biophys. Acta* **215**, 348–359.

Norman, A. W., Johnson, R. L., and Okamura, W. H. (1979). 24-Nor-25-hydroxyvitamin D$_3$: a specific antagonist of vitamin D$_3$ action in the chick. *J. Biol. Chem.* **254**, 11450–11456.

Norman, A. W., Frankel, B. J., Heldt, A. M., and Grodsky, G. M. (1980). Vitamin D deficiency inhibits pancreatic secretion of insulin. *Science* **209**, 823–825.

Norman, A. W., Roth, J., and Orchi, L. (1982). The vitamin D endocrine system: Steroid metabolism, hormone receptors, and biological response (calcium binding proteins). *Endocrinol. Rev.* **3**, 331–366.

Nseir, N. I., Szramowski, J., and Puschett, J. B. (1978). Mechanism of the renal tubular effects of 25-hydroxy and 1,25-dihydroxy vitamin-D$_3$ in the absence of parathyroid hormone. *Miner. Electrolyte Metab.* **1**, 48–56.

O'Doherty, P. J. A. (1979). 1,25-Dihydroxyvitamin D$_3$ increases the activity of the intestinal phosphatidylcholine deacylation-reacylation cycle. *Lipids* **14**, 75–77.

Ohnuma, N., and Norman, A. W. (1981). Studies on the metabolism of calciferol. XVIII. Production *in vitro* of 1,25-dihydroxyvitamin D$_3$-26,23-lactone from from 1,25-dihydroxy-vitamin D by rat small intestinal mucosa homogenates. *Arch. Bioch:m. Biophys.* **213**, 139–147.

Oldham, S. B., Smith, R., Hartenblower, D. L., Henry, H. L., Norman, A. W., and Coburn, J. W. (1979). The acute effects of 1,25-dihydroxycholecalciferol on serum immunoreactive parathyroid hormone in the dog. *Endocrinology* **104**, 248–254.

Olgaard, K., Schwartz, J., Finco, D., Arbalaez, M., Haddad, J., Avioli, L., Klahr, S., and Slatopolsky, E. (1982). Extraction of vitamin D metabolites by bones of normal adult dogs. *J. Clin. Invest.* **69**, 684–690.

Omdahl, J. L., Hunsaker, L. A., Evan, A. P., and Torrez, P. (1980). In vitro regulation of kidney 25-hydroxyvitamin D$_3$-hydroxylase enzyme activities by vitamin D$_3$ metabolites. *J. Biol. Chem.* **255**, 7460–7466.

Onisko, B. L., Schnoes, H. K., and DeLuca, H. F. (1979). 25-Azavitamin D$_3$, an inhibitor of vitamin D metabolism and action. *J. Biol. Chem.* **254**, 3493–3496.

Pansu, D., Bellaton, C., and Bronner, F. (1981). Effect of Ca intake on saturable and nonsaturable components of duodenal Ca transport. *Am. J. Physiol.* **240**, G32–G37.

Parfitt, A. M., Miller, M. J., Frame, B., Villanueva, A. R., Rao, D. S., Oliver, I., and Thomson, D. L. (1978). Metabolic bone disease after intestinal bypass for treatment of obesity. *Ann. Intern. Med.* **89**, 193–199.

Partridge, N. C., Frampton, R. J., Eisman, J. A., Michelangeli, V. P., Elms, E., Bradley, T. R., and Martin, T. J. (1980). Receptors for 1,25(OH)$_2$-vitamin D$_3$ enriched in cloned osteoblastic-like rat osteogenic sarcoma cells. *FEBS Lett.* **115**, 139–142.

Pettifor, J. M., Ross, P., Wang, J., Moodley, G. P., and Couper-Smith, J. (1978). Rickets in children of rural origin in South Africa: Is low dietary calcium a factor? *J. Pediatr.* **92**, 320–324.

Pettifor, J. M., Ross P., Moodley, G., and Shuenyane, E. (1979). Calcium deficiency in rural black children in South Africa: A comparison between rural and urban communities. *Am. J. Clin. Nutr.* **32**, 2477–2483.

Pettifor, J. M., Ross, F. P., Travers, R., Glorieux, F. H., and DeLuca, H. F. (1981). Dietary calcium deficiency: A syndrome associated with bone deformities and elevated serum 1,25-dihydroxyvitamin D concentrations. *Metab. Bone Dis. Rel. Res.* **2**, 301–305.

Piazolo, P., Schleyer, M., and Franz, I. E. (1971). Isolation and purification of a calcium binding protein from human tissues. *Hoppe-Seyler's Z. Physiol. Chem.* **352**, 1480–1486.

Pike, J. W. (1982). Interaction between 1,25-dihydroxyvitamin D_3 receptors and intestinal nuclei: Binding to nuclear constituents *in vitro*. *J. Biol. Chem.* **257**, 6766–6775.

Pike, J. W., Goozé, L. L., and Haussler, M. R. (1980). Biochemical evidence for 1,25-dihydroxyvitamin D receptor macromolecules in parathyroid, pancreatic, pituitary and placental tissues. *Life Sci.* **26**, 407–414.

Pleasure, D., Wyszinski, B., Sumner, A., Schotland, D., Feldmann, B., Nugent, N., Hitz, K., and Goodman, D. B. P. (1979). Skeletal muscle calcium metabolism and contractile force in vitamin D-deficient chicks. *J. Clin. Invest.* **64**, 1157–1167.

Poskitt, E. M. E., Cole, T. J., and Lawson, D. E. M. (1979). Diet, sunlight and 25-hydroxyvitamin D in healthy children and adults. *Br. Med. J.* **1**, 221–223.

Prader, A., Illig, R., and Heierli, E. (1961). Eine besondere Form der primaren vitamin D-resistenten Rachitis mit Hypocalcamie und autosomal-dominantem Erbgang: Die hereditare Pseudo-Mangelrachitis. *Helv. Paediatr. Acta* **16**, 452–468.

Preece, M. A., Tomlinson, S., Ribot, C. A., Pietrek, J., Korn, H. T., Davies, D. M., Ford, J. A., Dunnigan, M. G., and O'Riordan, J. L. H. (1975). Studies of vitamin D deficiency in man. *Q. J. Med.* **44**, 575–589.

Price, P. A., and Baukol, S. A. (1980). 1,25-Dihydroxyvitamin D_3 increases synthesis of the vitamin K-dependent bone protein by osteosarcoma cells. *J. Biol. Chem.* **255**, 11660–11663.

Procsal, D. A., Okamura, W. H., and Norman, A. W. (1975). Studies on the mode of action of calciferol IX: Structural requirements for the interaction of $1\alpha,25$-(OH)-vitamin D_3 with its chick intestinal receptor system. *J. Biol. Chem.* **250**, 8382–8388.

Prost, A., Hanniche, M., Bordier, P., Miravet, L., De Seze, S., and Rambaud, J. C. (1975). Osteomalacia in chromic pancreatitis. *Nouv. Presse Med.* **4**, 1561–1566.

Puschett, J. B., and Kuhrman, M. S. (1978). Renal tubular effects of 1,25-dihydroxy vitamin D_3: interactions with vasopressin and parathyroid hormone in the vitamin D-depleted rat. *J. Lab. Clin. Med.* **92**, 895–903.

Puzas, J. E., Turner, R. T., Howard, G. A., and Baylink, D. J. (1983). Cells isolated from embryonic intestine synthesize 1,25-dihydroxyvitamin-D_3 and 24,24-dihydroxyvitamin-D_3 in culture. *Endocrinology* **112**, 378–380.

Radparvar, S., and Mellon, W. S. (1982). Characterization of 1,25-dihydroxy-vitamin D_3-receptor complex interactions with DNA by a competitive assay. *Arch. Biochem. Biophys.* **217**, 552–563.

Raisz, L. G., Trummel, C. L., Holick, M. F., and DeLuca, H. F. (1972). 1,25-Dihydroxy-cholecalciferol: A potent stimulator of bone resorption in tissue culture. *Science* **175**, 768–769.

Raisz, L. G., Maina, D. M., Gworek, S. C., Deitrich, J. W., and Canalis, E. M. (1978). Hormonal control of bone collagen synthesis in vitro: Inhibitory effect of 1-hydroxylated vitamin D metabolites. *Endocrinology* **102**, 731–735.

Rasmussen, H., Fontaine, O., Max, E. E., and Goodman, D. B. P. (1979). The effect of 1α-

hydroxyvitamin D_3 administration on calcium transport in chick intestine brush border membrane vesicles. *J. Biol. Chem.* **254**, 2993–2999.

Rasmussen, H., Pecket, M., Anast, C., Mazur, A., Gertner, J., and Broadus, A. E. (1981). Long-term treatment of familial hypophosphatemic rickets with oral phosphate and 1alpha-hydroxyvitamin D_3. *J. Pediatr.* **99**, 16–25.

Reade, T., Scriver, C. R., Glorieux, F. H., Nogrady, B., Delvin, E., Poirier, R., Holick, M. F., and DeLuca, H. F. (1975). Response to crystalline 1-hydroxyvitamin D_3 in vitamin D dependency. *Pediatr. Res.* **9**, 593–599.

Reinhardt, T. A., Horst, R. L., Littledike, E. T., and Beitz, D. C. (1982). 1,25-dihydroxyvitamin D_3 receptor in bovine thymus gland. *Biochem. Biophys. Res. Commun.* **106**, 1012–1018.

Reinhold, J. G. (1971). High phytate content of rural Iranian bread: A possible cause of human zinc deficiency. *Am. J. Clin. Nutr.* **24**, 1204–1206.

Reinhold, J. G. (1976). Rickets in Asian immigrants. *Lancet* **2**, 1132.

Rhoten, W. B., and Christakos, S. (1981). Immunocytochemical localization of vitamin D-dependent calcium binding protein in mammalian nephron. *Endocrinology* **109**, 981–983.

Richards, P., Chamberlain, M. J., and Wrong, O. M. (1972). Treatment of osteomalacia of renal tubular acidosis by sodium bicarbonate alone. *Lancet* **2**, 994–997.

Riggs, B. L., Hamstra, A., and DeLuca, H. F. (1981). Assessment of 25-hydroxyvitamin D 1-hydroxylase reserve in postmenopausal osteoporosis by administration of parathyroid extract. *J. Clin. Endocrinol. Metab.* **53**, 833–835.

Riggs, B. L., Gallagher, J. C., DeLuca, H. F., and Zinsmeister, A. R. (1982). Studies on the mechanism of impaired calcium absorption in postmenopausal osteoporosis. *In* "Vitamin D, Chemical, Biochemical and Clinical Endocrinology of Calcium Metabolism" (A. W. Norman, K. Schaefer, D. v. Herrath, and H. G. Grigoleit, eds.), pp. 903–908. de Gruyter, Berlin.

Rinaldi, M. L., Haiech, J., Pavlovich, J., Rizk, M., Ferraz, C., Derancourt, J., and Demaille, J. G. (1982). Isolation and characterization of rat skin parvalbumin-like calcium-binding protein. *Biochemistry* **27**, 4805–4810.

Rizvi, S. N. A., Chawla, S. C., Sinha, S., Malhotra, P., Gulati, P. D., and Vaishnava, H. (1976). Some observations on the prevalence of vitamin D deficiency rickets amongst families of osteomalacics. *J. Assoc. Physicians India* **24**, 833–838.

Roberts, I. F., West, R. J., Ogilvie, D., and Dillon, M. J. (1979). Malnutrition in infants receiving cult diets; a form of child abuse. *Br. Med. J.* **1**, 296–298.

Robertson, I., Ford, J. A., McIntosh, W. B., and Dunnigan, M. G. (1981). The role of cereals in the aetiology of nutritional rickets: The lesson of the Irish National Nutrition Survey 1943–8. *Br. J. Nutr.* **45**, 17–22.

Rojanasathit, S., and Haddad, J. G. (1976). Hepatic accumulation of vitamin D_3 and 25-hydroxyvitamin D_3. *Biochim. Biophys. Acta* **421**, 12–21.

Rojanasathit, S., and Haddad, J. G. (1977). Ontogeny and effect of vitamin D deprivation on rat serum 25-hydroxyvitamin D binding protein. *Endocrinology* **100**, 642–647.

Rosen, J. F., Fleischman, A. R., Finberg, L., Hamstra, A., and DeLuca, H. F. (1979). Rickets with alopecia: An inborn error of vitamin D metabolism. *J. Pediatr.* **94**, 729–735.

Rosen, J. F., Chesney, R. W., Hamstra, A., DeLuca, H. F., and Mahaffey, K. R. (1980). Reduction in 1,25-dihydroxyvitamin D in children with increased lead absorption. *N. Engl. J. Med.* **302**, 1128–1131.

Roth, J., Thorens, B., Hunziker, W., Norman, A. W., and Orci, L. (1981). Vitamin D-dependent calcium binding protein: Immunocytochemical localization in chick kidney. *Science* **214**, 197–199.

Roth, J., Bonner-Weir, S., Norman, A. W., and Orci, L. (1982). Immunocytochemistry of vitamin D-dependent calcium binding protein in chick pancreas: Exclusive localization in B-cells. *Endocrinology* **110**, 2216–2218.

Rowe, D. W., and Kream, B. E. (1982). Regulation of collagen synthesis in fetal rat calvaria by 1,25-dihydroxyvitamin D_3. *J. Biol. Chem.* **257**, 8009–8015.

Russell, R. G. G., Monod, A., Bonjour, J. P., and Fleisch, H (1972). Relation between alkaline phosphatase and Ca^{2+}-ATPase in calcium transport. *Nature (London) New Biol.* **240**, 126–127.

Salimpour, R. (1975). Rickets in Teheran: Study of 200 cases. *Arch Dis. Child.* **50**, 63–66.

Salle, B. F., David, L., Glorieux, F. H., Delvin, E., Senterre, J., and Renaud, H. (1982). Early oral administration of vitamin D and its metabolites in premature neonates. Effect on mineral metabolism. *Pediatr. Res.* **16**, 75–78.

Sand N. N., and Kessler, R. H. (1971). Calcium binding component of dog kidney cortex and its relationship to calcium transport. *Proc Soc. Exp. Biol. Med.* **137**, 1267

Sato, K. A., Gray, R. W., and Leman J., Jr. (1982). Urinary excretion of 25-hydroxyvitamin D in health and the nephrotic syndrome. *J. Lab. Clin. Med.* **99**, 325–330.

Sauveur, B., Garabedian, M., Fellot, C., Mongin, P., and Balsan, S. (1977). The effect of induced metabolic acidosis on vitamin D_3 metabolism in rachitic chicks. *Calcif. Tissue Res.* **23**, 121–124.

Schacter, D., and Kowarski, S. (1982). Isolation of the protein IM Cal, a vitamin D-dependent membrane component of the intestinal transport mechanism for calcium. *Fed. Proc. Fed. Am. Soc. Exp. Biol.* **41**, 84–87.

Schmidt, T. J., Harmon, J. M., and Thompson, E. B. (1980). "Activation-labile" glucocorticoid-receptor complexes of a steroid-resistant variant of CEM-C7 human lymphoid cells. *Nature (London)* **286**, 507–510.

Scriver, C. R., Reade, T. M., DeLuca, H. F., and Hamstra, A. J. (1978). Serum 1,25-dihydroxyvitamin D levels in normal subjects and in patients with hereditary rickets or bone disease. *N. Engl. J. Med.* **299**, 976–979.

Scriver, C. R., Fraser, D., and Kooh, S. W. (1982). Hereditary rickets. *In* "Calcium Disorders" (D. Heath and S. J. Marx, eds.), pp. 1–46. Butterworth, London.

Seino, Y., Shimotsuji, T., Ishii, T., Ishida, M., Ikehara, C., Yamaoka, K., Yabuichi, H., and Dokoh, S. (1980). Treatment of hypophosphatemic vitamin D-resistant rickets with massive doses of 1α-hydroxyvitamin D_3 during childhood. *Arch. Dis. Child.* **55**, 49–53.

Sher, E., Eisman, J. A., Moseley, J. M., and Martin, T. J. (1981). Whole-cell uptake and nuclear localization of 1,25-dihydroxycholecalciferol by breast cancer cells (T47 D) in culture. *Biochem. J.* **200**, 315–320.

Shike, M., Sturtridge, W. C., Tam, C. S., Harrison, J. E., Jones, G., Murray, T. M., Husdan, H., Whitewell, J., Wilson, D. R., and Jeejeebhoy, K. N. (1981). A possible role of vitamin D in the genesis of parenteral-nutrition-induced metabolic bone disease. *Ann. Int. Med.* **95**, 560–568.

Silve, C., Lieberherr, M., Garabedian, M., Guillozo, H., Grosse, B., Thil, C. L., and Balsan, S. (1981). Somatostatin and vitamin D_3 metabolites in rat calvarium: In vitro evidence for physiological interaction. *Endocrinology* **109**, 1454–1462.

Simpson, R. U., and DeLuca, H. F. (1980). Characterization of a receptor-like protein for 1,25-dihydroxyvitamin D_3 in rat skin. *Proc. Natl. Acad. Sci. U.S.A.* **77**, 5822–5826.

Simpson, R. U., and DeLuca, H. F. (1982). Purification of chicken intestinal receptor for

1α,25-dihydroxyvitamin D_3 to apparent homogeneity. *Proc. Natl. Acad. Sci. U.S.A.,* **79,** 16–20.

Simpson, R. U., Franceschi, R. T., and DeLuca, H. F. (1980). Characterization of a specific, high affinity binding macromolecule for 1α,25-dihydroxyvitamin D_3 in cultured chick kidney cells. *J. Biol. Chem.* **255,** 10160–10166.

Slovik, D. M., Adams, J. S., Neer, R. M., Holick, M. F., and Potts J. T., Jr. (1981). Deficient production of 1,25-dihydroxyvitamin D in elderly osteoporotic patients. *N. Engl. J. Med.* **305,** 372–374.

Somjen, D., Somjen, G. J., Harell, A., Mechanic, G. L., and Binderman, I. (1982a). Partial characterization of a specific high affinity binding macromolecule for 24R,25 dihydroxyvitamin D_3 in differentiating skeletal mesenchyme. *Biochem. Biophys. Res. Commun.* **106,** 644–651.

Somjen, D., Somjen, G. J., Weisman, Y., and Binderman, I. (1982b). Evidence for 24,25-dihydroxycholecalciferol receptors in long bones of newborn rats. *Biochem. J.* **204,** 31–36.

Spencer, R. M., Charman, M., Emtage, J. S., and Lawson, D. E. M. (1976a). Production and properties of vitamin-D-induced mRNA for chick calcium binding protein. *Eur. J. Biochem.* **71,** 399–409.

Spencer, R. M., Charman, M., Wilson, P., and Lawson, E. (1976b). Vitamin D-stimulated intestinal calcium absorption may not invovle calcium-binding protein directly. *Nature (London)* **263,** 161–163.

Spencer, R. M., Charman, M., Wilson, P. W., and Lawson, D. E. M. (1978). The relationship between vitamin D-stimulated calcium transport and intestinal calcium-binding protein in the chicken. *Biochem. J.* **170,** 93–101.

Stamp, T. C. B. (1982). The Clinical Endocrinology of vitamin D. *In* "Endocrinology of Calcium Metabolism" (J. A. Parsons, ed.), pp. 363–422. Raven, New York.

Stamp, T. C. B., Round, J. M., Rowe, D. J. F., and Haddad, J. G., Jr. (1972). Plasma levels and therapeutic effects of 25-hydroxycholecalciferol in epileptic patients taking anticonvulsant drugs. *Br. Med. J.* **4,** 9–12.

Stamp, T. C. B., Haddad, J. G., and Twigg, C. A. (1977). Comparison of oral 25-hydroxycholecalciferol, vitamin D, and ultraviolet light as determinants of circulating 25-hydroxyvitamin D. *Lancet* **1,** 1341–1343.

Steichen, J. J., Tsang, R. C., Greer, F. R., Ho, M., and Hug, G. (1981). Elevated serum 1,25-dihydroxyvitamin D concentrations in rickets of very low-birth-weight infants. *J. Pediatr.* **99,** 293–298.

Stern, P. H., Trummel, C. L., Schnoes, H. K., and DeLuca, H. F. (1975). Bone resorbing activity of vitamin D metabolites and congeners *in vitro:* Influence of hydroxyl substituents in the A ring. *Endocrinology* **97,** 1552–1558.

Stumpf, W. E., Sar, M, Reid, F. A., Tanaka Y., and DeLuca, H. F. (1979). Target cells for 1,25-dihydroxyvitamin D_3 in intestinal tract, stomach, kidney, skin, pituitary, and parathyroid. *Science* **206,** 1188–1190.

Stumpf, W. E., Sar, M., Clark, S. A., Lieth, E., and DeLuca, H. F. (1980). Target neurons for 1,25(OH)$_2$vitamin D_3 in brain and spinal cord. *Neuroendocrinol. Lett.* **2,** 297–301.

Stumpf, W. E., Sar, M., Clark, S. A., and DeLuca, H. F. (1982). Brain target sites for 1,25-dihydroxyvitamin D_3. *Science* **215,** 1403–1405.

Svasti, J., and Bowman, B. H. (1978). Human group-specific component: Changes in electrophoretic mobility resulting from vitamin D binding and from neuraminidase digestion. *J. Biol. Chem.* **253,** 4188–4194.

Tanaka, H., Abe, E., Miyaura, C., Kuribayashi, T., Konno, K., Nishii, Y., and Suda, T.

(1982). 1α-25-dihydroxycholecalciferol and a human myeloid leukemia cell line (HL-60): The presence of a cytosol receptor and induction of differentiation. *Biochem. J.* **204,** 713–719.

Tanaka, Y., DeLuca, H. F., Omdahl, J., and Holick, M. F. (1971). Mechanism of action of 1,25-dihydroxycholecalciferol in intestinal transport. *Proc. Natl. Acad. Sci. U.S.A.* **68,** 1286–1288.

Tanaka, Y., and DeLuca, H. F. (1973). The control of 25-hydroxyvitamin D metabolism by inorganic phosphorus. *Arch. Biochem. Biophys.* **154,** 566–574.

Tanaka, Y., Lorenc, R. S., and DeLuca, H. F. (1975). The role of 1,25-dihydroxyvitamin D_3 and parathyroid hormone in the regulation of chick renal 25-hydroxyvitamin D_3-24-hydroxylase. *Arch. Biochem. Biophys.* **171,** 521–526.

Tanaka, Y., Castillo, L., and DeLuca, H. F. (1976). Control of renal vitamin D hydroxylases in birds by sex hormones. *Proc. Natl. Acad. Sci. U.S.A.* **73,** 2701–2705.

Tanaka, Y., Castillo, L., and DeLuca, H. F. (1977). The 24-hydroxylation of 1,25-dihydroxyvitamin D_3. *J. Biol. Chem.* **252,** 1421–1424.

Tanaka, Y., Castillo, L., Wineland, M. J., and DeLuca, H. F. (1978). Synergistic effect of progesterone, testosterone, and estradiol in the stimulation of chick renal 25-hydroxyvitamin D_3-1a-hydroxylase. *Endocrinology* **103,** 2035–2039.

Tanaka, Y., DeLuca, H. F., Kobayashi, Y., Taguchi, T., Ikekawa, N., and Morisaki, M. (1979). Biological activity of 24,24-difluoro-25-hydroxyvitamin D_3: Effect of blocking of 24-hydroxylation on the functions of vitamin D. *J. Biol. Chem.* **254,** 7163–7167.

Tanaka, Y., DeLuca, H. F., Schnoes, H. K., Ikekawa, N., and Eguchi, T. (1981). 23,25-Dihydroxyvitamin D_3: A natural precursor in the biosynthesis of 25-hydroxyvitamin D_3-26,23-lactone. *Proc. Natl. Acad. Sci. U.S.A.* **78,** 4805–4808.

Taylor, A. N., and Wasserman, R. H. (1967). Vitamin D_3 induced calcium binding protein: Partial purification, electrophoretic visualization and tissue distribution. *Arch. Biochem. Biophys.* **119,** 536–540.

Taylor, A. N., McIntosh, J. E., and Bourdeau, J. E. (1982). Immunocytochemical localization of vitamin D-dependent calcium-binding protein in renal tubules of rabbit, rat, and chick. *Kidney Int.* **21,** 765–773.

Taylor, C. M., Mawer, E. B., Wallace, J. E., St. John, J., Cochran, M., Russell, R. G. G., and Kanis, J. A. (1978). The absence of 24,25-dihydroxycholecalciferol in anephric patients. *Clin. Sci. Mol. Med.* **55,** 541–547.

Thomasset, M., Molla, A., Parkes, O., and Demaille, J. (1981). Intestinal calmodulin and calcium-binding protein differ in their distribution and in the effect of vitamin D steroids on their concentration. *FEBS Lett.* **127,** 13–16.

Thomasset, M., Desplan, C., and Parkes, O. (1982). Duodenal, renal and cerebellar vitamin D-dependent calcium-binding proteins in the rat. Specificity and acellular biosynthesis. *In* "Vitamin D: Chemical, Biochemical and Clinical Endocrinology of Calcium Metabolism" (A. W. Norman, K. Schaefer, D. v. Herrath, and H. G. Grigoleit, eds.) pp. 197–202. de Gruyter, Berlin.

Thorens, B., Roth, J., Norman, A. W. Percelet, A., and Orci, L. (1982). Immunocytochemical localization of the vitamin D-dependent calcium binding protein in chick duodenum. *J. Cell Biol.* **94,** 115–122.

Trechsel, U., Bonjour, J. P., and Fleisch, H. (1979). Regulation of the metabolism of 25-hydroxyvitamin D_3 in primary cultures of chick kidney cells. *J. Clin. Invest.* **64,** 206–217.

Trechsel, U., Eisman, J. A., Fischer, J. A., Bonjour, J. P., and Fleisch, H. (1980). Calcium-dependent, parathyroid hormone-independent regulation of 1,25-dihydroxyvitamin D. *Am. J. Physiol.* **239**, E119–E124.

Tsai, H. C., and Norman, A. W. (1973a). Studies on calciferol metabolism VIII. Evidence for a cytoplasmic receptor for 1,25-dihydroxyvitamin D_3 in the intestinal mucosa. *J. Biol. Chem.* **248**, 5967–5975.

Tsai, H. C., and Norman, A. W. (1973b). Studies on the mode of action of calciferol VI: Effect of 1,25-dihydroxyvitamin-D_3 on RNA synthesis in the intestinal mucosa. *Biochem. Biophys. Res. Commun.* **54**, 622–627.

Tsai, H. C., Midgett, R. J., and Norman, A. W. (1973). Studies on the calciferol metabolism. VII. The effects of actinomycin D and cycloheximide on the metabolism, tissue and subcellular localization and action of vitamin D_3. *Arch. Biochem. Biophys.* **157**, 339–347.

Tsuchiya, Y., Matsuo, N., Cho, H., Kumagai, M., Yasaka, T., Suda, T., Orimo, H., and Shimaki, M. (1980). An unusual form of vitamin D-dependent rickets in a child: Alopecia and marked end-organ hyposensitivity to biologically active vitamin D. *J. Clin. Endocrinol. Metab.* **51**, 685–690.

Tuan, R. S., Scott, W. A., and Cohn, Z. A. (1978). Calcium-binding protein of the chick chorioallantoic membrane: Immunohistochemical localization. *J. Cell Biol.* **77**, 743–751.

Turner, R. T., Puzas, J. E., Forte, M. D., Lester, G. E., Gray, T. K., Howard, G. A., and Baylink, D. J. (1980). In vitro synthesis of 1a,25-dihydroxycholecalciferol and 24,25-dihydroxycholecalciferol by isolated calvarial cells. *Proc. Nat. Acad. Sci. U.S.A.* **77**, 5720–5724.

Vaishnava, H. (1975). Vitamin D. deficiency in Northern India. *J. Assoc. Physicians India* **23**, 477–484.

Van Baelen, H., Bouillon, R., and DeMoor, P. (1980) Vitamin D-binding protein (G_c-globulin) binds actin. *J. Biol. Chem.* **255**, 2270–2272.

Walker, A. R. P. (1972). The human requirement of calcium: Should low intakes be supplemented? *Am. J. Clin. Nutr.* **25**, 518–530.

Walling, M. W. (1977). Intestinal Ca and phosphate transport: Differential responses to vitamin D_3 metabolites. *Am. J. Physiol.* **233**, E488–E494.

Walters, M. (1981). An estrogen-stimulated 1,25-dihydroxyvitamin D_3 receptor in rat uterus. *Biochem. Biophys. Res. Commun.* **103**, 721–726.

Walters, M. R., Hunziker, W., and Norman, A. W. (1980). Unoccupied 1,25 dihydroxyvitamin D_3 receptors: Nuclear/cytosol ratio depends on ionic strength. *J. Biol. Chem.* **255**, 6799–6805.

Walters, M. R., Rosen, D. M., Norman, A. W., and Luben, R. A. (1982). 1,25-dihydroxyvitamin D receptors in an established bone cell line, correlation with biochemical responses. *J. Biol. Chem.* **257**, 7481–7484.

Wark, J. D., and Tashjian, A. H., Jr. (1982). Vitamin D stimulates prolactin synthesis by GH4C1 cells incubated in chemically defined medium. *Endocrinology* **111**, 1755–1757.

Warner, M. (1982). Catalytic activity of partially purified renal 25-hydroxyvitamin D hydroxylases from vitaminD-deficient and vitamin D-replete rats. *J. Biol. Chem.* **257**, 12995–13000.

Wasserman, R. H., and Taylor, A. N. (1966). Vitamin D_3 in calcium binding protein in chick intestinal mucosa. *Science* **152**, 791–793.

Wasserman, R. H., Corradino, R. A., and Taylor, A. N. (1968). Vitamin D dependent calcium binding protein: Purification and properties. *J. Biol. Chem.* **243**, 3978–3986.

Wasserman, R. H., Taylor, A. N., and Fullmer, C. S. (1974). Vitamin D-induced calcium-binding protein and the intestinal absorption of calcium. *In* "The Metabolism and Function of Vitamin D" (D. R. Fraser, ed.), pp. 55–74. Biochemical Society, London.

Wasserman, R. H., Fullmer, C. S., and Taylor, A. N. (1978). The vitamin D-dependent calcium binding proteins. *In* "Vitamin D" (D. E. M. Lawson, ed.), pp. 133–166. Academic Press, New York.

Wecksler, W. R., and Norman, A. W. (1980). Biochemical properties of 1α,25-dihydroxy-vitamin D receptors. *J. Steroid Biochem.* **13,** 977–989.

Wechsler, W. R., Okamura, W. H., and Norman, A. W. (1978). Studies on the mode of action of Vitamin D: XIV. Quantitative assessment of the structural requirements for the interaction of 1α,25-dihydroxyvitamin D_3 with its chick intestine receptor system. *J. Steroid Biochem.* **9,** 929–937.

Wecksler, W. R., Ross, F. P., and Norman, A. W. (1979a). Studies on the mode of action of calciferol XX: Characterization of the 1α,25dihydroxyvitamin D_3 receptor from rat intestinal cytosol *J. Biol. Chem.* **254,** 9488–9491.

Wecksler, W. R., Mason, R. S., and Norman, A. W. (1979b). Specific cytosol receptors for 1,25-dihydroxyvitamin D_3 in human intestine. *J. Clin. Endocrinol. Metab.* **48,** 715–717.

Wecksler, W. R., Ross, F. P., Mason, R. S., and Norman, A. W. (1980). Biochemical properties of the 1α,25-dihydroxyvitamin D_3 cytosol receptors from chicken and human intestinal mucosa. *J. Clin. Endocrinol. Metab.* **50,** 152–157.

Weisman, Y., Vargas, A., Duckett, G., Reiter, E., and Root, A. W. (1978). Synthesis of 1,25-dihydroxyvitamin D_3 in the nephrectomized pregnant rat. *Endocrinology* **103,** 1992–1996.

Weisman, Y., Harell, A., Edelstein, S., David, M., Spirer, Z., and Golander, A. (1979). 1a,25-dihydroxyvitamin D_3 and 24,25-dihydroxyvitamin D_3 in vitro synthesis by human decidua and placenta. *Nature (London)* **281,** 317–319.

Whitsett, J. A., Ho, M., Tsang, R. C., Norman, E. J., and Adams, K. G. (1981). Synthesis of 1,25-dihydroxyvitamin D_3 by human placenta in vitro. *J. Clin. Endocrinol. Metab.* **53,** 484–488.

Wichman, J., Schnoes, H. K., and DeLuca, H. F. (1981a). Isolation and identification of 24(R)-hydroxyvitamin D_3 from chicks given large doses of D_3. *Biochemistry* **20,** 2350–2353.

Wichman, J. K., Schnoes, H. K., and DeLuca, H. F. (1981b). 23,24,25-Trihydroxyvitamin D_3, 24,25,26-trihydroxyvitamin D_3, 24-keto-25-hydroxyvitamin D_3 and 23-de-hydro-25-hydroxyvitamin D_3: New in vivo metabolites of vitamin D_3. *Biochemistry* **20,** 7385–7391.

Wiesner, R. H., Kumar, R., Seeman, E., and Go, V. L. W. (1980). Enterohepatic physiology of 1,25-dihydroxyvitamin D_3 metabolites in normal man. *J. Lab. Clin. Med.* **96,** 1094–1100.

Wilke, R., Harmeyer, J., Von Grabe, C., Hehrmann, R., and Hesch, R. D. (1979). Regulatory hyperparathyroidism in a pig breed with vitamin D dependency rickets. *Acta Endocrinol. (Copenhagen)* **92,** 294–308.

Wilson, P. W., and Lawson, D. E. M. (1981). Vitamin D-dependent phosphorylation of an intestinal protein. *Nature (London)* **289,** 600–602.

Winnacker, J. A., Yeager, H., Saunders, J. A., Russell, B., and Anast, C. (1977). Rickets in children receiving anticonvulsant drugs. *Am. J. Dis. Child.* **131,** 286–290.

Wolf, H., Rentschler, S., and Schmidt-Gayk, H. (1982). Effect of mode of administration on the absorption of vitamin D and 25-(OH)-D_3 in low birth weight infants. *In* "Vitamin D, Chemical, Biochemical and Clinical Endocrinology of Calcium Metabolism" (A. W. Norman, K. Schaefer, D. v. Herrath, and H. G. Grigoleit, eds.), pp. 591–593. de Gruyter, Berlin.

Wong, G. L., Luben, R. A., and Cohn, D. V. (1977). 1,25-Dihydroxycholecalciferol and parathormone: Effects on isolated osteoclast-like and osteoblast-like cells. *Sicence* **197,** 663–665.

Yoon, P. S., and DeLuca, H. F. (1981). Resolution and reconstitution of soluble components of rat liver microsomal vitamin D_3-25-hydroxylase. *Arch Biochem. Biophys.* **203,** 529–541.

Zerwekh, J. E., Lindell, T. J., and Haussler, M. R. (1976). Increased intestinal chromatin template activity: Influence of 1α,25-dihydroxyvitamin D_3 and hormone-receptor complexes. *J. Biol. Chem.* **251,** 2388–2394.

Zerwekh, J. E., Glass, K., Jowsey, J., and Pak, C. Y. C. (1979). A unique form of osteomalacia associated with end organ refractoriness to 1,25-dihydroxyvitamin D and apparent defective synthesis of 25-hydroxyvitamin D. *J. Clin. Endocrinol. Metab.* **19,** 171–175.

Zerwekh, J. E., McPhaul, J. J., Parker, T. F., and Pak, C. Y. C. (1982). Effect of acute 25-hydroxyvitamin D_3 therapy on vitamin D metabolite concentrations in chronic renal failure: Evidence for extrarenal production of 24,25-dihydroxyvitamin D. *In* "Vitamin D, Chemical, Biochemical and Clinical Endocrinology of Calcium Metabolism" (A. W. Norman, K. Schaefer, D. v. Herrath, and H. G. Grigoleit, eds.), pp. 641–643. de Gruyter, Berlin.

Index

Date Due